Nursing Diagnoses and Process in Psychiatric Mental Health Nursing

Gertrude K. McFarland,
RN, DNSc, FAAN
Health Scientist Administrator
Nursing Research Study Section
Division of Research Grants
National Institutes of Health
U.S. Department of Health and Human Services
Bethesda, Maryland

Evelyn L. Wasli,
RN, DNSc
Chief Nurse
Emergency Psychiatric Response Division
Community Mental Health Services
D.C. Commission of Mental Health Services
Washington, DC

Elizabeth Kelchner Gerety,
RN, MS, CS
Clinical Nurse Specialist, Psychiatry
Psychiatry Consultation Service
Portland Veterans Affairs Medical Center
Instructor, Department of Mental Health Nursing
School of Nursing
Oregon Health Sciences University
Portland, Oregon

Nursing Diagnoses and Process in Psychiatric Mental Health Nursing

Second Edition

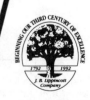

J. B. Lippincott Company

Philadelphia

New York   London   Hagerstown

Sponsoring Editor: Ellen M. Campbell
Production Manager: Janet Greenwood
Production: Bermedica Production, Ltd.
Compositor: Maryland Composition Company
Printer/Binder: R. R. Donnelley & Sons

Second Edition

6 5 4 3 2 1

The opinions expressed herein are those of the authors and do not necessarily reflect those of the US Department of Health and Human Services, the National Institutes of Health, or the Department of Veterans Affairs.

Library of Congress Cataloging-in-Publication Data

McFarland, Gertrude K., 1941–
    Nursing diagnosis and process in psychiatric mental health nursing
  / Gertrude K. McFarland, Evelyn L. Wasli, Elizabeth Kelchner Gerety.
  —2nd ed.
        p.   cm.
    Includes bibliographical references and index.
    ISBN 0-397-54758-7
    1. Psychiatric nursing.   2. Mental illness—Diagnosis.   I. Wasli,
  Evelyn L.   II. Gerety, Elizabeth Kelchner.   III. Title.
    [DNLM: 1. Mental Disorders—diagnosis—outlines.   2. Nursing
  Assessment—outlines.   3. Nursing Process—outlines.   4. Psychiatric
  Nursing—outlines.   WY 18 M4777n]
  RC440.M32 1992
  616.89′075—dc20
  DNLM/DLC
  for Library of Congress   91-44529
                                                                                CIP

The authors and publisher have exerted every effort to ensure that drug selection and dosage set forth in this text are in accord with current recommendations and practice at the time of publication. However, in view of ongoing research, changes in government regulations, and the constant flow of information relating to drug therapy and drug reactions, the reader is urged to check the package insert for each drug for any change in indications and dosage and for added warnings and precautions. This is particularly important when the recommended agent is a new or infrequently employed drug.

Consultants /

Cheryl Forchuk, RN, MScN, PhD Candidate

Clinical Nurse Specialist
Hamilton Psychiatric Hospital
Hamilton, Ontario, Canada

Fellow of the Ontario Ministry of Health
Health Research Personnel Development Program
Ontario, Canada

Robert Keisling, MD

Director, Emergency Psychiatric Response Division
D.C. Commission of Mental Health Services
Washington, D.C.

Suzanne Beverlee Millar, Pharm D

Clinical Pharmacist Specialist
Portland Veterans Affairs Medical Center
Portland, Oregon

Assistant Professor of Clinical Pharmacy
Oregon State University, College of Pharmacy
Corvallis, Oregon

Jeannette Y. Wick, RPh

Chief Pharmacist
D.C. Commission of Mental Health Services
Washington, D.C.

Preface /

While practicing in an era of cost containment, every nurse should have the goal of providing the highest quality nursing care. This text contains the concepts and principles essential to caring for clients who have behavioral problems. Content is presented in as practical a format as possible so that nurses can be guided in caring for the client who is experiencing behavioral or mental health problems in whatever setting care is being rendered.

The authors have presented updated information that is necessary for the understanding of mental health and mental illness. The major schools of psychiatric thought are concisely described. Techniques and concepts useful in developing the therapeutic nurse–patient relationship and in facilitating communication are illustrated with examples. The nursing process is introduced, a systems theory–based conceptual model for the practice of psychiatric nursing is illustrated, and a chapter on psychosocial assessment is provided.

The authors have selected from the most current North American Nursing Diagnoses Association (NANDA) listing those nursing diagnoses that are most relevant to the psychosocial care of clients. (The entire official NANDA listing of nursing diagnoses is provided in the text.) Based on extensive literature review, research, clinical observation and practice, and colleague input, a number of nursing diagnoses have been added where there appear to be gaps in the current listing developed by NANDA. Provided for each nursing diagnosis presented is a definition, general principles, related factors, defining characteristics, strategies for nursing assessment, suggested patient outcomes and nursing interventions, content on health education and health promotion, and evaluation criteria. A chapter on major nursing interventions has been added, also based on extensive literature review, clinical experience, and observation, as well as expert colleague input. Separate chapters cover knowledge about selected psychiatric disorders and related psychiatric treatment modalities and administration of drug therapy.

The authors envision that as these nursing diagnoses continue to be tested and utilized in clinical practice, additional knowledge will be generated that will provide input to NANDA's ongoing development work. In addition, nurses are encouraged to continue to identify and develop major nursing interventions and build on the present knowledge base.

The authors wish to acknowledge their families—Al McFarland and parents John and Emma Ramseier; Arne Wasli and sons Kevin and Eric; and Dick Gerety and John and Danica Kelchner, for their support and patience during the preparation of this project.

Our appreciation is also extended to all those nurses who are working to identify, develop, clinically utilize, and research nursing diagnoses and nursing interventions.

Contents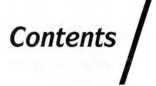

1
Concepts of Mental Health and Mental Illness — 1

Major Views of Mental Health
   and Mental Illness   1
The Problem   2
Neurobiological Approach   3
Stress-Adaptation Approach   4
Psychodynamic Approach   5
Interpersonal Approach   9
Ego Development Approach   10
Behaviorist Approach   12
Humanistic-Existential Approach   13
Family Approach   13
Group Approach   15

2
Therapeutic Relationship — 19

The One-To-One Nurse-Patient
   Relationship   19
Definition and Characteristics   19
Definition of Related Terms   19
Phases of the Nurse-Patient
   Relationship   20

Phase I (Beginning or Orientation
    Phase)   *20*
Phase II (Middle or Working
    Phase)   *21*
Phase III (Termination or Resolution
    Phase)   *22*
Principles and Strategies for Developing
    and Maintaining a Therapeutic
    Nurse-Patient Relationship   *23*

3
Initial Psychiatric Assessment of the Adult   33

Conceptual Framework for Psychiatric
    Mental Health Nursing Practice   *33*
The Nursing Process   *33*
Assessment   *35*
Nursing Diagnosis   *35*
Psychiatric Assessment of the Adult
    Patient   *36*
Planning   *40*
Intervention   *40*
Evaluation   *40*
The Mental Status Examination   *40*
The Multiaxial Evaluation System of the
    DSM-III-R   *44*
Psychological Testing   *45*

4
Nursing Diagnoses in Caring for the Psychiatric Patient   49

Definition and Characteristics of Nursing
    Diagnoses   *49*
Nursing Diagnosis Definition   *49*
NANDA Approval List of Nursing
    Diagnoses   *49*

Framework for Discussing Nursing
  Diagnoses   *52*
Aggression (mild, moderate, extreme/
  violence)   *53*
Anxiety (mild, moderate, severe,
  extreme/panic)   *65*
Communication, Impaired   *73*
Coping, Defensive (denial, ineffective
  denial)   *79*
Coping, Ineffective Individual   *84*
Crisis, Situational   *92*
Decisional Conflict (specify)   *98*
Depression   *102*
Family Processes, Altered   *108*
Grieving, Anticipatory   *114*
Grieving, Dysfunctional   *116*
Manipulation   *123*
Powerlessness   *127*
Ritualistic Behavior   *133*
Self-Esteem Disturbance   *136*
Sexual Dysfunction   *141*
Social Interaction, Impaired   *148*
Suicide, Potential   *152*
Thought Processes, Altered   *160*
  Acute Confusion   *160*
  Delusions   *166*
  Hallucinations   *170*
  Suspiciousness   *174*

5
Major Nursing Interventions   179

Advocacy   *179*
Assertiveness Training   *180*
Communication Techniques   *181*
Contracting   *183*

Crisis Intervention *184*
Decision-Making *185*
Discharge Planning *187*
Education *188*
   Patient Education *188*
   Family Education *191*
Milieu Therapy *194*
Protective Interventions *195*
   Activity Area Restriction *195*
   Observation for Suicide
     Prevention *196*
   Seclusion *197*
   Restraints *199*
   Seizure Management *201*
Reality Orientation *203*
Social Skills Training *204*
Stress Management *206*
Supportive Therapy *209*
   Grief Counseling *209*
   Offering Hope *210*
   Presence *211*
Group Treatment *223*

6
Major Psychiatric Disorders   *231*

Organic Mental Syndromes and
   Disorders *231*
Psychoactive Substance Use
   Disorders and Psychoactive
   Substance-Induced Organic Mental
   Disorders *238*
Schizophrenia *252*
Mood Disorders and Adjustment
   Disorder with Depressed
   Mood *260*

Delusional (Paranoid) Disorder and
   Psychotic Disorders Not Elsewhere
   Classified   *266*
Anxiety Disorders and Adjustment
   Disorders with Anxious
   Features   *268*
Somatoform Disorders   *273*
Dissociative Disorders   *275*
Personality Disorders   *277*

7
Administration of Drug Therapy   *283*

Areas for Nursing Assessment   *283*
Antipsychotic Drugs   *285*
Anticholinergic/Antiparkinsonian
   Drugs   *293*
Antidepressant Drugs   *294*
Antimanic Drugs   *301*
Antianxiety Drugs   *305*

Index   *311*

Concepts of Mental Health and Mental Illness

/

1

1. *Mental health*—"A state of being, relative rather than absolute. The best indices of mental health are simultaneous success at working, loving, and creating with the capacity for mature and flexible resolution of conflicts between instincts, conscience, important other people, and reality."[52]

2. *Jahoda's six cardinal aspects of mental health*[26]—These aspects include a positive attitude toward self, active growth and development toward self-actualization, integration, autonomy and independence from social influences, accurate perception of reality, environmental mastery.

3. *Roger's process of self-actualization*[40]—The person engaging in the process exhibits openness to experience, lack of defensiveness, accuracy in symbolization, congruency, flexibility, unconditional self-regard, creative adaptation, effective reality testing, harmony with others.

4. *Maslow's*[31] *view of health* is the achievement of self-actualization, including an understanding of self and reality, the expression of emotionality and spontaneity, and the achievement of life goals.

5. *Mental illness*—"An illness with psychologic or behavioral manifestations and/or impairment in functioning due to a social, psychologic, genetic, physical/chemical, or biologic disturbance. The disorder is not limited to relations between people and society. The illness is characterized by symptoms and/or impairment in functioning."[45] Some common indicators of mental illness are depression, feelings of anxiety that are not proportionate to a possible cause, physical complaints having no organic cause, any sudden change of behavior or mood, unreasonable and unrealistic expectations of self or others, and failure to achieve potential.

6. *Insanity*—This is a legal concept describing a mental disturbance affecting a person with the consequence that the individual is not crim-

inally responsible for an act. Rules and criteria for insanity are set by legal process.

   a. Mc Naughten Rule declared a person insane and not responsible for the criminal act if the person had a disease of the mind that impaired the ability to distinguish right from wrong.
   b. Durham Rule said that the accused is not guilty if the unlawful act was done as a product of mental illness or deficit.
   c. American Law Institute test stated that if the defendant has a mental disease or deficit and consequently lacks the capacity to appreciate the criminality of own behavior or to conform own behavior to the law, the individual is not responsible for the criminal act.

7. Mental disorders[1]—The American Psychiatric Association's Diagnostic and Statistical Manual of Mental Disorders (DSM-III-R) provides a classification of mental disorders (see Chapter 6). There are five axes on which each individual is evaluated. The first three represent the official diagnostic assessment.

   Axis 1—Clinical Syndrome and V codes
   Axis 2—Developmental Disorders and Personality Disorders
   Axis 3—Physical Disorders and Conditions
   Axis 4—Severity of Psychosocial Stress
   Axis 5—Global Assessment of Functioning

■ THE PROBLEM[1-53]

1. Mental health problems that are widespread and identified by the World Health Organization[52] are mental retardation, acquired conditions of the central nervous system, peripheral neuropathy, psychoses, epilepsy, conduct disorder, psychoactive substance abuse, and conditions of life that lead to mental disease, violence, excessive risk-taking behavior in young, and family breakdown.
2. There is a prevalence rate of 15–20% for mental disease in the world.[52]
3. Twenty percent of the U.S. population experiences a mental disorder.[39]
4. The major mental disorders in the U.S.[35] are

alcohol abuse or dependency	13.6%
phobia	11.3%
drug abuse and dependency	5.6%
depression	5.0%

5. The number of chronically mentally ill in the U.S.[30] ranges from 1.7 to 2.4 million. Diagnoses include

schizophrenia	500,000–900,000
depression	600,000–800,000
organic mental disorders	600,000–1,250,000.

6. There is an increase in community-based care as compared to hospital-based care.[39]
7. Chronically mentally ill patients are found in nursing homes (750,000), in the community- and hospital-based area (800,000), and in a variety of residential facilities in the community (700,000).
8. Personnel offering treatment to the person with a mental disorder are mostly mental health workers who do not have bachelor's degrees; 30% of personnel are from the four professional groups.[39]

—— Neurobiological Approach

This approach emphasizes a scientific approach to the study of the nervous system, to explain and treat mental disorders. *Illness* is defined as a disturbance in the neurobiological system.

A. Theoretical basis: genetics.
1. Family risk, twin, and adoption studies have found increased risk for relatives of persons with mental illness.(See discussion of specific mental disorder).
2. *Diathesis stress theory*—Offers an explanation that the genetic disease produces an intrauterine metabolic disorder that causes changes in the central nervous system. The infant has problems in sensing and in perceiving and constructing his or her world and is thus more vulnerable to environmental stress.
3. *Monogenic bioamine theory*—This is a genetic disorder that produces an abnormal metabolite that affects the arousal system, making the world appear new and confusing and the symptoms of schizophrenia appear.
4. *Defective hedonic capacity theory*—There is a genetic impairment of the capacity to experience pleasure. The infant is further hampered by an inadequate pain/pleasure response in learning adaptive behavior.

B. Theoretical basis: neurotransmitters
1. Each neuron receives information through its many dendrites from thousands of other axons of neurons. Consequently, each neuron sends messages by its network of axons. The gap between the axon of one neuron and the dendrite of another neuron is the synapse; the transaction occurring is the synaptic transmission.
2. Chemical substances called neurotransmitters are active in the synapse. The neurotransmitter is released from the endings of the axon. Other neurons are specifically sensitive to the chemical and dendrites respond.
3. The transmitters produce an excitatory or inhibitory effect at the synapse. One neuron has many synapses, with excitatory forces firing the neuron and inhibitory forces decreasing the firing. An imbalance of these forces may result in aggressiveness, rage, or lethargy.
4. Thousands of these chemical reactions are occurring at any one time and are the biological basis for thinking and feeling.
5. Characteristics of the neurotransmitter are
   a. synthesis and storage of substance in neuron;
   b. release of substance upon stimulation of neuron;
   c. termination of activity by enzymes and uptake process.
6. The cell bodies of neurons containing certain transmitters—norepinephrine, dopamine, and serotonin—have been located in brain stem, and their pathways extending to the brain and spinal cord have been identified by histochemical fluorescence method. Further study of the pathways or tracts will explain seemingly unrelated symptoms.
7. Selected neurotransmitters:
   a. *Dopamine.* Tracts are found in the substantia nigra, hypothalamus, neocortex, and limbic system. Overactivity of the dopaminergic system (tracts and receptors at synapses) is associated with schizophrenia and mood disorders.

    b. *Norepinephrine and epinephrine.* Tracts are found mostly in the pons with pathways to the brain stem, limbic system, thalamus, hypothalamus, and spinal cord. Tricyclic antidepressant and monoamine oxidase inhibitor effects have been related to this system.

    c. *Serotonin.* Tracts are found in pons and midbrain with pathways to basal ganglia, limbic system, cerebral cortex, and spinal cord. Decreased concentrations of serotonin in the synapse have been associated with schizophrenia, mood disorders, anxiety disorders, and episodes of violence.

    d. *Acetylcholine* (produced at the cholinergic synapse). Tracts are found in nucleus basalis with pathways to the cerebral cortex, limbic system, thalamus, and hypothalamus. Dementia has been associated with degeneration of these neurons. Disruption in the physiology of the cholinergic system has been associated with movement disorders—i.e., the parkinsonian side effects of antipsychotics.

C. Therapy

Diagnostic aids such as computed tomography (CT) scans, electroencephalograms (EEGs), laboratory studies, radiographs, history of present illness, history of familial incidences of disorders, physical examination, and behavior observations are used to determine areas of dysfunction. Drugs that effect change in the neurobiological system are prescribed, and changes are monitored. Genetic counseling is provided.

—— Stress-Adaptation Approach

This method emphasizes the role of stress in the increased incidence of illness. Illness is viewed as a human reaction pattern to stress or maladaptation.

A. Theoretical basis

1. Examples of risk factors that have been identified by various writers as being associated with the development of mental disorders are prematurity, poor diet, chromosomal disorders, accidents, and racial discrimination.

2. Life events that are stressors and contribute to development of crises include death of a spouse, divorce, and marital separation. There remains controversy how stress mechanisms affect a person. If a person receives adequate support, the risk of illness is less.

3. Crisis exists when a person is unable to cope with a threat and experiences an increase in anxiety; tries other coping mechanisms and the problem is resolved. If the problem is not resolved, the anxiety increases and a variety of symptoms can emerge, such as suicidal and homicidal thoughts, somatic symptoms, confusion, depression, isolation, and nonproductivity. Crises can be divided into three groups: maturational (e.g., transition into retirement), situational (e.g., loss of a job), and adventitious (e.g., earthquake).

4. The competence of a person in adapting to crisis affects the adaptation process.

    a. A person makes a cognitive appraisal of the stressor. For example, a situation can be viewed as a challenge by one individual and as a catastrophe by another.

b. Many coping behaviors, mechanisms, and strategies exist and are classified in various ways.
    c. Vaillant offers a hierarchy of ego defenses based on the Grant Study of Adult Development.[50,51]
        (1) Psychotic mechanisms: denial, distortion, delusional projection
        (2) Immature ego defenses: fantasy, projection, passive aggression, hypochondriasis, acting out
        (3) Neurotic ego defenses: intellectualization, repression, displacement, dissociation, reaction formation
        (4) Mature ego defenses: sublimation, altruism, suppression, humor, anticipation
5. The presence of social support assists a person in problem solving and offers sustenance during a crisis period.

B. Therapy
The focus is on establishing a working relationship with the client, problem identification and steps in resolution, support of coping strategies, enhancement of self-esteem, anticipatory guidance, and preventive interventions (e.g., assisting a mother in parenting techniques). For further discussion, see the section on ineffective individual coping in Chapter 4.

—— Psychodynamic Approach

This approach emphasizes the influences of intrapsychic forces on observable behavior. *Illness* is defined in terms of behavior disorders that originate in conflicts occurring before 6 years of age among the id, ego, superego, and/or environment. Anxiety is then experienced as a result of these conflicts. Excessive use of mental defense mechanisms leads to serious behavioral disturbances.

A. Theoretical basis[8,12,20,27–29,41]
1. Freud is recognized as the founder of the psychoanalytic school of thought.
2. Psychic activity is influenced by two drives: sexual and aggressive.
3. The psyche is divided into levels of consciousness:
    a. *Conscious*—the awareness of self and environment that occurs when a person is awake
    b. *Preconscious*—contains memories and thoughts that are easily recalled
    c. *Unconscious*—contains memories and thoughts that ordinarily do not enter consciousness
4. Structural aspects of the psyche are
    a. *Id*—the part containing instinctual drives and impulses. The ego and superego develop from the id.
        (1) *Pleasure principle*—The id seeks immediate release from tension or pleasure and avoids displeasure without regard for consequences.
        (2) *Primary process thinking*—Mental activity of the id is characterized by a collapse of time periods and by images mistaken for reality, occurring naturally in infants and during dreams and in some mental illnesses.

    b. *Ego*—The part that assists the psyche in relating to the environment through such functions as memory and thinking and in resolving psyche conflicts. One of the more important functions is reality testing (the ego's function in sorting perceptions coming from the id and from the environment). Its primary growth period is 6 months to 3 years of age. It is the "I."

        (1) *Reality principle*—states that the ego tends to delay satisfaction by accommodation to situational factors

        (2) *Secondary process thinking*—mental activity of the ego characterized by reason, logic, and differentiating among people, situations, and things

    c. *Superego*—the part that evaluates thought and actions, rewarding the good and punishing the bad

5. *Anxiety*—an automatic response occurring when the psyche is flooded with uncontrollable stimulation

    a. *Signal anxiety or reality anxiety*—a type of anxiety produced by the ego in anticipation of danger, such as loss of a loved one or disapproval of superego

    b. *Moral anxiety*—type of anxiety from overwhelming feelings of guilt or shame about an act or thought

    c. *Neurotic anxiety*—type of anxiety in which impulses from the id, such as aggressive or sexual impulses, threaten to overpower the ego

B. Psychosexual stages of development

These stages are crucial because they are periods during which unconscious conflicts among id, ego, and superego develop. Fixation, or arrest of development, at any stage may occur as a result of excessive gratification or deprivation.

1. *Oral stage* (birth to $1\frac{1}{2}$ years)

    a. The infant obtains relief from biological and psychological tensions through his or her mouth and lips.

    b. Learns to depend on external objects

    c. Sucks, swallows, takes in, bites, chews, spits, and cries

    d. Experiences a warm, trusting, and dependent pattern of relating

    e. Gratifies needs and begins to delay immediate satisfaction

    f. Ego development begins primarily through the process of identification.

    g. Problems and/or traits related to oral stage: over-dependency, clinging behavior, pessimism, optimism, narcissism (self-love), "world-owes-me-a-living" attitudes, alcoholism, smoking, overeating, drug addiction, refusal to eat, vomiting, gullibility

2. *Anal stage* ($1\frac{1}{2}$ to 3 years)

    a. The infant achieves control over anal sphincter and gives up some control as he or she experiences toilet training.

    b. The infant and the parents are involved in issues of control over defecation.

        (1) The infant may give the feces as a gift or keep them or expel them violently.

        (2) The infant may control the time of defecation or do what he or she wants with the feces.

(3) The infant may relinquish control or comply with the control imposed.

c. The sense of "I" becomes well developed.

d. Problems and/or traits related to anal stage are compliance, defiance, perfectionism, obsessive-compulsiveness, antagonism, negativism, sadomasochism (pleasure from inflicting pain on others or self), procrastination, miserliness, stuttering, phobias, compulsions, constipation, bedwetting, overconformity, competitiveness, generosity, creativity, possessiveness.

3. *Phallic stage* (3 to 6 years)

  a. Child experiences the genitals, particularly the penis, as the main source of pleasurable sensation and interest.

  b. Parents are vital in the process of the child's developing sexual identity.

  c. *Oedipus complex*—Refers to the emotional attachment of boy for mother and ambivalent feelings toward father. The boy fears retaliation and possible loss of penis (*castration fear*) and he has wishes of killing father.

  d. *Electra complex*—Describes a girl's wishes for penis of father and hopes to take the place of mother, whom she blames for not having penis.

  e. The complex is resolved by girl or boy in the identification of the child with the parent of the same sex.

  f. The superego is strengthened as the child accepts the standards of the parent.

  g. Problems and/or traits related to phallic stage are homosexuality, transsexuality, problems with authority, overinvolvement in being sexually attractive.

4. *Latency stage* (6 to 12 years)

  a. Child experiences a quiet period during which the sexual drive is dormant.

  b. Sexual and aggressive drives are channeled into school activities, play, and work.

  c. Relationships are mostly with peers of same sex.

  d. Problems noted in latency stage are delinquency, rebelliousness, tics, restlessness, hysteria, anxiety states, anorexia.

5. *Genital stage* (12 years to adulthood)

  a. The person experiences onset of puberty, renewed interest in sexual activity, and conflicts that were unresolved in past developmental stages.

  b. The person learns to develop mature relationships with males and females.

  c. The person begins to stop depending on parents.

  d. Problems arising in the genital stage can include conflicts, character disorders, and other mental disorders.

C. Defense mechanisms

The following are mental processes used by the ego to reduce anxiety and conflict by modifying, distorting, or rejecting reality. The most frequently used defense mechanisms include

1. *Repression*—Response keeps painful thoughts, feelings, and impulses from consciousness.
2. *Denial*—Response acknowledges no awareness of a painful event.
3. *Reaction formation*—Response expresses feelings opposite to those being experienced.
4. *Projection*—Response ascribes the unacceptable thoughts and feelings to another person.
5. *Rationalization*—Response justifies behavior by an attempt to explain it logically.
6. *Undoing*—Response cancels the effect of another response just made.
7. *Displacement*—Response misdirects from original person or object to safer target.
8. *Sublimation*—Response partially substitutes socially acceptable activities for unacceptable impulses.
9. *Regression*—Response involves behaving at a level more appropriate to an earlier age.
10. *Identification*—Response involves acting and feeling in the same manner as a significant other.
11. *Introjection*—Response involves taking an aspect of behavior or thought of another into the ego structure.
12. *Isolation*—Response involves blocking the feeling associated with an unpleasant, threatening situation or thought.
13. *Suppression*—Response involves consciously and deliberately forcing certain ideas from thought and action.

D. Grouping of defense mechanisms[50,51]
1. **Psychotic mechanisms**
    a. Denial of external reality
    b. Distortion of external reality
2. **Immature mechanisms**
    a. Autistic fantasy
    b. Projection
    c. Dissociation
    d. Devaluation, idealization, splitting
    e. Passive-aggressive behavior
    f. Acting out
3. **Intermediate defenses**
    a. Intellectualization
    b. Repression
    c. Reaction-formation
    d. Displacement
    e. Somatization
4. **Mature mechanisms**
    a. Sublimation
    b. Altruism
    c. Suppression
    d. Humor

E. Therapy
1. *Psychoanalysis* is an intense relationship with a psychoanalyst for a period of time for the purpose of helping the person establish conscious control of affect and behavior.

2. Through dream analysis, free association, interpretation, analysis of resistance and *transference* (ascribing to the analyst the thoughts and feelings associated with parents or other important people), and neutrality, the analyst assists the patient in reducing the anxiety associated with thought.
3. Conflicts are brought into awareness and thus resolved.

—— Interpersonal Approach

This approach emphasizes the importance of interpersonal relationships and communication on behavior. *Behavior disorders* are a result of patterns of avoidance, use of substitutive processes, and experiences with significant adults.

A. Theoretical basis
1. Sullivan is noted for interpersonal theory of psychiatry.[46]
2. *Satisfaction* is achieved through interaction to obtain relief from tension from biological drives or needs.
3. *Security* is achieved when basic needs are satisfied in relationship to a mothering person without the presence of anxiety.
4. *Self system* develops from the dynamic interplay of the basic needs and the interpersonal process to achieve satisfaction and security and to avoid or decrease anxiety.
   a. Modes of experiencing describe one's perception and thoughts.
      (1) *Prototaxic mode*—Person identifies with the whole world; thoughts and responses are undifferentiated.
      (2) *Parataxic mode*—Person recognizes that things go together, but there is no logic. Things are put together only because one event occurs and is followed by another.
      (3) *Syntaxic mode*—Person is able to use logic in explaining events.
   b. Person appraises self through significant others' reactions and organizes the appraisals in terms of
      (1) bad me—acts that result in anxiety;
      (2) good me—acts that cause no anxiety;
      (3) not me—acs that are totally disapproved; severe anxiety is experienced.

B. Stages of growth and development
   These stages reflect emphasis of interpersonal approach.
1. Infancy—lasts until the appearance of speech, which enables infant to change environment
2. Childhood—lasts until emergence of need for peers
3. Juvenile—lasts until need for close relationship
4. Preadolescence—lasts until puberty and beginning interest in opposite sex
5. Early adolescence—lasts until development of relationships with opposite sex
6. Late adolescence—lasts until the establishment of a stable love relationship with another

C. Anxiety
1. First develops as infant experiences tension or insecurity of mother.
2. Later it is experienced whenever a threat of disapproval from a significant person occurs.
3. Avoidance behaviors develop to deal with anxiety:
   a. Physically avoiding the situation
   b. Changing the interaction in the situation
   c. Using selective inattention, which is the process the person employs to not attend to that which causes anxiety
   d. Using substitutive processes in which the person dissociates certain aspects of interpersonal system. The term *security operations* also is used to describe these processes; these are similar to the defense mechanisms described by Freud.

D. Therapy
1. The therapist is a participant observer and not a neutral object.
2. *Elucidation* is a principle that states that a behavior change can occur when one can identify, conceptualize, and evaluate behavior.
3. Focus of the interview is on exploring the avoidance behaviors, anxiety experiences, and the interpersonal context in which the avoidance behaviors and anxiety occur.

—— Ego Development Approach

This method emphasizes the development of ego identity throughout the life span; it was developed by Erikson. *Illness* is characterized by problems with self, relationships, or society that may cause extension of the developmental period. Behavioral disorders result from unresolved conflicts during the stages of the life cycle.

A. Theoretical basis
1. Human beings progress through a series of eight psychosocial developmental stages.
2. The growth plan is governed by both social experiences and innate capacities, the epigenetic principle.
3. In each developmental stage, the potential exists for the person to develop a new task that serves as a building block for subsequent stages. Physical and psychosocial hazards may thwart the person from achieving the task central to a given developmental stage. The lack of achievement of the task has a negative affect on subsequent developmental stages and may lead to maladaptive behavioral patterns.

B. Erikson's eight developmental stages[14–19]
1. *Infancy* (birth to 18 months)
   a. During this stage, the infant learns to *trust* self and others, provided his or her needs have been met in a consistent and satisfying manner.
   b. Confidence, realistic trust, hope, optimism, and the ability to form relationships in later life stem from such an attitude of trust.
   c. Subject to hazards such as mistreatment, the infant may develop *mistrust* that is later reflected in hostility, suspiciousness, and a general feeling of dissatisfaction.

2. *Early childhood* (18 months to 3 years)
    a. In this stage, *autonomy* results from reassuring, constructively guided experiences in which the child is allowed to exercise self-control of behavior without being subjected to experiences beyond the child's capabilities.
    b. Socially acceptable behaviors of holding and letting go, on which toilet training focuses during this stage, become generalized to other aspects of living.
    c. The development of autonomy leads to self-control without loss of self-esteem, a sense of pride and good will, the ability to initiate activities yet be cooperative, and appropriate generosity and withholding.
    d. Difficulties, such as from external overcontrol, can lead to *shame and doubt* (i.e., feelings of being exposed, lack of a belief in being able to control one's life, and a lack of self-worth).
3. *Late childhood* (3 to 5 years)
    a. The child develops *initiative*, the ability to undertake and plan tasks, the pleasure of being active, and the experience of a sense of purpose.
    b. Pleasure in attack and conquest aid in developing sexual identity and roles.
    c. Initiative is controlled by a developing conscience. The person grows to develop and strives to utilize potentials in a socially appropriate manner.
    d. *Guilt*, accompanied by self-restriction and denial, can result from an unsuccessful negotiation of this stage. The person fails to develop potential.
4. *School age* (6 to 12 years)
    a. The major task is *industry*, characterized by involvement in the world, construction and planning, development of relationships with peers, development of specific skills, and identification with admired others.
    b. A sense of competence and the pleasure of diligence develops.
    c. *Inferiority*, the feeling that one is unworthy and inadequate, can result from hindrances.
5. *Adolescence* (12 to 20 years)
    a. The developmental task is *identity*, a confident sense of self, commitment to a career, and finding one's place in society.
    b. Successful resolution leads to the ability to work toward long-term goals, self-esteem, and emotional stability.
    c. The danger is *role* confusion, characterized by feelings of confusion, lack of confidence, indecision, alienation, and possibly acting-out behavior.
    d. Unsuccessful resolution may require the adult to spend life-long energies attempting to resolve remaining conflicts.
6. *Young adulthood* (18 to 25 years)
    a. *Intimacy* is the major developmental task. The person develops the ability to love, to develop commitments to other persons, and to enter true mutual relationships.
    b. *Isolation* is the danger. The person remains distant from others, withdraws, enters into superficial relationships, or develops prejudices.

7. *Adulthood* (28 to 65 years)
    a. *Generativity* is the task. The adult becomes responsible for guiding children or for the creation and development of productive and constructive tasks.
    b. Failure leads to *stagnation*, personal impoverishment, and self-indulgence.
8. *Old age* (65 years to death)
    a. The last stage is characterized by feelings of acceptance, importance, and self-worth about the value of one's life—*integrity*.
    b. *Despair*, the negative outcome of this stage, is the sense of loss, a feeling of life's meaninglessness, and the feeling that life's goals have not been achieved and that it is too late to start over.

C. Therapy
Focus is on establishing trust not obtained early in life and helping patient gain insight into unconscious motivations, thus reducing anxiety.

— Behaviorist Approach

This approach emphasizes observable and measurable behavioral processes. *Maladaptive behavior* can be classified as behavior excess, behavioral deficit, distortion of reinforcing stimuli, distortion of discrimination stimuli, and aversive behavior.

A. Theoretical basis[4,8,12,20,28,41]
1. Watson, Pavlov, and Skinner contributed to the development of the behaviorist school of thought.
2. Two schools of thought have developed.
    a. *Behaviorism*—All behavior follows learning principles; therefore, behavior may become maladaptive but is not considered abnormal.
        (1) *Respondent conditioning*—concept that states that a specific stimulus elicits a certain response.
        (2) *Operant conditioning*—concept that states that behavior responses are influenced by what follows the response.
        (3) *Reinforcement*—concept that states that a behavior response can be influenced by positive and negative rewards.
    b. *Cognitive behaviorism*—Behavior is influenced by cognition, independently of the stimulus.
        (1) Important variables determining behavior include plans, beliefs, expectancies, encodings, and competencies.
        (2) Feelings are believed to follow thoughts.

B. Therapy
1. *Functional analysis* is analysis of the manifest behavior.
    a. What behaviors are problematic?
    b. Under what conditions does the behavior occur?
    c. What are the positive reinforcers?
    d. What are the negative reinforcers?
    e. What are the effective behaviors that could be used as substitutes or as reinforcers?
2. Techniques frequently used in behavioral therapy are systematic desensitization, flooding, implosion, positive reinforcement, programs

such as assertiveness training, relaxation exercises, token economy, and sex therapy.
3. Cognitive therapy focuses on changing the internal contingencies, such as expectancies, distortions, self-injunctions, self-reproaches, and sequence of thoughts, to effect a behavior change.
4. Techniques in cognitive therapy include verbal probing, reality testing, thought substitution, role playing, self-monitoring, assignment of tasks, use of humor, and reflection.

—— Humanistic-Existential Approach

This approach emphasizes the holistic view of man, man's individuality and intrinsic worth, the importance of experiencing the present, and the personal meanings of experience. According to Rogers, Maslow, and Frankl, abnormal behavior is a consequence of the following:

Rogers—An incongruence exists between one's self-image and experience.[40]

Maslow—Basic needs are not satisfied (air, food, water, safety, love, belonging, self-actualization).[31]

Frankl—Lack of meaning of life may result in illness.[21]

A. Theoretical basis: Rogers
1. *Self* is a central concept because one's evaluation of life is related to views of the self: Who am I? What I can do? What am I able to do? What do I want to be? Man strives for self-actualization.
2. Incongruence can develop between the ideal self and the real self and/or reality. This causes dissatisfaction, anxiety, and activation of a self-defense mechanism.
3. Continuous feedback about behavior is being given to the child by others. These experiences are integrated, denied, or accepted as truth by the child, thus affecting the self.
4. The importance of accepting one's feelings and not denying them and of recognizing one's own values and beliefs and not generally accepting the values of others is stressed.

B. Therapy
Therapist demonstrates unconditional positive self-regard (genuine acceptance), empathetic understanding (ability to perceive another's world), correctness, and congruence to assist patient in exploring his uniqueness and worth.

—— Family Approach[23]

Differing conceptual views of family theory and family therapy exist. There is no accepted typology or diagnostic view of families.

A. Structural framework
1. Minuchin[33] views the family as a social system with structure and organization in which the individual lives and responds. Transactional patterns develop that control the interaction and behavior of family members.
2. Maladaption is noted in the transactional patterns (i.e., disengagement

with no or minimal contact among the family members and enmeshment with an overinvolvement between and/or among members.

3. Therapy is directed toward initiating change in the family structure by clarifying boundaries, rules, and expectations.

B. Interactional framework: Satir[42] and Haley[24,25]
1. The double bind theory offers a way to view the development of dysfunction in a family system. Its characteristics are as follows:
    a. The individual is in an important relationship that involves being able to understand what is communicated.
    b. The other person in the relationship is communicating two orders of messages and they are contradictory.
    c. The individual is unable to make a comment about either order of the messages and therefore is in a double bind.
2. Dysfunctional communication is produced by denying, rejecting, or disqualifying the relationship aspect as the message aspects of the communication; by differing punctuation in the interactions between two persons, which results in greater and greater differences; and by having symmetrical or rigid interaction patterns.
3. Problems are viewed as consequences of using a solution that obviously is not working. Mishandling occurs as
    a. steps are not taken and action is needed;
    b. steps are taken and no action is needed; or
    c. steps are taken at every level of communication.
4. Therapy is directed toward change in the individual interaction patterns in the family system (e.g., Satir) and/or change in the structure or transaction pattern (e.g., Haley) by setting goals, giving tasks, symptom prescription, advertising symptoms, reframing behavior, and so on.

C. Bowen system theory[9,32,36]
The Bowen system presents a conceptualization of the emotional system over several generations. It emphasizes variables of anxiety and level of integration and their influence on the family system. Illness is viewed as an aspect of human adaptation in which a person experiences a level of undifferentiation resulting from the transmission of low levels of differentiation from past generations.
1. Theoretical basis
    a. *Sibling position*—Personality characteristics are related to sibling position (10 have been identified) and provide predictive data.
    b. *Triangles*—the basic unit of the emotional system (i.e., a twosome and an outsider). When tension is experienced, each person will attempt to obtain the outside position. If the tension increases, one of the persons will triangle another; a larger and larger interlocking system is thus formed.
    c. *Family projection process*—Anxiety is experienced by the mother, who may respond by becoming sensitive to the child and overconcerned. The mother's overattachment to the child is supported by the father. The child becomes anxious, demanding, and unable to function alone. Schizophrenia may develop following several generations of lower levels of differentiation as a result of the family projection process.
    d. *Multigenerational transmission process*—The family projection process

involves multiple generations, with one child in each generation becoming less differentiated and less able to function.

e. *Emotional cut-off*—This concept describes the process of separation from parents as people attempt to resolve the emotional attachments. The more intense the cut-off from parents, the more likely that the person and the person's children will have similar problems in life.

f. *Differentiation*—This concept is related to a state of being and to the process of becoming more responsible for oneself at emotional and intellectual levels. Profiles are developed for different levels of differentiation.

g. *Nuclear family emotional system*—Patterns of functioning of mother, father, and children are identified. Major patterns include marital conflict, dysfunction in one spouse, projection of problems to a child, and/or a combination of these patterns.

h. *Societal regression*—When a society is exposed to chronic anxiety, it responds with emotionality to relieve the anxiety; thus, functioning regresses. An example of regression response is overuse of drugs in society.

2. Therapy

a. Therapy focuses on reducing reactivity and increasing one's differentiation.

b. Expression of feelings is not encouraged or interpreted, but person is assisted in thinking about processes.

c. Exploration of family's past history is encouraged.

d. Reestablishment of contact with family is supported.

e. Therapist remains out of the interlocking triangles, thereby increasing flexibility and ability to decrease anxiety.

—— Group Approach: Types of Groups Based on Theoretical Frameworks[6,11,12,27,44,53]

A. Client-centered groups
Based on theories of Carl Rogers.[40]

1. *Goals*—increased awareness and acceptance of oneself and others, self-actualization, self-responsibility

2. *Role of therapist*—nondirective; shows genuineness, unconditional positive regard, and empathy; focuses on being with the individuals in group and on group process

B. Transactional analysis groups
These groups are based on theories of Eric Berne.

1. *Goals*—increased insight; reconstruction of personality structure; assumption of self-responsibility; autonomy in spontaneity and intimacy

2. *Role of therapist*—identifies ego states, transactions, and games used by members of group and facilitates more adaptive behaviors; relates openly and honestly in a manner that is free from personal games; serves as teacher and facilitator

C. Interpersonal groups
These groups are based on the theories of Harry S. Sullivan.[46]

1. *Goals*—increased insight and personality reconstruction

2. *Role of therapist*—serves as participant observer, catalyst, and facilitator; supports enhancement of self-esteem; focuses on link between current problems and prior distorted experiences; encourages consenual validation of behavior in order to correct developmental distortions

D. Psychoanalytic groups
   These groups are based on theories of Sigmund Freud.
   1. *Goals*—reconstruction of personality structure
   2. *Role of therapist*—serves as neutral sounding board and authority figure; listens actively; focuses on analyzing individual in group dealing with transferences, dream content, resistance, and past traumatic relationships and link to present behavior; focuses on needs of group by identifying group processes that are operant

E. Gestalt groups
   Gestalt groups are based on theories of Frederick Perls.
   1. *Goals*—assuming responsibility for self; increasing awareness of personal feelings and behavior; increasing awareness of the behavior and feelings of others; completing unfinished business (e.g., by experiencing past experiences in the present)
   2. *Role of therapist*—Confronts, supports, and takes an active role in directing structured exercises; works with individual group member on the "hot seat" in the "here and now"

F. Existential groups
   These groups are based on such theorists as Rollo May.
   1. *Goals*—fully experiencing and relating to others; self-actualization
   2. *Role of therapist*—shares self intimately with group as whole; nondirective but guiding when appropriate

■ REFERENCES

1. American Psychiatric Association: Diagnostic and Statistical Manual of Mental Disorders, 3rd ed., revised. Washington DC, American Psychiatric Association, 1987
2. Andrews G, Pollack C, Stewart G: The determination of defense style by questionnaire. Arch Gen Psychiatry 46(5):455–460, 1989
3. Bachrach LL: The homeless mentally ill and mental health services: an analytical review of the literature. In Lamb HR (ed): The Homeless Mentally Ill. A task Force Report of the American Psychiatric Association. pp 20–21. Washington, DC, American Psychiatric Association, 1984
4. Bandura A: Principles of Behavior Modification. New York, Holt, Rinehart & Winston, 1969
5. Beck A: Cognitive Therapy and Emotional Disorders. New York, International Universities Press, 1976
6. Bion W: Experiences in Groups, and Other Papers. New York, Basic Books, 1961
7. Bloom BL: Community Mental Health: A General Introduction, 2nd ed. Monterey CA, Brooks Cole, 1984
8. Bootzin RR, Acocella JR: Abnormal Psychology: Current Perspectives, 5th ed. New York, Random House, 1988

9. Bowen M: Family Therapy in Clinical Practice. New York, Jason Aronson, 1978
10. Bowlby J: Developmental psychiatry comes of age. Am J Psychiatry 145(1):1–10, 1988
11. Cartwright D, Zander A: Group Dynamics: Research and Theory. New York, Harper & Row, 1968
12. Corsini RJ, Wedding D: Current Psychotherapy, 4th ed. Itasca IL, FE Peacock Publishers, 1989
13. Ellis A, Dryden W: Rational-emotive therapy; an excellent counseling theory for NP's. Nurse Pract 12(7):16–37, 1987
14. Erikson E: Childhood and Society. New York, WW Norton, 1964
15. Erikson E: Identity and the Life Cycle. New York, WW Norton, 1979
16. Erikson E: Identity: Youth and Crisis. New York, WW Norton, 1968
17. Erikson E: Insight and Responsibility. New York, WW Norton, 1968
18. Erikson E: The Life Cycle Completed: A Review. New York, WW Norton, 1982
19. Erikson E: Toys and Reasons: Stages in the Ritualization of Experience. New York, WW Norton, 1977
20. Ford DH, Urban HB: Systems of Psychotherapy. New York, John Wiley & Sons, 1963
21. Frankl VE: Man's Search for Meaning: An Introduction to Logotherapy. Boston, Beacon Press, 1963
22. Green RK, Schaefer AB: Forensic Psychology: A Primer for Legal and Mental Health Professionals. Springfield IL, Charles C Thomas, 1984
23. Gurman AS, Kniskern DP (eds): Handbook of Family Therapy. New York, Brunner-Mazel, 1981
23a. Hales RE, Yudofsky SC (eds): The American Psychiatric Press Textbook of Neuropsychiatry. Washington, D.C., American Psychiatric Press, 1987
24. Haley J: Leaving Home. New York, McGraw-Hill, 1980
25. Haley J: Problem Solving Therapy. San Francisco, Jossey-Bass, 1977
26. Jahoda M: Current Concepts of Positive Mental Health. New York, Basic Books, 1958
27. Kaplan H, Sadock B (eds): Comprehensive Group Psychotherapy. Baltimore, Williams & Wilkins, 1983
28. Kaplan HI, Sadock BJ: Synopsis of Psychiatry: Behavioral Sciences, Clinical Psychiatry. Baltimore, Williams & Wilkins, 1988
29. Mackenzie KR: Recent developments in brief psychotherapy. Hosp Community Psychiatry 39(7):742–752, 1988
30. Manderscheid RW, Barrett SA (eds): Mental Health, United States, 1987. DHHS Pub No.(ADM) 87-1518. Washington DC, U.S. Government Printing Office, 1987
31. Maslow AH (ed): Motivation of Personality, 2nd ed. New York, Harper & Row, 1970
32. McFarlane AJ: A nursing reformulation of Bowen's family systems theory. Arch Psychiatr Nurs 2(5):319–324, 1988
33. Minuchin S: Families and Family Theory. Cambridge, MA, Harvard University Press, 1974
34. Myers JK, et al: Six-month prevalence of psychiatric disorders in three communities, 1980–1982. Arch Gen Psychiatry 41(10):906, 1984
35. National Center for Health Statistics: Health, U.S. 1986. DHHS Pub No. (PHS) 86-1232. Washington, DC, U.S. Gov Printing Office, 1986

36. Novotny PC: Bowen family systems theory and psychoanalysis—echo or metamorphosis. Bull Menninger Clin 51(4):323–337, 1987

37. Perry S, Cooper AM, Michels R: The psychodynamic formulation: its purpose, structure, and clinical application. Am J Psychiatry 144(5):543–550, 1987

38. Pollack WS: Schizophrenia and the self: contributions of psychoanalytic self-psychology. Schizophr Bull 15(2):311–321, 1989

39. Reamer FG: The contemporary mental health system: facilities, services, personnel, and finances. In Rochefort DA (ed): Handbook on Mental Health Policy in U.S. New York, Greenwood Press, 1989

40. Rogers C: A theory of therapy, personality and interpersonal relationships as developed in the client-centered framework. In Koch S (ed): Psychology, a Study of Science. New York, McGraw-Hill, 1963

40a. Rowland LP (ed): Merritt's Textbook of Neurology, 8th ed. Philadelphia, Lea & Febiger, 1989

41. Sarason IG, Sarason BR: Abnormal Psychology: The Problem of Maladaptive Behavior, 6th ed. New Jersey, Englewood Cliffs, 1989

42. Satir V: Conjoint Family Therapy, revised ed. Palo Alto CA, Science and Behavior Books, 1967

43. Siegel GJ, et al (eds): Basic Neurochemistry, 4th ed. New York, Raven Press, 1989

44. Slater P: Microcosm, Structural, Psychological, and Religious Evolution in Groups. New York, John Wiley & Sons, 1966

45 Subcommittee of the Joint Commission on Public Affairs. Werner A (chairman), et al: A Psychiatric Glossary, 5th ed. Washington, DC, American Psychiatric Association, 1984

45a. Sudarsky L: Pathophysiology of the Nervous System. Boston, Little, Brown, & Co., 1990

46. Sullivan HS: The Interpersonal Theory of Psychiatry. New York, WW Norton, 1953

47. Task Force Report of American Psychiatric Association. Treatment of Psychiatric Disorders. Vols 1 and 2. Washington DC, American Psychiatric Association, 1989

48. Taube CA, Barrett SA (eds): Mental Health, United States, 1983. DHHS Publication No. (ADM)83-1275. p 10. Rockville MD, The National Institute of Mental Health, 1983

49. Uhlenhutt et al: Symposium checklist syndrome in the general population. Arch Gen Psychiatry 40(11):167–173, 1983

50. Vaillant GE: Adaptation to Life. Boston, Little, Brown, 1977

51. Vaillant GE: Defense mechanisms. In Nicholi AM (ed): The New Harvard Guide to Psychiatry. Cambridge MA, Harvard University Press, 1988

52. World Health Organization: World Health Statistical Manual. Geneva, World Health Organization, 1986

53. Yalom I: Inpatient Group Psychotherapy. New York, Basic Books, 1983

Therapeutic Relationship

/2

■ THE ONE-TO-ONE NURSE-PATIENT RELATIONSHIP[3,4,17,39,40,41,64]

A. Definition and characteristics of the one-to-one relationship include
1. A mutually defined professional relationship that focuses attention on the patient's emotional, cognitive, and behavioral responses and concerns.
2. A series of purposeful and mutually determined, goal-directed nurse-patient interactions occurring over time.
3. Goal-directed interpersonal techniques, including active listening, are used in order to foster exploration of problem areas, learning, change, and personal growth.
4. Scope can range from brief interactions and counseling by a generalist in psychiatric mental health nursing who uses psychotherapeutic interventions to individual psychotherapy by a psychiatric mental health clinical nurse specialist.

B. Definition of terms related to the one-to-one nurse-patient relationship.
1. *Psychotherapeutic intervention*—"A specific, time-limited interaction of a nurse with a client who has a problem that presents an immediate and ongoing difficulty related to health or well-being. The difficulty is investigated through use of a problem-solving approach so that the experience may be understood more fully and integrated with other life experiences. Counseling by the nurse may include regularly scheduled brief and short-term interviewing in a variety of settings, such as homes, hospitals, clinics, and schools."[3,p.26;4,p.20]
2. *Psychotherapy*—"All generally accepted and respected methods of treatment, specifically including individual therapy; play; brief, goal-oriented therapy; behavioral therapy; group therapy; and family therapy.

It is a structured, contractual relationship between the therapist and client for the exclusive purpose of effecting changes in the client. This modality attempts to alleviate emotional disturbance, to reverse or change maladaptive behavior, and to facilitate personality growth and development.[3,p.26;4,p.20]

3. *Generalist in psychiatric mental health nursing*—"A nurse who is educated at the basic level for entry into professional nursing practice, who practices . . . psychiatric and mental health nursing, and who refines clinical skills through ongoing supervision of practice in a clinical setting."[3,p.26]

4. *Psychiatric mental health nurse clinical specialist*—"A nurse who holds a minimum of a master's degree . . . in psychiatric and mental health nursing, has had supervised clinical experience at the graduate level, and demonstrates depth and breadth of knowledge, competence, and skill in the practice of . . . psychiatric and mental health nursing."[3,p.26]

C. Phases of the nurse-patient relationship (phases are overlapping and interlocking throughout the nurse-patient relationship)[1,5–7,9,11,12,14,16, 21–28,31,33–35,43,45,47,48,50,55,59,64]

1. Phase I (beginning, or orientation, phase)
   a. Common patient characteristics and behaviors include the following. The patient
      (1) experiences a felt (but sometimes poorly understood) need for assistance and seeks assistance for this need;
      (2) experiences tension or anxiety which is not always observable;
      (3) frequently bases preconceptions and expectations of current nurse-patient relationship on past experiences;
      (4) may reach a certain point or state where there is nothing more to say;
      (5) tests parameters of the nurse-patient relationship, including behaviors that the nurse will tolerate—i.e., unexpected tardiness or absence or the extent to which the nurse will go to meet the patient's needs;
      (6) raises questions with the nurse;
      (7) uses cognitive words and phrases to describe situations and events, with minimal focus on identification and description of feelings.
   b. Therapeutic nursing tasks during orientation phase:
      (1) Assess, identify, and clarify patient's current needs and problems.
      (2) Formulate initial nursing diagnoses.
      (3) Begin to formulate health pattern profiles.
      (4) Clarify own preconceptions and expectations.
      (5) Establish a mutually agreed-upon therapeutic contract for the one-to-one nurse-patient relationship. This contract includes
         (a) explanation of the nurse's role and responsibilities in the relationship;
         (b) description of the overall purpose of the one-to-one nurse-patient relationship;
         (c) identification of mutually defined cognitive, emotional, and behavioral goals;

(d) agreement on place, time, and length of meetings.

(e) establishment of fee/reimbursement (if applicable);

(f) statement of actual or tentative length of therapy/nurse-patient relationship (preparation for termination phase);

(g) statement on policy for cancellation of appointments;

(h) discussion of parameters regarding the role of family/significant others;

(i) discussion of the patient's responsibilities in the one-to-one nurse-patient relationship;

(j) verbalization of patient's understanding of orientation information, explanations, and the therapeutic contract.

(6) Discuss confidentiality of information shared by patient.

(a) Inform patient that progress in therapy will be shared with the health care team members in general terms.

(b) Inform patient if written progress reports by the nurse will be shared with the patient prior to being placed in the patient's record.

(c) If the situation warrants, inform patient that harmfulness to self or others will be shared with appropriate professional staff, family, or significant others who would need to be informed in case of danger to self or others. Give patient rationale for this action.

(d) Avoid making promises in response to patient requests to not share information (i.e., suicidal or homicidal ideation, alcohol and drug use) with other health team members. Emphasize that the sharing of specific patient information with the health team is a decision that is based upon the nurse's professional judgment.

(7) Build trusting relationship by maintaining the stipulations of the contract and informing the patient of any changes, such as unavoidable absences.

2. Phase II (middle or working phase)

a. Common patient characteristics and behaviors: The patient

(1) responds to offers of help from the nurse;

(2) identifies and describes problems;

(3) decreases testing maneuvers that were evident during the orientation phase—e.g., asking personal information about nurse; questioning focus, length, and frequency of interviews;

(4) fluctuates in the need for dependency, independence, and interdependency in the nurse-patient relationship;

(5) demonstrates increased ability to discuss problems and to identify, describe, and explore feelings;

(6) imitates or copies behaviors or appearance of the nurse in an attempt to convey identification with or wishing to be like the nurse;

(7) demonstrates movement toward therapeutic goals that were formulated during the orientation phase;

(8) makes full use of the services offered by the nurse and attempts to obtain maximum benefits from the nurse-patient relationship.

b. Therapeutic nursing tasks during the working phase:

(1) Recognize behavioral manifestations of ambivalence and resistance—i.e., rejection, avoidance, denial, hostility, and reaching a plateau in therapy.

(2) Attend to frequency of patient's use of affective words and phrases and to the patient's descriptions of behavioral trends and patterns.

(3) Encourage expression and analysis of emotional concerns and self-defeating behavioral patterns and trends.

    (a) Mutually determine the behavioral dynamics of the patient and explore the origin, operation, and consequences of behavioral patterns.

    (b) Facilitate patient's own assessment of self-defeating behavioral patterns.

(4) Periodically devote a portion of the nurse-patient interaction to a mutual review (by the patient and the nurse) of the progress which has been made in the achievement of the goals which were formulated during the orientation phase. Use the findings from this review to determine the need for reformulation of therapeutic goals.

(5) Avoid making observations about the patient's copying or imitating the nurse's appearance or behaviors, in order to minimize the patient's being able to recognize things about the nurse that the patient does *not* wish to copy.

(6) Facilitate resolution of emotional conflicts, reduction in self-defeating behavioral patterns, and attainment of the mutually defined behavioral goals of the patient.

    (a) Identify, with the patient, forces that hinder behavioral change.

    (b) Facilitate problem-solving strategies to formulate behavioral alternatives, and to select a behavioral alternative for testing.

    (c) Make assignments for the patient to work on between counseling sessions, to help the patient change undesirable cognitive and behavioral patterns.

    (d) Create an atmosphere in which the patient can test new behaviors and work through any associated anxiety.

(7) Begin preparation for termination by periodically reminding the patient of the remaining length of time that the nurse and patient will be meeting together.

3. Phase III (termination or resolution phase)

    a. Common patient characteristics and behaviors: The patient

        (1) responds to the actual termination with the nurse according to prior termination experiences, type of treatment, present problems, actual and perceived rationale for termination, and patient's personality; reactions to impending loss of the nurse-patient relationship can include grief, sadness, depression, displacement of feelings, ambivalence, reaction formation, dependency, regression, frank hostility, missed appointments, rejection of the nurse;

        (2) maximizes learning which has occurred throughout the one-to-one relationship;

        (3) participates in evaluation of the progress made toward achievement of the goals identified during the orientation phase;

(4) demonstrates increased ability to use cognitive words and themes in relation to the ending of the nurse-patient relationship and in the formulation of future plans.

b. Therapeutic nursing tasks during the termination phase:
(1) Establish the reality of the ending of the relationship.
(2) Determine the extent of the patient's readiness for termination by evaluating factors such as progress toward resolution of identified problems, constructive use of defense mechanisms, and attainment of planned treatment goals.
(3) When possible, mutually determine actual termination date.
(4) Anticipate own reactions to ending of relationship.
(5) Assist patient to identify feelings and reactions to impending loss of nurse.
(6) Encourage patient to express feelings.
(7) Help patient tolerate the discomfort involved in termination.
(8) Acknowledge own feelings and reactions in a manner which does not place a burden on the patient.
(9) Help patient to discuss and resolve feelings about the impending separation from the nurse.
(10) Encourage patient to describe and evaluate observations of experiences throughout the one-to-one relationship.
(11) Facilitate patient's review and evaluation of the therapeutic contract.
(12) Encourage and support patient's emotional investment in other relationships.
(13) Convey recognition of patient's accomplishments during the relationship.
(14) Summarize observations of areas for further growth for patient to consider.
(15) Teach prevention measures—i.e., recognizing early signs of relapse and use of available community resources for continuation of medications or individual therapy.

■ PRINCIPLES AND STRATEGIES FOR DEVELOPING AND MAINTAINING A THERAPEUTIC NURSE-PATIENT RELATIONSHIP

A. Develop effective communication skills[5,7,15,16,21,22,30,39–42,44,49,52,61,65]
1. Definition and elements
a. *Communication*—This is a dynamic, complex, constantly changing process that occurs over time in which human beings send and receive verbal and nonverbal messages in order to understand and to be understood by others, adapt to the environment, and transfer ideas to another.
b. It is impossible not to communicate, because all behavior communicates something.
c. Communication includes
(1) content aspect of message—verbal message;
(2) relationship aspect of message—verbal and/or nonverbal aspect of message about the relationship between the sender and the receiver. Nonverbal communication can qualify or disqualify verbal message.

      d. Elements of communication include
         (1) Sender—message transmitter of message
         (2) Message—meaning that is communicated, intentionally or un-intentionally
         (3) Code, channel, or media—the way in which a message is sent
         (4) Receiver—recipient of message
         (5) Response of feedback—behavior of receiver (verbal and non-verbal) in relation to message received

2. Types of communication
    a. Verbal—use of written or spoken words
    b. Nonverbal—use of facial expression; eye contact; posture; bodily movements; touch; appearance and dress; pitch, rate, and volume of voice; gestures
    c. Digital—the verbal mode of communication
    d. Analogic—the nonverbal mode of communication including the context
    e. Symmetrical—communication characterized by equality in the right to initiate communication, to criticize, and to offer advice
    f. Complementary—communication characterized by one person giving and the other receiving in the interaction

3. Factors affecting communication
    a. Culture, customs, education, social background, physical attributes, mental well-being, body image, self-esteem, intellectual ability, and past experiences of the participants
    b. Channel, language, and words used to transmit message
    c. Context in which communication occurs
    d. Perceptions, feelings, thoughts, and motivations of receiver and sender prior to communication
    e. Nature of the relationship between sender and receiver
    f. Intentions or goals of sender and receiver
    g. Self-concept or self-perception of sender and receiver
    h. Anxiety or stress level of sender or receiver
    i. Sensory organ impairment or physical disorder interfering with mechanical ability to produce or to hear sound
    j. Disorders interfering with cognitive functioning and/or information processing
    k. Discrepancies between the sender's and receiver's punctuation of the communication sequence of events—that is, the particular aspect of the communication on which each focuses

B. Develop an understanding of the causes of communication breakdown or distortion[5,7,15,16,18,21–23,27,30,42,44,49,52,61,62,65]
1. Unintelligible messages—using terms the patient does not understand, especially psychiatric or medical terminology or jargon
2. Incomplete messages—assuming that the patient already has the knowledge and therefore leaving the patient's questions unanswered
3. Inadvertent messages—unintentionally transmitting a message, such as by giving too much detail, which the patient then misinterprets
4. Omitted messages—failing to explain something the patient should know
5. Contradictory messages—transmitting a message in which the verbal

and nonverbal aspects are contradictory, or several different staff members giving different messages to the patient

6. Unfulfilled messages—making promises that are not kept
7. Failure to listen actively
8. Failure to interpret the message accurately
9. Failure to focus on the patient's concerns
10. Ineffective or inappropriate reassurance
11. Lecturing, moralizing, pep talks
12. Switching topic of conversation to superficial aspects
13. Judgmental attitude, prejudice, stereotyping
14. Stress perceived or faced by nurse in work situation
15. Culturally incongruent verbal or nonverbal behavior
16. High level of fear and anxiety patient may have about illness and its treatment (Items 1 through 15 can increase patient's anxiety.)

C. Develop and improve self-awareness[5,7,8,13,16,18,19,22,29,31,32,38,40,47,51,52,54,60,62,63]

1. Develop awareness of own verbal and nonverbal communication patterns.
2. Recognize, explore origin, and attempt to work through stereotyping, prejudices, and negative attitudes.
3. Develop awareness of own cultural and subcultural values and customs and their influence on personal behavior as well as on one's own perception and interpretation of another's behavior.
4. Identify common personal stressors and typical behavioral responses.
5. Identify and increase own adaptive coping patterns in response to stress.
6. Identify and develop constructive personal ethical values in relation to care of the adult psychiatric patient and health care in general.
7. Validate perceptions and interpretations of patient's behavior with patient or with professional colleague as indicated.
8. Examine own motives, feelings, and behavior.
   a. Develop self-acceptance, self-esteem, and self-respect.
   b. Develop ability to differentiate clearly between own feelings and those belonging to the patient.
   c. Recognize, accept, and analyze origin of negative feelings.
9. Operate on facts rather than on assumptions or misperceptions.
10. Identify awareness of anxiety developed in self during a nurse-patient interaction and seek to gain information about the patient's anxiety level, using self as guide.
11. Assume responsibility for continuing education to increase self-awareness—i.e., institutional inservices, regional and national continuing education, postgraduate courses, graduate and doctoral programs.[3,4]

D. Use clinical consultation/supervision in the one-to-one nurse-patient relationship to improve self-awareness[2,19,20,23,32,42,47,56–58,61,63]

1. Definition and characteristics of clinical consultation/supervision
   a. *Clinical consultation/supervision*—an interpersonal process between a mental health professional, preferably a certified psychiatric mental health clinical nurse specialist or a nurse who has a doctoral

degree in psychiatric mental health nursing, and a psychiatric mental health nurse, for the purpose of focusing on the empathic process and treatment issues in the one-to-one nurse-patient relationship, in order to facilitate the consultee/supervisee's clinical competence.

b. The consultation/supervision process is cognitive and didactic, emphasizing the cultivation of therapeutic use of self, psychotherapeutic skills, and psychotherapeutic interventions.

c. The focus is on the treatment of the patient and not the nurse's personal needs, unless these needs are directly related to issues in the one-to-one relationship.

d. The consultant/supervisor serves as a mentor to guide the application of theory in the practice of psychotherapeutic nursing interventions.

2. Phases of consultation/supervision:

a. Beginning (honeymoon)—The consultant/supervisor focuses on establishing a learning alliance; and the nurse strives to be open to suggestions, to learn more about the therapeutic use of self, and to gain knowledge about the nurse-patient relationship.

b. Mid-phase (working)—The nurse may experience feelings of anger and confusion during the process of identifying with the consultant/supervisor's expertise and of attempting to incorporate new clinical information. The consultant/supervisor avoids personalization of these feelings and evaluates the nurse's anxiety to determine the extent to which new material can be processed.

c. Integration phase—The consultant/supervisor facilitates the nurse to move towards becoming an autonomous clinical practitioner. The nurse demonstrates the ability to integrate clinical knowledge and psychotherapeutic interventions that are consistent with the nurse's personality and treatment preferences.

d. End phase—The consultant/supervisor and the nurse mutually review and evaluate the consultation/supervisory process. Recognition of accomplishments and recommendations for future learning are discussed. Successful termination of the consultation/supervisory relationship is dependent upon the consultant/supervisor and the nurse working through this evaluation process.

E. Develop trust[5,8,22,31,37,42,52,53,62,63]

1. Establish a sense of confidence and security in the reliability of oneself and others.

2. Be consistently truthful.

3. Offer the patient a clear understanding of the purpose of the nurse-patient relationship or one-to-one nurse therapy.

4. Be consistent, reliable, and open.

5. Demonstrate genuine interest in and commitment to the patient over a period of time.

6. Be sensitive to the patient's needs.

7. Create an interpersonal relationship in which the patient can freely communicate feelings, needs, and problems.

8. Communicate a warm, positive regard for the patient.

9. Don't make promises unless they can be kept.

10. Try to respond to reasonable requests.

F. Be congruent[5,7,10,16,18,22,38,60,63,67]
1. Strive for an expression of consistency between actual feelings, thoughts, verbalization, and behavior.
2. Be natural, spontaneous, real, open, sincere, and nondefensive.
3. Admit one's own errors to patient, when appropriate.
4. Communicate negative feelings to patient if
   a. it can be done within the context of a therapeutic objective;
   b. they are truly generated by the patient, not from the nurse's own past;
   c. the patient is capable of distinguishing the feedback as an aspect of the patient's behavior and not as the patient's total being.
5. Share one's own personal reactions and feelings with patient, if this serves a therapeutic purpose.
   a. Avoid constant and total disclosure of feelings.
   b. Express negative feelings to the patient in a nondestructive way that encourages further discussion.
6. Be as natural and spontaneous as possible in the use of therapeutic interventions. Avoid artificial, mechanical use of interpersonal techniques.

G. Use personal self-disclosure appropriately[5,15,22,61,63]
1. Avoid self-disclosure to meet nurse's personal needs
2. Understand that if the nurse or patient discloses self at a certain level in the relationship, the other person tends to respond with a similar or greater degree of self-disclosure.
3. Recognize that the higher the level of trust, the higher the level of self-disclosure.
4. Recognize that inappropriate disclosure can be incorporated into the patient's delusions or fantasies.

H. Provide consistency of experience[22,31,52,55,63]
1. Enforce consistent restrictions.
2. Provide consistency in attitude.
3. Meet with patient at agreed-upon time(s).
4. Give the patient information about changes in the patient's schedule or surroundings.

I. Demonstrate sensitivity to and respect for patient[22,37,42]
1. Support healthy parts of the patient's personality.
2. Use words that the patient can understand to explain and provide information about the patient's condition and the health care setting in which the patient is being treated. Use informational booklets and other teaching material as appropriate.
3. Permit expression of negative feeling. Avoid retaliation and punishment for expression of these feelings.
4. Focus on strengths and potential of patient.
5. Avoid increasing anxiety unnecessarily.

J. Express empathy[5,7,8,15,36,46,47,61,63,66,67]
"The emergence of a particular affective state" in which the nurse experiences both "the patient's conscious and unconscious emotional states. . . ."[8, p. 421]

1. Use empathy as a therapeutic tool to make clinical observations about the patient's internal state in a manner that helps the patient feel understood and soothed and to promote the achievement of the mutually determined goals in the nurse-patient relationship.
2. Perceive and recognize patient's private, inner experiences and feelings.
    a. Use open-ended questions focusing on feelings.
    b. Reflect patient's feelings.
    c. Focus on "being with" patient.
3. Develop awareness of own responses to patient.
    a. Recognize interaction of one's own experiences and those described by patient.
    b. Develop awareness of one's own responses to assist in grasping dynamic meaning, significance, and purpose of patient's experiences and feelings.
    c. Develop a sense of meaning for that which the patient is not fully aware.
    d. Achieve an ongoing awareness of perceptual, cognitive, and affective aspects of patient.
4. Communicate accurate, sensitive understanding.
    a. Selectively use self-disclosure: Share experiences that model the patient's expression of feelings and help patient recognize that the patient is not alone.
    b. Communicate understanding of the feelings expressed by patient.
    c. Communicate understanding of underlying feelings and assumptions implied by patient.

K. Demonstrate unconditional positive regard and acceptance of the uniqueness of the patient[7,15,22,52,60–63]
1. Communicate value of the patient's being and potential.
    a. Preserve patient's individuality, opinions, uniqueness, and feelings.
    b. Be nonevaluative and nonjudgmental.
    c. Avoid reducing self-esteem of patient.
2. Demonstrate sincere and nonpossessive caring and concern.
3. Communicate openness and willingness to engage in a therapeutic nurse-patient relationship.
4. Convey acceptance of patient's uniqueness, but do not convey approval of inappropriate behavior.
5. Remain objective in observing and identifying reasons for patient's behavior.
6. Make self available.
    a. Do not communicate indifference or rejection.
    b. Offer presence and spend time with patient.
7. Don't attempt to negate patient's perception of an experience by comments such as, "Oh, it can't be that bad!"
8. Attempt to understand patient's perspective and feelings.

L. Use confrontation appropriately[7,10,30,61]
1. Consider the possible outcomes of confrontation—i.e., the risks and benefits.
2. Use appropriate timing when using confrontation; confrontation is seldom used during orientation phase; it should only be used after basic trust has been established, which is usually during the working phase.

3. Avoid overuse of nurse-initiated confrontation.
4. Use empathy, authenticity, and respect to facilitate self-confrontation.
5. Communicate to the patient growth-defeating discrepancies in the patient's feelings, perceptions, and thinking.
6. Assist the patient to become fully aware of a specific aspect of behavior or problem.
7. Encourage the patient to examine and to begin to acquire new strategies for choosing options.

▰ REFERENCES

1. Aggleton P, Chalmers H: Peplau's development model. Nurs Times 86(2):38–40, 1990
2. Alonso A: The Quiet Profession: Supervisors of Psychotherapy. New York, Macmillan, 1985
3. American Nurses' Association Council on Psychiatric and Mental Health Nursing: Standards of Child and Adolescent Psychiatric and Mental Health Nursing Practice. Kansas City, American Nurses' Association, 1985
4. American Nurses' Association Division on Psychiatric and Mental Health Nursing Practice: Standards of Psychiatric and Mental Health Nursing Practice. Kansas City, American Nurses' Association, 1982
5. Arnold E, Boggs K: Interpersonal Relationships: Professional Communication Skills for Nurses. Philadelphia, WB Saunders, 1989
6. Belcher JR, Fish LJB: Hildegard E. Peplau. In The Nursing Theories Conference Group. Nursing theories: The Base for Professional Nursing Practice. New Jersey, Prentice-Hall, 1980
7. Benjamin A: The Helping Interview: With Case Illustrations. Boston, Houghton Mifflin Co, 1987
8. Book HE: Empathy: misconceptions and misuses in psychotherapy. Am J Psychiatry 145(4):420–424, 1988
9. Boulanger G: Working with the entitled patient. J Contem Psychother 18(2):124–144, 1988
10. Bromley GE: Confrontation in individual psychotherapy. J Psychosoc Nurs Ment Health Serv 19(5):15–18, 1981
11. Busch P: Therapy with the noninvolved client. J Psychosoc Nurs Ment Health Serv. 25(11):21–25, 1987
12. Campaniello JA: The process of termination. J Psychiatr Nurs 18(2):29–32, 1980
13. Campbell J: The relationship of nursing and self-awareness. Adv Nurs Sci 2(4):15–25, 1980
14. Carey ET, Noll J, Rasmussen L, Searcy B, Stark NL: Hildegard E. Peplau: psychodynamic nursing. In Marriner-Tomey A: Nursing Theorists and Their Work, 2nd ed. St. Louis, CV Mosby, 1989
15. Cassell EJ, Coulehan JL, Putnam SM: Making good interview skills better. Patient Care 23(6):145–148, 155–166, 1989
16. Chapman AH: The Treatment Techniques of Harry Stack Sullivan. New York, Brunner/Mazel, 1978
17. Church OM, Hardin SB, Durham JD: Introducton and historical perspective: the nurse psychotherapist as private practitioner. In Durham JD, Hardin SB (eds): The nurse psychotherapist in private practice. New York, Springer Publishing Co., 1986

18. Colson DB, Allen JG, Coyne L, et al: An anatomy of countertransference: staff reactions to difficult psychiatric hospital patients. Hosp Community Psychiatry 37(9):923–928, 1986
19. Critchley DL: Clinical supervision. In Critchley DL, Maurin JT (eds): The Clinical Specialist in Psychiatric Mental Health Nursing. New York, John Wiley & Sons, 1985
20. Critchley DL: Clinical supervision as a learning tool for the student therapist in milieu settings. J Psychosoc Nurs Ment Health Serv 25(8):18–22, 1987
21. Emdon T: The basics of therapy, fresh out of miracles. Nurs Times 85(48):36–38, 1989
22. Field WF: The Psychotherapy of Hildegard E. Peplau. New Braunfels Texas, PSF Productions, 1979
23. Fiore RJ: Toward engaging the difficult patient. J Contem Psychother 18(2):87–106, 1988
24. Forchuk C, Beaton S, Crawford L, Ide L, Voorberg N, Bethune J: Incorporating Peplau's theory and case management. J Psychosoc Nurs Ment Health Serv 27(2):35–38, 1989
25. Forchuk C, Brown B: Establishing a nurse-client relationship. J Psychosoc Nurs Ment Health Serv 27(2):30–34, 1989
26. Gerace LM: The patient needing long-term supportive therapy. In Durham JD, Hardin SB (eds): The Nurse Psychotherapist in Private Practice. New York, Springer Publishing Co., 1986
27. Goldman SB. To be or not to be a real object: monitoring the therapeutic relationship. J Contem Psychother 18(2):164–178, 1988
28. Hale SL, Richardson JH: Terminating the nurse-patient relationship. AJN 63(9):116–119, 1963
29. Hardin SB, Halaris AL: Nonverbal communication of patients and high and low empathy nurses. J Psychosoc Nurs Ment Health Serv 21(1):14–20, 1983
30. Hedlund N: Therapeutic communication. In Beck CK, Rawlins RP, Williams SR (eds): Mental Health-Psychiatric Nursing: A Holistic Life-Cycle Approach, 2nd ed. St. Louis, CV Mosby, 1988
31. Holmberg S. Trust-mistrust: In Beck CK, Rawlins RP, Williams SR (eds): Mental Health-Psychiatric Nursing: A Holistic Life-Cycle Approach, 2nd. St. Louis, CV Mosby, 1988
32. Hughes CM: Supervising clinical practice in psychosocial nursing. J Psychosoc Nurs Health Serv 23(2):27–32, 1985
33. Kasch CR: Interpersonal competence and communication in the delivery of nursing care. Advances Nurs Sci 6(2):71–88, 1984
34. Kasch CR, Kasch JB, Lisnek P: Women's talk and nurse-client encounters: developing criteria for assessing interpersonal skill. Scholarly Inquiry Nurs Prac 1(3):241–255, 1987
35. Kirkman MB, Bell SK: AIDS and confidentiality. Nurs Forum 24(3,4):47–51, 1989
36. Krouse HJ, Roberts SJ: Nurse-patient interactive styles: power, control, and satisfaction. West J Nurs Res. 11(6):717–725, 1989
37. Krouse HJ, Krouse JH, Roberts SJ: Preliminary validation of a nurse-patient interaction tool. Percept Mot Skills 67:281–282, 1988
38. Krikorian DA, Paulanka BJ: Self-awareness—the key to a successful nurse-patient relationship? J Psychosoc Nurs Ment Health Serv 20(6):19–21, 1982

39. Lego S. The one-to-one nurse-patient relationship. Perspect Psychiatr Care. 18:67–69, 1980
40. Lego S. Individual therapy. In Lego S (ed): The American Handbook of Psychiatric nursing. Philadelphia, JB Lippincott, 1984
41. Lego S. Psychoanalytically oriented individual and group therapy with adults. In Critchley DL, Maurin JT (eds): The Clinical Specialist in Psychiatric Mental Health Nursing. New York, John Wiley & Sons, 1985
42. Limandri BJ: The theapeutic relationship with abused women: nurses responses that facilitate or inhibit change. J Psychosoc Nurs Ment Health Serv 25(2):8–16, 1987
43. Marriner-Tomey A, Mills DI, Sauter MK: Ida Jean Orlando (Pelletier): nursing process theory. In Marriner-Tomey A: Nursing Theorists and Their Work, 2nd ed. St. Louis, CV Mosby, 1989
44. McFarland GK, Leonard HS, Morris MM: Nursing Leadership and Management: Contemporary Strategies. New York, John Wiley & Sons, 1984
45. McHale MD: Mumbling: a defense mechanism in therapy resistance. J Psychosoc Nurs Ment Health Serv 26(9):27–30, 1988
46. Morath J: Empathy training: development of sensitivity and caring in hospitals. Nurs Management. 20(3):60–62, 1989
47. Moore JC, Hartman CR: Developing a therapeutic relationship. In Beck CK, Rawlins RP, Williams SR (eds): Mental Health-Psychiatric Nursing: A Holistic Life-Cycle Approach, 2nd ed. St. Louis, CV Mosby, 1988
48. Moscato B: The one-to-one relationship. In Wilson HS, Kneisl CR: Psychiatric Nursing, 3rd ed. Menlo Park, California, Addison-Wesley, 1988
49. Naschinski C: The communication process. In McFarland GK, Thomas MD: Psychiatric Mental Health Nursing: Application of the Nursing Process. Philadelphia, JB Lippincott, 1991
50. Orlando IJ: The Dynamic Nurse-Patient Relationship: Function, Process and Principles. New York, Putnam, 1961
51. O'Toole AW: Elements of a graduate curriculum to prepare nurse psychotheapists. In Durham JD, Hardin SB (eds): The Nurse Psychotherapist in Private Practice. New York, Springer Publishing Co., 1986
52. O'Toole AW, Welt SR (eds): Interpersonal Theory in Nursing Practice: Selected Works of Hildegard E. Peplau. New York, Springer Publishing Co., 1989
53. Peplau HE: Interpersonal Relations in Nursing. New York, GP Putnam's Sons, 1952
54. Peplau HE: Talking with patients. AJN 60(7):964–966, 1960
55. Peplau HE: Basic Principles of Patient Counseling: Extracts from Two Clinical Nursing Workshops in Psychiatric Hospitals, 2nd ed. Philadelphia, Smith Kline & French Laboratories, 1964
56. Pesut DJ, Williams CA: The nature of clinical supervision in psychiatric nursing: a survey of clinical specialists. Arch Psychiatric Nurs 4(3):188–194, 1990
57. Platt-Koch LM: Clinical supervision for psychiatric nurses. J Psychosoc Nurs Ment Health Serve 26(1):6–15, 1986
58. Rankin DJ: Therapy supervision; the phenomena and the need. Clin Nurse Specialist 3(4):204–208, 1989

59. Schmieding NJ: Orlando's theory. In Winstead-Fry P (ed): Case Studies in Nursing Theory. New York, National League for Nursing, 1986
60. Schroder PJ: Recognizing transference and countertransference. J Psychosoc Nurs Ment Health Serv 23(2):21–26, 1985
61. Stuart GW, Sundeen SJ: Principles and Practice of Psychiatric Nursing, 3rd ed. St. Louis, CV Mosby, 1987
62. Thomas MD: Cultural concepts and psychiatric mental health nursing. In McFarland GK, Thomas MD: Psychiatric Mental Health Nursing: Application of the Nursing Process. Philadelphia, JB Lippincott, 1991
63. Thomas MD: Therapeutic relationships with clients. In McFarland GK, Thomas MD: Psychiatric Mental Health Nursing: Application of the Nursing Process. Philadelphia, JB Lippincott, 1991
64. Thompson L: Peplau's theory: an application to short-term individual therapy. J Psychosoc Nurs Ment Health Serv 24(8):26–31, 1986
65. Topf M, Dambacher B: Teaching interpersonal skills: a model for facilitating optimal interpersonal relations. J Psychosoc Nurs Ment Health Serv 19(12):29–33, 1981
66. Wheeler K: A nursing science approach to understanding empathy. Arch Psychiatric nurs 2(2):95–102, 1988
67. Young JC: Rationale for clinician self-disclosure and research agenda. Image J Nurse Scholarship. 20(4):196–199, 1988

Initial Psychiatric Assessment of the Adult

3

■ CONCEPTUAL FRAMEWORK FOR PSYCHIATRIC MENTAL HEALTH NURSING PRACTICE[1-40]

A. Human beings are in continuous interplay with their environment.

B. Human beings possess the potential ability to cope with stressors, meet needs, and attain goals through adaptive strategies, skills, and processes.

C. Adaptive strategies, skills, and processes include the following:
1. *Interaction*—exchanging, interchanging, or linking matter, energy, persons, or objects between the person and the environment
   a. *Exchanging*—matter and energy interchange
   b. *Communicating*—information interchange
   c. *Relating*—person or object linkage(s) and interaction
2. *Action*—assigning value, selecting alternatives, and taking action
   a. *Valuing*—assigning value, worth, or meaning
   b. *Choosing*—setting priorities and selecting alternatives
   c. *Moving*—taking action within one's environment
3. *Awareness*—alertness, feeling, knowing/perception
   a. *Waking*—level of alertness
   b. *Feeling*—sensation and mood
   c. *Knowing*—ability to perceive, store, and use information accurately
See Figure 3-1.

— The Nursing Process[1-40]

The nursing process is an interactive, systematic, problem-solving process that is used to assist the client to achieve a maximum level of wellness. It should be utilized throughout the one-to-one nurse-patient relationship.

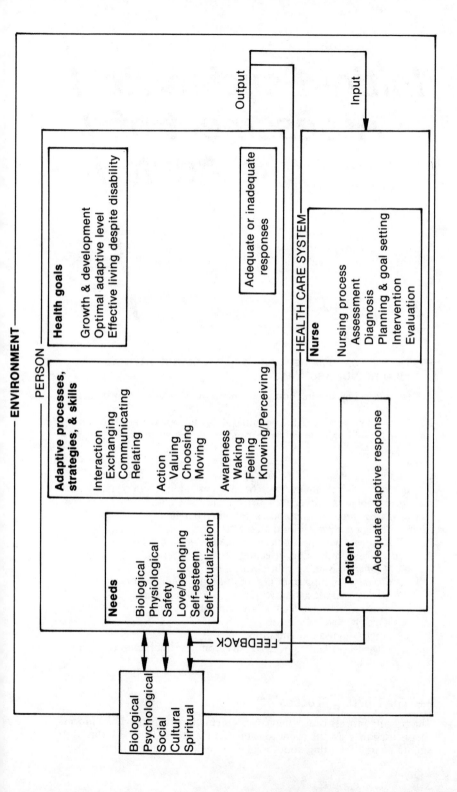

A. Assessment

Assessment is the systematic and continuous collection of data about the health status of the client.

1. Guidelines for structuring the process and content of the interview
   a. Utilize a nursing history guide during the interview to collect data. Use open-ended questions.
   b. Provide for privacy, physical comfort, and freedom from interruption during the interview.
   c. Conduct interview with sensitivity so as to facilitate the beginning of a positive nurse-patient relationship. Use pauses to allow for full disclosure.
   d. Explain the purpose, nature, and length of the interview.
   e. Inform patient that information gained will be utilized to assist in treatment and will be shared with appropriate staff.
   f. Ask about the nature of the patient's problem and current life situation. Show interest and allow patient to fully express all concerns.
   g. Observe for both verbal and nonverbal expressions, changes in mood, and difficulties in answering any questions.
   h. Ask questions in a concrete and simple way. Use narrowly focused questions to test hunches.
   i. Repeat and also summarize periodically what patient says.
   j. Utilize a conceptual framework for nursing practice to guide observations, interviewing, and assessment.
   k. Follow health care agency guidelines for charting observations and assessment.

2. *Process recordings*—written records of the communication of both the nurse and the patient, especially during individual nurse psychotherapy when indicated
   a. May be used by a nurse expert to review and supervise the one-to-one nurse-patient relationship developed by the nurse or nursing student being supervised
   b. Can include an analysis of
      (1) The nurse's thoughts, observations, feelings, and interventions (including the treatment goal)
      (2) The patient's responses
      (3) The total interaction

B. Nursing diagnosis

The diagnosis is formulated from an analysis of patient assessment and the data collected. According to Shoemaker,[18] a nursing diagnosis is a clinical judgment about an individual, family, or community and is derived through

←————————

FIGURE 3-1. *A conceptual framework for psychiatric nursing practice.* (Adapted from Maslow A: Toward a Psychology of Being. New York, Van Nostrand Rheinhold, 1968; Riehl JP and Roy C: Conceptual Models for Nursing Practice, 2nd ed. New York, Appleton-Century-Crofts, 1980; Kim M, Moritz D: Classification of Nursing Diagnoses: Proceedings of Third and Fourth National Conference. New York, McGraw-Hill, 1982; Kim M, McFarland G, McLane A [eds]: Classification of Nursing Diagnoses: Proceedings of the Fifth National Conference. St Louis, CV Mosby, 1984)

(text continued on p. 40)

Initial Psychiatric Nursing Assessment of the Adult Patient[1-40]

1. General Information

   Name: _____

   Address: _____

   Phone: _____

   Age: _____ Sex: _____ Race: _____

   Marital status: _____ Religion: _____

   Name of spouse, relative, or friend: _____

   Occupation/Education: _____

   Hobbies and use of leisure time: _____

   General appearance: _____

   Patient's statement of current health problem:

   _____

2. Initial Assessment Parameters

   Vital signs: _____

   Allergies: _____

   Neurological status _____

      Level of consciousness: _____

      History of seizures: _____

      History of blackouts: _____

      Presence of tardive dyskinesia: _____

   Suicidal thoughts/behavior: _____

   Homocidal thoughts/behavior: _____

   Current medications: _____

   Use of street drugs or alcohol: _____

   Weight (loss or gain): _____

   Dentures/dental problems: _____

   Skin condition: _____

Initial Psychiatric Nursing Assessment of the Adult Patient (*continued*)

Vision: _____

Hearing: _____

3. Interaction (exchanging, communicating, relating)
   Document observations about self-care abilities or limitations in each area.

Eating/drinking: _____

Eliminating: _____

Breathing: _____

Circulation: _____

General grooming/hygiene: _____

Current physical problems: _____

Current treatments and medications: _____

Previous and current use of health care resources: ____

Previous mental or physical illness: _____

General level of growth and development: _____

Communication skills: _____

   With staff: _____

   With spouse: _____

   With children: _____

   With others (specify): _____

Relating: _____

   Ability to trust: _____

   Expression of sexuality: _____

   Self-control: _____

   Manner of expression of needs/goals: _____

   Degree of social interation: _____

   Style of social interaction: _____

   Attitude toward perceived current role status: _____

(Continued)

Initial Psychiatric Nursing Assessment of the Adult Patient (*Continued*)

Social network: _____

Relationship with spouse and/or significant other(s): _____

History of abuse, including sexual abuse: _____

Significant others' reponse to patient's illness: _____

Work history and current status: _____

Recreational activities and hobbies: _____

Arrests, court dates, probation: _____

4. Action (valuing, choosing, moving)
   Patient's perception/understanding of current mental illness and cause(s): _____
   _____

   Beliefs about illness and health and personal health goals: _____
   _____

   Patient's attitudes/beliefs toward hospitalization and health care personnel: _____
   _____

   Patient's expectations and goals for current hospitalization: _____
   _____
   _____
   _____

   Past and current compliance with prescribed treatment and health instructions: _____
   _____

   Coping skills used: _____
   _____

   Religion/spiritual beliefs: _____

   Attitudes toward future worth/value of own life: _____

   Decision-making abilities/limitations: _____

   Influence of cultural factors: _____

   Values and beliefs about mental health: _____

   Values and beliefs about mental illness: _____

   Customs related to verbal and non-verbal communication: _____
   _____

Initial Psychiatric Nursing Assessment of the Adult Patient (*Continued*)

Customs related to decision making: _____

Religious customs: _____

Customs related to foods: _____

Customs related to family roles: _____

Social structure components (family structures, religion, economics, available health systems): _____
_____

Physical environment: _____

Cultural change: _____

Activities/habits detrimental to health: _____

Activity pattern: _____

5. Awareness (alertness, feeling, knowing/perception)

Orientation to time, place, person: _____

Arousal level: _____

Level of energy: _____

Sleep/rest pattern: _____

Anxiety: _____

Degree and nature of ambivalence: _____

Guilt and source: _____

Type and change of mood or affect: _____

Frequency and types of physical complaints: _____

Patient's adjustment to types, number, and recency or stressors: __
_____

Type and use of defense mechanisms: _____

Patient's opinion of self (identity, self-worth, etc.): _____
_____

Patient's awareness of concerns about physical appearance: _____
_____

Knowledge about present illness (prevention, treatment, self-care reponsibilities): _____

Initial Psychiatric Nursing Assessment of the Adult Patient (*Continued*)

   Knowledge about current medications: _____

   Unusual beliefs: _____

   Unusual sensations and perceptions: _____

6. Discharge planning: _____

   Resources: _____

      Financial resources: _____

   Outpatient appointments: _____

   Home environment: _____

   Community environment: _____

---

a deliberate, systematic process of data collection and analysis. It provides the basis for prescriptions for definitive therapy for which the nurse is accountable.

C. Planning
1. Develop patient outcomes after adequate assessment and formulation of the nursing diagnosis.
2. Plan with input from patient, as much as possible.

D. Intervention
1. Intervention strategies should be designed to help the patient achieve formulated behavioral outcomes.
2. A conceptual framework for nursing practice serves to guide planning and design intervention strategies.

E. Evaluation
1. Determine the extent to which patient outcomes have been met.
2. Data resulting from evaluation are used to plan and redesign intervention strategies to meet, revise, or formulate new patient outcomes, as necessary.

■■■ THE MENTAL STATUS EXAMINATION

The mental status review is usually performed by the psychiatrist, psychiatric clinical nurse specialist, or psychologist. It serves as only one component of the overall assessment of mental health.

A. Objective
The objective is to assess the mental functioning and present emotional state of the patient.

B. General appearance
Observe the following about the patient:
1. Grooming and dress (slovenly, neat, unkempt, overly meticulous, disheveled, inappropriate, unusual)
2. Facial expression (calm, perplexed, stressed, tense, alert, dazed)
3. Physical appearance (noticeable physical deformities, thin, obese, average weight)
4. Posture (normal, rigid, slouching)
5. Eye contact (eyes closed, eyes open, good contact, avoids contact, stares)

C. Motor behavior
Observe for unusual bodily movements, such as the following:
1. *Choreiform movements*—irregular, involuntary actions of muscles of face and extremities
2. *Waxy flexibility*—holding body posture that is imposed by another person for a long time
3. *Hyperkinesia*—excessive movement; destructive or assaultive activity
4. *Compulsive*—unwanted repetitive actions
5. *Automatism*—not consciously controlled, automatic, undirected motor activity
6. *Cataplexy*—temporary loss of muscle tone precipitated by strong emotions
7. *Catalepsy*—a trancelike state with loss of voluntary motion
8. *Stereotypy*—repetitive, persistent motor activity or speech
9. *Echopraxia*—repetitive imitation of another person's movements
10. *Psychomotor retardation*—decreased, slowed activity
11. *Catatonic stupor*—extreme underactivity
12. *Catatonic excitement*—extreme overactivity
13. *Impulsiveness*—outbursts of activity that are unpredictable and sudden
14. *Tics and spasms*—involuntary twitching and jerking of muscles, usually above the shoulders

D. Speech
Observe for speech activity, normal and unusual patterns, or unusual use of words, such as the following:
1. *Verbigeration*—repetitive, meaningless expression of sentences, phrases, or words
2. *Rhyming*—interjecting into the conversation regular, recurring, corresponding sounds at the end of phrases or sentences, as in poetry
3. *Punning*—interjecting into the conversation the clever and humorous use of a word or words
4. *Mutism*—no expression of words or lack of communication over a period of time
5. *Aphasia*—partial or total loss of the ability to express self through language or the ability to understand the verbal communication of another person
6. *Neologisms*—words created by the patient that are not easily understood by others
7. Unusual rate of speech, volume of voice, intonation, or modulation.

E. Functioning
Assess the patient for the following:
1. Orientation
   a. Orientation to time
      Ask the patient to name the month, day of the week, and time, and to state how long the patient has been in the hospital.
   b. Orientation to place
      Ask the patient: Where are you now located? What is the name of this place?
   c. Orientation to person
      Does patient know own name? Does patient know who the person conducting the interview is?
2. Memory
   a. Memory for remote events—Ask the patient the following:
      (1) Date(s) of marriage(s) and divorce(s), if any
      (2) Birthdate(s) of child(ren), if any
      (3) Own birthdate
      (4) Name of grade school, high school, and/or college attended
      (5) Type of position and month and year of employment of first job after high school or college graduation
   b. Memory for recent past events—Ask the patient the following:
      (1) Where did the patient live during past 3 months? With whom did the patient live? Where did the patient work?
      (2) Which types of recreational activities was patient involved in?
   c. Memory for recent events—Ask the patient the following:
      (1) What the patient ate for breakfast, lunch, and dinner today.
      (2) Activities of yesterday and today.
   d. Immediate memory and recall
      (1) Give patient the names of three unrelated objects, ask patient to repeat; wait 3–5 minutes, and ask patient to repeat again.
      (2) Administer digit span test. Ask patient to repeat numbers in sequence, increasing to as large a span as patient can repeat. Repeat process, asking patient to repeat numbers in reverse order.
      (3) Other assessment techniques include asking patient the same question several times during the interview to determine whether the same or a different answer is given.
      (4) Determine for presence of impaired memory, such as amnesia, anterograde amnesia, psychogenic amnesia.
3. Level and fund of knowledge
   a. To determine fund of knowledge, ask such questions as: What are the names of three countries in Europe? The colors in the American flag? The distance between any two major U.S. cities?
   b. Request listing of three items in different categories, such as U.S. state capitols and fruits.
   c. Overall responses to total interview questions are used to assess level of knowledge appropriate patient's age and socioeconomic, cultural, occupational, and educational background.
4. Attention and calculation
   Instruct to patient to subtract 7 from 100 and to keep subtracting 7s, allowing up to 30 seconds between calculations. If the patient is unable

to complete this activity, have the patient spell "world" forward and backwards.
5. Ability to think abstractly or to make generalizations
   a. Ask patient to interpret a proverb, or to identify the similarity inherent in two objects, e.g., a bicycle and a train.
   b. Use object sorting test by having patient group toy objects according to use.

F. Perception
Observe for signs of altered or abnormal awareness of self or environment, such as the following:
1. *Hallucinations*—false sensory experiences, based on unreality, that may be triggered by external or internal stimuli. These can be visual, olfactory, auditory, tactile, gustatory, or kinesthetic
2. *Hypnagogic hallucinations*—misperceptions occurring as patient is falling asleep for which there is no basis in reality
3. *Hypnopompic hallucinations*—misperceptions occurring as patient is waking up for which there is no basis in reality
4. *Illusion*—misinterpretation of an actual, existing external stimuli by any of the senses
Observe for changes in the patient's general manner of feeling, thinking, or behavior during the interview as evidenced by the patient's being any one or more of the following: cooperative, outgoing, withdrawn, evasive, sarcastic, aggressive, perplexed, hostile, arrogant, dramatic, ingratiating, submissive, fearful, seductive, uncooperative, impatient, remote, resistant, unfeeling, apprehensive, or apathetic.

G. Affective state
Observe for unusual mood or expression of emotions, such as the following:
1. *Euphoria*—excessive feeling of emotional and physical well-being inappropriate for actual environmental stimuli
2. *Flat affect*—less than normal expression of feelings
3. *Blunting*—loss of affective expression
4. *Elation*—high degree of confidence, boastfulness, uncritical optimism, and joy, accompanied by increased motor activity
5. *Exultation*—affective reaction extending beyond elation and accompanied by feelings of grandeur
6. *Ecstasy*—overpowering feeling of joy and rapture
7. *Anxiety*—apprehensive, uneasy, and worried feeling usually of unconscious, intrapsychic origin
8. *Fear*—apprehensive, uneasy, and worried feeling related to a known source of danger, usually externally based
9. *Ambivalence*—expression of the existence of two opposing feelings or emotions at the same time
10. *Depersonalization*—feeling that oneself or one's environment is unreal
11. *Irritability*—feeling characterized by impatience, annoyance, and easy provocation to anger
12. *Rage*—furious, uncontrolled anger
13. *Lability*—quick change of expression of mood or feelings
14. *Depression*—feeling characterized by sadness, dejection, and helplessness, hopelessness, worthlessness, and gloom.

H. Thought processes and content
Observe for the following:
1. *Blocking*—sudden cessation of flow of thinking and speech related to strong emotions
2. *Flight of ideas*—rapid conversation with logically unconnected shifting of topics
3. *Word salad*—combination of phrases, words, and sentences that are disconnected and incoherent
4. *Perseveration*—pathological repetition of a sentence, phrase, or word
5. *Neologisms*—use of new expressions, phrases, or words or creation of a new meaning for accepted expressions, phrases, or words (See speech)
6. *Circumstantiality*—interjection of great detail and incidental material that have no primary significance to the central idea of the conversation
7. *Tangentiality*—deviation from central theme of conversation
8. *Echolalia*—repetitive imitation of another person's speech
9. *Condensation*—process of reducing several ideas into one symbol
10. *Delusion*—false belief kept despite nonsupportive evidence
11. *Phobia*—strong, persistent, abnormal fear of an object or situation
12. *Obsession*—persistent, unwanted, recurring thought
13. *Hypochondriasis*—morbid concern for one's health and feeling ill without any actual medical basis

I. Judgment
Observe patient's ability to solve problems and choose among alternatives based on reality.

J. Alertness
Observe patient for levels of alertness (drowsiness, hyperalertness, somnolence, intermittent alertness, drowsiness, and stupor).

■ THE MULTIAXIAL EVALUATION SYSTEM OF THE DIAGNOSTIC AND STATISTICAL MANUAL OF MENTAL DISORDERS (THIRD EDITION, REVISED) (DSM-III-R)

A. The purpose of the DSM-III-R "is to provide clear descriptions of diagnostic categories in order to enable clinicians and investigators to diagnose, communicate about, study, and treat the various mental disorders."[2,p.xxix]

B. The DSM-III-R recommends the evaluation of a patient's psychological and physical functioning, stressors contributing to the development of a psychological disorder, and strengths and limitations.

C. In using the DSM-III-R, the clinician looks at specific behaviors and takes into consideration prior history of illness and family history. In order to arrive at a differential diagnosis, the clinician views the patient both longitudinally and cross-sectionally.

D. The five axes of the DSM-III-R on which the patient is evaluated are as follows[2,pp.15,16]:

1. Axis I—clinical syndromes and conditions not attributable to a mental disorder that are a focus of attention or treatment
2. Axis II—developmental disorders and personality disorders
3. Axis III—physical disorders and conditions
4. Axis IV—severity of psychosocial stressors
5. Axis V—global assessment of functioning during past year

■ PSYCHOLOGICAL TESTING
— Intelligence Testing

A. The purpose of such testing is to assess cognitive and intellectual abilities; it is usually administered by a psychologist.
1. *Wechsler Adult Intelligence Scale (WAIS)*—most widely used standardized test of general intelligence

B. Personality testing
   This testing assesses personality functioning and psychodynamics and is usually administered by a psychologist.
1. *Thematic Apperception Test (TAT)*—a projective test consisting of a series of pictures that are presented to the patient with instructions that a story be constructed or created about the picture
2. *Rorschach Test*—a projective test consisting of a set of 10 inkblots. The patient is asked to respond to what is seen in the inkblot, what it looks like, and what it suggests.
3. *Draw a Person Test (DAP)*—The patient is asked to draw one or more persons and possibly a house, a tree, the family, or an animal. The clinician may also question the patient about the drawing. It is a projective test used for personality analysis and in screening for organic brain damage.
4. *Bender-Gestalt Test*—the patient is presented with nine cards, one at a time, and is asked to copy the geometric designs on them. The test is used to detect organic pathology and is also employed as a projective technique to assess personality functioning.
5. *Sentence Completion Test (SCT)*—The patient is presented with a series of sentence stems that are to be completed with the first response that comes into mind. The test taps much conscious data and can identify the patient's preoccupations, concerns, fears, and goals.
6. *Minnesota Multiphasic Personality Inventory (MMPI)*—a 500-item questionnaire designed to measure major aspects of personality related to hypomania, paranoia, hypochondriasis, hysteria, psychopathic deviation, psychasthenia, schizophrenia, masculinity/femininity, and depression

■ REFERENCES

1. Abraham IL, Fox JM, Harrington DP, et al: A psychogeriatric nursing assessment: protocol for use in multidisciplinary practice. Arch Psychiatric Nurs IV(4):242–259, 1990
2. American Psychiatric Association: Diagnostic and Statistical Manual of Mental Disorders, (3rd ed. Revised). Washington DC, American Psychiatric Association, 1987

3. Berthot BD, Lapierre ED: What does it mean? A new scale for rating patient's behavior. J Psychosoc Nurs Ment Health Serv 27(10):25–28, 1989

4. Blumenthal SJ: Suicide: a guide to risk factors, assessment, and treatment of suicidal patients. Medical Clinics of North America. 72(4):937–971, 1988

5. Blumenthal SJ: Youth suicide: risk factors, assessment, and treatment of adolescent and young adult suicidal patients. Psychiatr Clin N Am 13(3):511–556, 1990

6. Bryant SO, Kopeski LM: Psychiatric nursing assessment of the eating disorder client. Top Clin Nurs 8(1):57–66, 1986

7. Campinha-Bacote J: Culturological assessment: an important factor in psychiatric consultation-liaison nursing. Arch Psychiatr Nurs 2(4):244–250, 1988

8. Cassell EJ, Coulehan JL, Putnam SM: Making good interview skills better. Patient Care 23(6):145–148, 155–166, 1989

9. Catherman A: Biopsychosocial nursing assessment: a way to enhance care plans. J Psychosoc Nurs Ment Health Serv 28(6):31–33, 1990

10. Coler MS, Vincent KG: Psychiatric mental health assessment: a new look at the concept. Arch Psychiatr Nurs 1(4):258–263, 1987

11. Coler MS: Diagnoses for child and adolescent psychiatric nursing: combining NANDA and the DSM-III-R. J Child Adolesc Psychiatr Ment Health Nurs 2(3):115–119, 1989

12. Forchuk C: Assessing the environment. In Baumann A, Johnston NE, Antai-Otong D: Decision Making in Psychiatric and Psychosocial Nursing. Philadelphia, BC Decker, 1990

13. Gerety EK, McKim JD, Sosnovec PA, Cowan ME: Instructor's manual to accompany McFarland and Thomas's Psychiatric Mental Health Nursing. Philadelphia, JB Lippincott, 1991

14. Grebb JA: Psychiatric rating scales. In Kaplan HI, Sadock BJ (eds): Comprehensive Textbook of Psychiatry. 5th ed. Vol I. Baltimore, Williams & Wilkins, 1989

15. Gryfinski JJ, Lampe SS: Implementing focus charting: process and critique. Clin Nurs Specialist 4(4):201–205, 1990

16. Hagerty B: Psychiatric-Mental Health Assessment. St Louis, CV Mosby, 1984

17. Hall JM, Stevens PE: AIDS: a guide to suicide assessment. Arch Psychiatr Nurs II (2):115–120, 1988

18. Kim MJ, Mc Farland GK, McLane A (eds): Classification of Nursing Diagnoses: Proceedings of the Fifth National Conference. St Louis, CV Mosby, 1984

19. Kim MJ, Moritz D (eds): Classification of Nursing Diagnoses: Proceedings of Third and Fourth National Conference. New York, McGraw-Hill, 1982

20. King J, McSwain K, Reid S: A nursing family assessment program. Can J Psychiatr Nurs 27(3):12–14, 1986

21. Kirch DG. Medical assessment and laboratory testing in psychiatry. In Kaplan HI, Sadock BJ (eds): Comprehensive Textbook of Psychiatry, 5th ed. Vol 1. Baltimore, Williams & Wilkins, 1989

22. Leon RI, Bowden CI, Faber RA: The psychiatric interview; history and mental status examination in Kaplan HI, Sadock BJ (eds): Compre-

hensive Textbook of Psychiatry. 5th ed. vol 1. Baltimore, Williams & Wilkins, 1989

23. Leopold B, Lion JR: The diagnostic process. In Lion JR, Adler WN, Webb WL (eds): Modern Hospital Psychiatry. New York, WW Norton, 1988
24. Levin RF, Crosley JM: Focused data collection for generation of nursing diagnoses. J Nurs Staff Dev 4:56–64, 1987
25. Levin HS, Benton AL, Fletcher JM, Satz P: Neuropsychological and intellectual assessment of adults. In Kaplan HI, Sadock BJ. (eds): Comprehensive Textbook of Psychiatry. 5th ed. vol 1. Baltimore, Williams & Wilkins, 1989
26. Maslow A; Toward a Psychology of Being. New York, Van Nostrand Rehinhold, 1968
27. Merker MS: Psychiatric emergency evaluation. Nurs Clin North Amer 21(3):387–396, 1986
28. Morrison EG: Nursing assessment: what do nurses want to know? West J Nurs Res 11(4):469–476, 1989
29. Mulhearn S: The nursing process: improving psychiatric admission assessment. J Adv Nurs 14(10):808–814, 1989
30. Palmateer LM, McCartney JR: Do nurses know when patients have cognitive deficits? J Gerontol Nurs 11(2):7, 10–12, 15–16, 1985
31. Riehl J, Roy C: Conceptual Models for Nursing Practice, 2nd ed. New York, Appleton-Century-Croft, 1980
32. Sanger E, Thomas MD, Whitney JD: A guide for nursing assessment of the psychiatric inpatient. Arch Psychiatr Nurs 2(6):334–338, 1988
33. Talley S, King MC. Psychiatric Emergencies: Nursing Assessment and Interventions. New York: Macmillan, 1984
34. Tardiff K: Assessment and Management of Violent Patients. Washington DC, American Psychiatric Press, 1989
35. Tripp-Reimer T, Brink PJ, Saunders JM: Cultural assessment: content and process. Nurs Outlook 32(2):78–82, 1984
36. Thomas MD, Sanger E, Whitney JD: Nursing diagnosis of depression. J Psychosoc Nurs Ment Health Serv 24(8):6–12, 1986
37. Tilley S, Weighill VE: How nurse therapists assess and contribute to the management of alcohol and sedative drug use among anxious patients. J Adv Nurs. 11(5):499–503, 1986
38. Webster M: Assessing suicide potential. In Lego S (ed): The American Handbook of Psychiatric Nursing. Philadelphia, JB Lippincott, 1984
39. Webster M: Psychiatric nursing assessment. In: Lego S (ed). The American Handbook of Psychiatric Nursing. Philadelphia, JB Lippincott, 1984
40. Yazdanfar DJ: Assessing the mental status of the cognitively impaired elderly. J Gerontol Nurs 16(9):32–36, 1990

Nursing Diagnoses in Caring for the Psychiatric Patient / 4

The nursing diagnoses selected for discussion in this chapter relate primarily to the care of the individual psychiatric patient. However, these nursing diagnoses can be applied to other patients whose nursing care is enhanced by the appropriate diagnoses and by the planning and implementation of psychosocial interventions.

The majority of nursing diagnoses outlined in this chapter were selected from the approved list of the North American Nursing Diagnoses Association (NANDA). A few labels have been modified, and some have been added as a result of ongoing clinical observation, colleague input, research, and literature review. For example, the authors use the nursing diagnosis label *impaired communication* instead of the label on the NANDA list *impaired verbal communication*.

Other nursing diagnoses labels (e.g., *situational crisis*) have been added because there are gaps in the current NANDA list as developed for the nursing care of psychiatric patients. It must be understood that NANDA's work is developmental and ongoing. As nursing diagnostic labels are developed, utilized, and tested in clinical practice, it is important that input be provided to NANDA's ongoing developmental work.

—— Definition and Characteristics of Nursing Diagnoses

1. *Nursing diagnosis* is a clinical judgment about individual, family, or community responses to actual and potential health problems/life processes. Nursing diagnoses provide the basis for selection of nursing interventions to achieve outcomes for which the nurse is accountable.[14a, p.5]
2. Nursing diagnoses approved by the North American Nursing Diagnoses Association (NANDA)[14a] are as follows:
   Activity intolerance
   Activity intolerance, potential

Adjustment, impaired
Airway clearance, ineffective
Anxiety
Aspiration, potential for
Body image disturbance
Body temperature, potential, altered
Bowel incontinence
Breastfeeding, effective
Breastfeeding, ineffective
Breathing pattern, ineffective
Cardiac output, decreased
Communication, impaired verbal
Constipation
Constipation, colonic
Constipation, perceived
Coping, defensive
Coping, family: potential for growth
Coping, ineffective family: compromised
Coping, ineffective family: disabling
Coping, ineffective individual
Decisional conflict (specify)
Denial, ineffective
Diarrhea
Disuse syndrome, potential for
Diversional activity deficit
Dysreflexia
Family processes, altered
Fatigue
Fear
Fluid volume deficit (1)
Fluid volume deficit (2)
Fluid volume deficit, potential
Fluid volume excess
Gas exchange, impaired
Grieving, anticipatory
Grieving, dysfunctional
Growth and development, altered
Health maintenance, altered
Health-seeking behaviors (specify)
Home maintenance management, impaired
Hopelessness
Hyperthermia
Hypothermia
Incontinence, functional
Incontinence, reflex
Incontinence, stress
Incontinence, total
Incontinence, urge
Infection, potential for
Injury, potential for

Knowledge deficit (specify)
Mobility, impaired physical
Noncompliance (specify)
Nutrition, altered: less than body requirements
Nutrition, altered: more than body requirements
Nutrition, altered: potential for more than body requirements
Oral mucous membrane, altered
Pain
Pain, chronic
Parental role conflict
Parenting, altered
Parenting, potential, altered
Personal identity disturbance
Poisoning, potential for
Post-trauma response
Powerlessness
Protection, altered
Rape-trauma syndrome
Rape-trauma syndrome: compound reaction
Rape-trauma syndrome: silent reaction
Role performance, altered
Self-care deficit, bathing/hygiene
Self-care deficit, dressing grooming
Self-care deficit, feeding
Self-care deficit, toileting
Self-esteem disturbance
Self-esteem, chronic low
Self-esteem, situational low
Sensory perceptual alterations (specify) (visual, auditory, kines-
    thetic, gustatory, tactile, olfactory)
Sexual dysfunction
Sexuality patterns, altered
Skin integrity, impaired
Skin integrity, potential, impaired
Sleep pattern disturbance
Social interaction, impaired
Social isolation
Spiritual distress (distress of the human spirit)
Suffocation, potential for
Swallowing, impaired
Thermoregulation, ineffective
Thought processes, altered
Tissue integrity, impaired
Tissue perfusion, altered (specify type: renal, cerebral, cardiopul-
    monary, gastrointestinal, peripheral)
Trauma, potential for
Unilateral neglect
Urinary elimination, altered
Urinary retention
Violence, potential for: self directed or directed at others

—— Framework for Discussing Nursing Diagnoses Within this Section

1. *Definition*—a brief description of the diagnostic label
2. *General principles*—relevant principles discussed when appropriate
3. *Related factors*—the contributing factor(s) or cause(s)
4. *Defining characteristics*—includes the empirical indicators or behavioral manifestations
5. *Nursing assessment*—initial or ongoing diagnosis-specific assessment factors supplemental to the overall assessment parameters outlined in Chapter 3. The questions and statements listed serve as guidelines for assessment and should be adapted as necessary.
6. *Patient Outcomes and Nursing Interventions*—includes patient outcomes followed by nursing interventions designed to achieve each specific patient outcome.
   a. In designing an individual patient care plan, the nurse can restate outcomes in more specific patient behavioral outcome terms.
   b. The nurse selects interventions from among those listed to individualize the nursing care plan for a specific patient.
   c. Specific content useful in patient teaching or as preventive measures is included in this section.
   d. Selected major nursing interventions are more fully described in Chapter 5 and, as such, are cross-referenced.
7. *Evaluation*—Outcome criteria are specified.
8. There are differences in the conceptual level of abstraction of the listed diagnoses. The best diagnosis(es) for a patient should be determined on the basis of an analysis of the available assessment data collected.
9. Nursing diagnosis can be changed as more data warranting the change become available.
10. The established nursing diagnosis(es) for a patient gives direction to the next phases of the nursing process—planning, intervention, and evaluation.
    a. The related factor(s) should be identified, if possible, and added to the main phrase of the nursing diagnosis.
    b. The two parts are linked with the words "related to."

■ REFERENCES

1. American Psychiatric Association: Diagnostic and Statistical Manual of Mental Disorders, 3rd ed. Revised. Washington DC, American Psychiatric Association, 1987
2. Carroll-Johnson RM (ed): Classification of Nursing Diagnoses: Proceedings of the Eighth Conference. Philadelphia, JB Lippincott, 1989
3. Gebbie KM: Summary of the Second National Conference—Classification of Nursing Diagnoses. St Louis, The Clearinghouse, St Louis University, 1976
4. Gebbie K, Lavin M: Classifying nursing diagnoses. AJN 74(2):250–253, 1974
5. Gebbie K, Lavin M (eds): Classification of Nursing Diagnoses. St Louis, CV Mosby, 1975
6. Gebbie KM, Lavin MA: Classification of Nursing Diagnoses: Proceedings of the First National Conference. St Louis, CV Mosby, 1975

7. Gordon M: Nursing diagnoses: Process and Application. New York, McGraw-Hill, 1987
8. Hurley ME (ed): Classification of Nursing Diagnoses: Proceedings of the Sixth Conference. St Louis, CV Mosby, 1986
9. Kim MJ, McFarland GK, McLane AM (eds): Classification of Nursing Diagnoses: Proceedings of the Fifth National Conference. St Louis: CV Mosby, 1984
10. Kim MJ, McFarland GK, McLane AM: Pocket guide to nursing diagnoses, 4th ed. St Louis, CV Mosby, 1991
11. Kim M, Moritz D (eds): Classification of Nursing Diagnoses: Proceedings of the Third and Fourth National Conference. New York, McGraw-Hill, 1981
12. McFarland GK, McFarlane EA: Nursing Diagnosis and Intervention: Planning for Patient Care. St Louis, CV Mosby, 1989
13. McLane AM (ed): Classification of Nursing Diagnoses: Proceedings of the Seventh Conference. St Louis, CV Mosby, 1987
14. Meldman M, McFarland G, Johnson E: The Problem-oriented Psychiatric Index and Treatment Plans. St Louis, CV Mosby, 1976
14a. North American Nursing Diagnosis Association. Taxonomy I–Revised 1990. St. Louis, The North American Nursing Diagnosis Association, 1990
15. Roy C: A diagnostic classification system for nursing. Nurs Outlook 23(2):90–94, 1975

■ AGGRESSION (MILD, MODERATE, EXTREME/VIOLENCE)

— Definition[1-67]

Aggression (Mild, moderate, extreme/violence) is a forceful, generally inappropriate and nonadaptive verbal or physical action that may result from such feelings as anger, anxiety, tension, guilt, and hostility, in turn resulting from a variety of precipitating factors.

Mild—actions conveying displeasure or tension, e.g., sarcasm

Moderate—more forthright expression of anger or displeasure, e.g., verbal degradation or harassment; threats of physical violence, using abusive language

Extreme/violence—physical acting out of verbal threats, anger, or displeasure; engaging in behavior which endangers others or destroys property; use of physical force; at extreme end of aggression continuum.

— General Principles[1-67]

Aggression (mild, moderate, extreme/violence) may be:

- Learned and perpetuated by motives, attitudes, and rationalizations, supported by subculture;
- Produced or perpetuated by social structure (e.g., coercion, regimentation, personal space invasion).

See Table 4-1 Model of Aggression.

TABLE 4-1   Model of Aggression

Possible Causes	Possible Resulting Feelings	Possible Resulting Responses
Frustration Loss of dignity Fear Need to test reality Physical impairment (e.g., minimal brain dysfunction) Inferiority and low self-esteem Repressed resentment, hate, or hostility Grief (anger phase) Perceived threat Threat of intimacy Perceptual or cognitive distortion Social milieu (e.g., rejection from significant others or subculture expression of aggression) Helplessness Thwarting of goals as career progression Thwarting of needs for power, control, authority, attention Ward milieu (e.g., staff conflict, overcrowding, etc.)	Anxiety Guilt Tension Anger Hostility	***Adaptive Response*** Use of coping skills and strategies resulting in resolution, including constructive expression of aggression as in problem solving or realistic defense. OR ***Inadequate Adaptive Response— (mild, moderate, extreme/ violence)*** Defensive actions: designed to meet personal needs, achieve goals, and protect self, including both inappropriate verbal or physical expression of aggression. Offensive actions: designed to punish or destroy, including verbal hostility, physical assault, or violence. Direct action against target: includes other-directed physical or verbal aggression, such as hitting or pushing others, starting fights, biting. Indirect action against target: includes scapegoating; acting out; overuse of displacement, projection, introjection, reaction-formation, or somatization; or passive-aggressive behavior, such as gossiping, roundabout derogation, derogatory jokes, slamming doors, temper tantrums, negativism, resentment, irritability, or postponements. Withdrawal: includes withdrawal behavior and internalization of feelings; includes lack of involvement with others or programs; lack of direct communication; maintaining communication on superficial level; passivity

— Related Factors[1-67]

Fear
Guilt
Increasing anxiety or frustration
Increasing anger or hostility
Repressed resentment
Grief
Powerlessness
Threatened goal progression or achievement
Threat to need satisfaction
Threatened or poor self-concept
Poor impulse control
History of violence
Lack of trust
Difficulty in learning from past mistakes
Availability of weapon
Aggressive trait
History of family violence
Invasion of personal space
Use of disinhibiters (e.g., alcohol or drugs)
Delusions, e.g., persecutory delusions
Misinterpretation of environment/interpersonal stimuli
Interpersonal conflicts
Acceptance of aggressive behavior as a norm by members of
    subculture
Disturbed relationship with significant other(s)
Environmental factors, e.g., staff conflict that is conveyed to patient
Physical disorder, e.g., temporal lobe epilepsy.
Auditory hallucinations, e.g., command hallucinations

— Defining Characteristics[1-67]

- Inappropriate forceful verbal action, without consideration of
  rights of others; e.g., derogatory jokes, gossiping, cursing,
  sarcasm, verbal threats.
- Inappropriate forceful physical action, directed to self or others,
  including assault/injury of persons or animals, or inappropriate
  defensive actions.
- Inappropriate forceful physical action against property; e.g.,
  damaging physical objects, slamming doors.
- Passive aggressive behavior
- Nonverbal body language; e.g., glaring eyes, angry facial
  expression, clenched fists, strained or raised voice.
- Increased motor tension, e.g., pacing, agitation.
- Scapegoating
- Negativism
- Irritability
- Temper tantrums
- Resentment
- Intimidation

- Physical threat
- Homicidal ideation.

— Nursing Assessment[1-67]

What is the nature of the patient's aggressive behavior? What are the preceding events, precipitants, place of occurrence, actual behavior—including intensity, target(s), degree of inner controls, and degree of unpredictability? What is the patient's perception of self, others, and environment? What is the meaning behind the aggressive behavior? Determine patient's prior methods of coping with stress-producing situations and socially acceptable ways used to express emotions.

How does the patient cope with anger?
- Internalizes, becomes depressed?
- Unable to identify source, displacement?
- Able to identify source but unable to express directly? Passive-aggressive? Passive?
- Identifies source along with direct and appropriate or inappropriate expression?

How has the patient coped with frustrations in the past?

Assess potential for violent behavior by considering factors such as the following:
- Past history of arrests, violent behavior, types and pattern of aggressive behavior
- History of life stressors resulting in bitterness
- Unstable family situation characterized by quarreling
- Violence displayed by significant others, especially parental brutality
- History of battering relationship
- High interest in, and availability of, weapons; attempts to use weapons
- Low self-esteem
- Disinhibiting state from alcohol or drug abuse
- Presence of persecutory delusions
- History of physical impairment, such as minimal brain dysfunction
- Increased erratic, impulsive, or unpredictable behavior
- Marked changes in values that are out of character for person
- Organization and rehearsal of plans for violent act
- Absence of dependable significant other(s)
- Degree of reversibility of predisposing conditions
- Methods of dealing with similar past situations
  Continue observations for
- Behavioral changes indicating increasing anxiety, guilt, anger
- Homicidal or suicidal ideation
- Level of aggression (mild, moderate, extreme/violence)
    - What were the preceding events, including ward milieu?
    - What were the precipitating factors?
    - What actually happened?
    - How does the patient perceive the event?
- Ward milieu, including staff ability to cope with own emotions
- Possession of any weapons

- Change in ability to resolve anxiety, anger, tension or guilt in an acceptable way
- Other acts of aggression on ward that seem unrelated.
- Ability to respond to directions, questions, suggestions

—— Patient Outcomes and Nursing Interventions[1-67]

Patient Outcome: Identify and Express Feelings such as Anger and Hostility Appropriately

- Assist patient in dealing with anger and hostility
  - Provide feedback on nonverbal behavior to help patient identify anger or hostility, as well as sources of such feelings
  - Develop relationship in which patient can be angry and can learn to differentiate thoughts and feelings from actions
  - Have patient practice verbalizing angry or hostile feelings in a minimally threatening situation
  - Assist patient to identify sources of anger or hostility
  - Explore and aid in developing alternate methods of expressing anger or hostility
- Assist patient in reducing aggression
  - After having developed positive relationship, use gentle confrontation and set firm, clear limits, linking behaviors and their consequences
  - Set limits and give positive reinforcement for appropriate behavior.
- Assist patient to identify cause(s) of aggression.
- For clients with organic mental disorder, provide structured environment oriented to person, place, time. Provide simple directions. Use calm approach.
- For young children, (a) redirect the child toward appropriate behavior by means of a verbal prompt; e.g., "You can beat the drum instead of kicking the table"; or, (b) use contingency statements by verbally calling attention to a rule or limitation, permitting free play within a restricted area with freedom to remain in restricted area, and limiting the contingency statement to about where the play can take place.
- For children who are aggressive and out of control, institute therapeutic holding (physical restraint by two nursing personnel) as soon as feasible, which minimizes view of adult as rejecting and punitive. After therapeutic holding has calmed child, encourage child to express feelings associated with aggressive act, using art materials, journal entries, and verbal discussions.
- For elderly, (a) assist staff to assess personal beliefs, values, and nursing practice in relation to elderly who are aggressive; (b) determine elderly patient's perception and meaning of the aggressive episode; (c) reinforce and augment constructive coping strategies in patient's repertoire for dealing with specific related factors; (d) teach patient new coping skills within his or her ability to learn.
- Develop and use therapeutic ward milieu. (See Chapter 5.)

- Provide opportunity through group meetings for staff and patients to discuss reactions and feelings about moderate or extreme aggression and to resolve patient-staff conflict.
  - Resolve conflict.
  - Work through phases of planned change.
  - Decrease confusion in environment.
- Mutually develop goals with patient for more appropriate expression of anger, hostility, anxiety, tension, or guilt. Seek alternatives that can be used after discharge.
- Analyze own perceptions of patient. Avoid stereotyping or "expecting" physical aggression.
- Use time-out procedure in which patient is removed from environment.
- Assist patient to reduce cognitive distortion by developing alternative perspectives about self and the causes of aggression.
- Help reduce anxiety.
- Point out consequences of aggression.
- Prevent suicide or homicide.
- Evaluate need for and patient's ability to participate in group, family, or individual therapy.
- Provide outlets for feelings engendered (e.g., activity groups, punching bags, clay, sports, art, music).
- Help patient recognize relationship between precipitating factors and aggressive behavior displayed.
- Develop behavior-modification approaches for selected aggressive behaviors.
- Explore patient's past experiences with aggressive behavior and the rewards that current aggressive behavior achieves.
- Provide peer role models who demonstrate more adaptive behavioral responses.
- Allow patient maximum autonomy and control over own situation within openly communicated behavioral limits (e.g., behavior injurious to others not tolerated).

Patient Outcome: Not injure self or others and recognize potential consequences of extreme aggression/violence

- Do not ignore threats of physical aggression.
- Use specific behavior contracts regarding not injuring self or others. At times of risk, maintain regular observation (e.g., constant, every 15 minutes, or every 30 minutes, depending on degree of risk and institutional policy).
- If patient possesses a weapon (other than gun)
  - Don't attempt to grab it, unless there are enough staff members present.
  - Request that weapon be deposited in a neutral place.
  - If threatened with weapon, place protective barrier between self and weapon, such as mattress or chair.
- If weapon is gun
  - Evacuate others from area.
  - Notify security/police.

- Maximize patient's ego strengths.
  - Use honest, emphatic, firm approach.
  - Avoid accusatory approach and increasing guilt.
- Recognize potential for moderate and extreme aggression and intervene prior to expression.
- Be cautious and avoid facade of bravado. Convey a sense of personal control and security.
- Avoid overt communication of feelings of fear or panic.
- Provide opportunity for verbalization of feelings, especially anger; attempt to "talk down."
- Avoid premature attempts to uncover precipitants. Acknowledge recognition of patient's tension.
- State desire to help patient regain control.
- Set consistent limits on type and degree of aggression that is tolerated.
- Clearly verbalize expectation that patient will not be permitted to lose control and physically harm others.
- Pose well-timed questions about what the patient may be experiencing.
- Be aware of potentially stressful situations for patients, and document and communicate any change in behavior.
- If physical aggression is imminent or occurring, approach patient quietly with staff and, if indicated, use a well-planned method of physical restraint. (See Chapter 5.)
- For violent nonpsychotic adolescents, carefully evaluate use of neuroleptics prior to seclusion. (Administering medications prior to seclusion may teach adolescent avoidance since uncomfortable feelings are blocked by medication.)
  - Institute crisis intervention protocol if difficulty maintaining control is experienced by adolescent. (See Chapter 5.)
  - If seclusion is necessary, use seclusion without administering neuroleptics.
  - After seclusion without neuroleptics, assist adolescent in identifying and examining feelings and precipitating factors to violence and exploring alternative behaviors.
- Do not ignore threats of physical aggression.
- Be available to patient during periods of increasing tension.
- Respect patient's need for personal space and freedom from undesired physical intrusion.
- Provide consistent set of expectations for patient to develop self-control.
- Assist staff in dealing with feelings aroused by patients who are aggressive. (Aggressive patients are more subject to patient abuse by caregivers than patients who are passive.)
- Assist staff victims of extreme aggression in dealing with feelings of self blame, hostility towards patient, or role conflict.
  - Administer the Assault Response Questionnaire[34] to determine impact of assault on staff member. Refer to Peer Support Program if available.
- Explore options for more constructive outlets for aggression.
- Be as truthful as possible.
- Remove external object that patient fears, if possible.

- Recognize need for clearcut staff-patient boundaries.
- When therapist is verbally threatened
  - Continue patient contact.
  - Explore precipitants of threat.
  - Permit verbalizations of feelings associated with threat.
  - Assist patient in realizing link between cause of aggression, subsequent feelings, and verbal threat.
- When verbal and nonverbal cues indicate potential for physical aggression
  - Do not avoid but interact early with patient.
  - Convey acceptance of person but not of physical aggression.
  - Avoid retaliatory behaviors.
  - Permit verbalization of feelings.
  - Suggest constructive physical outlets, such as use of punching bag.
  - Suggest use of a quiet area until self-control is fully regained.
- Maintain stable, therapeutic ward milieu for brain-damaged patients.
- Develop and implement well-planned, orderly method of restraint for violent patient.
- Be aware of potential target for patient's physical aggressions.
- Determine and anticipate need for medications, physical restraint, seclusion, or mechanical restraints, and utilize these interventions, according to institutional protocol. (See also Chapter 5.)
- Ask patient whether medications are desired and encourage patient to take them to prevent further agitation.
- If medications are refused, offer them again a short time later.
- If agitation continues and patient refuses to accept medications, administer medications after patient has been physically restrained in flat position. (See Chapter 5.)
- Discuss violence and physical aggression with patient after the episode.
- Communicate that staff members are attempting to solve the immediate problem.
- Avoid sudden movements with a violent patient.
- To avoid injury from violence
  - Observe, plan, and act.
  - Give one staff member final authority on method of restraint to be used.
  - Give staff specific instructions.
  - Use agency policy as guideline.
  - Have more staff present than needed to communicate strength.
  - Do not use excessive force.
  - Use pillows, mattress, or chair to ward off blows.
  - Remove other patients from potentially dangerous area.
- Use self-protective devices to deal with *actual physical aggression*: Do not inflict pain or injury.
  - Controlled breathing—Inhale and exhale deeply and sharply before physical action to protect self.

- Movement—Move while speaking to agitated patient so he can't predict exact location.
- Stance—Place feet shoulder-width apart, forward foot in front, and back foot at 90° angle from forward foot.
- Utilize protective fall.
- Observation—Observe patient's eyes because he will observe body part that will be attacked.
- Protective actions
    - Deflect patient action by self-defense techniques.
    - Use counterpressure.
    - Use body pressure points.
    - Seek assistance as soon as possible.
- To *prevent* inappropriate expression of aggression, teach patient to
    - Recognize warning signs, symptoms, and feelings preceding occurrence.
    - Avoid disinhibiting substances, such as alcohol and drugs, which can impair judgment.
    - Practice self-control and appropriate expression of feelings and aggression, beginning with precipitants that evoke minor tension, anger, guilt, or anxiety.
    - Seek psychiatric assistance when patient feels need for help in establishing self-control.
    - Refer to group therapy or individual therapy as appropriate.
- List phone numbers of hot line and professionals who can be contacted when need arises.
- Teach use of relaxation techniques. (See Chapter 5.)
- Teach assertive communication skills. (See Chapter 5.)
- Teach family member or significant other ways to assess patient's level of aggression and potential for dangerousness.
- Teach family members about resources of domestic crisis centers.

—— Evaluation/Outcome Criteria

- Engages in problem solving
- Engages in realistic and constructive self-defense
- Uses appropriate techniques to control aggression, respecting the personal integrity of others
- Utilizes assertive communication skills
- Does not verbally attack others
- Identifies angry feelings
- Asks for help in controlling angry feelings
- Demonstrates ability to control aggression
- Does not injure self or others
- Does not damage property

▄▄ REFERENCES

1. Alexander D: Aggression (mild, moderate, sever, extreme/violence). In McFarland G, Thomas MD: Psychiatric Mental Health Nursing. Philadelphia, JB Lippincott, 1991

2. Balderston C, Negley EN, Kelly GR, Lion JR: Data-based interventions to reduce assaults by geriatric inpatients. Hosp Community Psychiatry 41(4):447–449, 1990

3. Barlow D: Therapeutic holding, effective intervention with the aggressive child. J Psychosoc Nurs Ment Health Serv 27(1):10–14, 1989

4. Barnes DM: The origins of violent behavior: what research strategies will emerge? J NIH Res 1:27–29, 1989

5. Billowitz A, Pendleton L: Successful resolution of threats to a therapist. Hosp Community Psychiatry 39(7):782–785, 1988

6. Boettcher EG: Preventing violent behavior, an integrated theoretical model for nursing. Perspect Psychiatr Care 21(2):54–58, 1983

7. Brizer DA: Psychopharmacology and the management of violent patients. Psychiatr Clin North Am 11(4):551–568, 1988

8. Carmel H, Hunter M: Staff injuries from inpatient violence. Hosp Community Psychiatry 40(1):41–45, 1989

9. Carmel H, Hunter M: Compliance with training in managing assaultive behavior and injuries from inpatient violence. Hosp Community Psychiatry 41(5):558–560, 1990

10. Carpenito LJ: Nursing Diagnosis: Application to Clinical Practice, 2nd ed. Philadelphia, JB Lippincott, 1987

11. Cowgill G, Doupe G: Recognizing and helping victims of torture. Can Nurse 81(11):19–22, 1985

12. Craig C, Ray F, Hix C: Seclusion and restraint: decreasing the discomfort. J Psychosoc Nurs Ment Health Serv 27(7):16–19, 1989

13. Csernansky JG, Maddock RJ, Hollister LE: Pharmacologic treatment of aggression. Hosp Formul 20(10):1091–1104, 1985

14. Davis DL, Boster L: Multifaceted therapeutic interventions with the violent psychiatric inpatient. Hosp Community Psychiatry 39(8):867–869, 1988

15. Dawson J, Johnston M, Kehiayan N, Kyanko S, Martinez R: Response to patient assault, a peer support program for nurses. J Psychosoc Nurs Ment Health Serv 26(2):8–15, 1988

16. Fernandex TM: How to deal with overt aggression. Issues Ment Health Nurs 8:79–83, 1986

17. Foster LA, Veale CM, Fogel CI: Factors present when battered women kill. Issues Ment Health Nurs 10:273–284, 1989

18. Fromm E: The Anatomy of Human Destructiveness. New York, Holt, Rinehart & Winston, 1973

19. Gerety EK, McKim JD, Sosnovec PA, Cowan ME: Instructor's Manual for McFarland/Thomas's Textbook of Psychiatric Mental Health Nursing. Philadelphia, JB Lippincott, 1991

20. Gerlock A, Solomons HC: Factors associated with the seclusion of psychiatric patients. Perspect Psychiatric Care. 21(2):46–53, 1983

21. Glenn MB: Update on pharmacology, a pharmacologic approach to aggressive and disruptive behaviors after traumatic brain injury. J Head Trauma Rehabil 2(1):71–73, 1987

22. Glynn SM, Bowen LL, Barringer DM, Banzett LK: Compliance with less restrictive aggression control procedures. Hosp Community Psychiatry 40(1):82–84, 1989

23. Gondolf EW, Mulvey EP, Lidz CW: Characteristics of perpetrators of family and nonfamily assaults. Hosp Community Psychiatry 41(2):191–193, 1990

24. Grant CA, Burgess AW, Hartman CR, Burgess AG, Shaw ER, MacFarland G: Juveniles who murder: insights for intervention. J Psychosoc Nurs Ment Health Serv 27(12):4–11, 1989
25. Greenfield T, McNiel D, Binder R: Violent behavior and length of psychiatric hospitalization. Hosp Community Psychiatry 40(8):809–814, 1989
26. Helping angry and violent people manage their emotions and behavior. Hosp Community Psychiatry 38(11):1207–1210, 1987
27. Henson TK; Medicolegal role in detection and prevention of human abuse. Holistic Nurs Pract 1(2): 75–84, 1987
28. Holden RJ: Aggression against nurses. Aust Nurses J 15(3):44–48, 1985
29. Janofsky JS, Spears S, Neubauer DN: Psychiatrists' Accuracy in predicting violent behavior on an inpatient unit. Hosp Community Psychiatry 39(10):1090–1094, 1988
30. Kim MJ, McFarland GK, McLane AM: Pocket guide to nursing diagnoses, 4th ed. St Louis, CV Mosby, 1991
31. Kirkpatrick H: A descriptive study of seclusion: the unit environment, patient behavior, and nursing interventions. Arch Psychiatr Nurs 3(1):3–9, 1989
32. Krakowski M, Convit A, Jaeger J, Lin S, Volavka J: Neurological impairment in violent schizophrenic inpatients. Am J Psychiatry 146(7):849–853, 1989
33. Krakowski M, Volavka J, Brizer D: Psychopathology and violence; a review of literature. Compr Psychiatry 27(2):131–148, 1986
34. Landenburger K: A process of entrapment in and recovery from an abusive relationship. Issues Ment Health Nurs 10:209–227, 1989
35. Lanza ML: Assault response questionnaire. Issues Ment Health Nurs 9:17–29, 1988
36. Lanza ML: Factors relevant to patient assault. Issues Ment Health Nurs 9:239–257, 1988
37. Lanza ML: The relationship of the severity of assault to blame placement for assault. Arch Psychiatr Nurs 1(4):269–278, 1987
38. Lanza ML, Milner J, Riley E: Predictors of patient assault on acute inpatient psychiatric units: a pilot study. Issues Ment Health Nurs 9:259–270, 1988
39. Larson LA: Potential for violence: self-directed or directed at others. In McFarland GK, McFarlane EA: Nursing Diagnosis and Intervention: Planning for Patient Care. St Louis, CV Mosby, 1989
40. Leiba PA: Violence: the community nurse's dilemma. Health Visitor 5(11):361–362, 1987
41. Limandri BJ: The therapeutic relationship with abused women. J Psychosoc Nurs Ment Health Serv 25(2):9–16, 1987
42. Lion JR: Violence and suicide within the hospital. In Lion JR, Adler WN, Webb WL (eds): Modern Hospital Psychiatry. New York, WW Norton, 1988
43. Lorenz K: On aggression. New York, Harcourt, Brace & World, 1966
44. Lowenstein M, Binder RL, McNiel DE: The relationship between admission symptoms and hospital assaults. Hosp Community Psychiatry 41(3):311–313, 1990
45. Martin ML, Kirkpatrick H: Nursing assessment of the aggressive elderly. Perspect Psychiatr Nurs Fall:8–10, 1987

46. May R: Power and Innocence: A Search for the Sources of Violence. New York, WW Norton, 1972
47. McGuire MT, Troisi A: Aggression. In Kaplan HI, Sadock BJ (eds): Comprehensive Textbook of Psychiatry. Baltimore, Williams & Wilkins, 1989
48. McNiel DE, Binder RL: Relationship between preadmission threats and later violent behavior by acute psychiatric inpatients. Hosp Community Psychiatry 40(6):605–608, 1989
49. Meddaugh DI: Reactance: understanding aggressive behavior in long-term care. J Psychosoc Nurs Ment Health Serv 28(4):28–33, 1990
50. Miller D, Walker MC, Friedman D: Use of a holding technique to control the violent behavior of seriously disturbed adolescents. Hosp Community Psychiatry 40(5):520–524, 1989
51. Minden P: The victim care service: a program for victims of sexual assault. Arch Psychiatr Nursing 3(1):41–46, 1989
52. Moehling KS: Battered women and abusive partners: treatment issues and strategies. J Psychosoc Nurs Ment Health Serv 26(9):9–16, 1988
53. Morrison EF: Instrumentation issues in the measurement of violence in psychiatric inpatients. Issues Ment Health Nurs 9:9–16, 1988
54. Morrison EF: Theoretical modeling to predict violence in hospitalized psychiatric patients. Res Nurs Health 12:31–40, 1989
55. Newbern VB: Caregiver perceptions of human abuse in health care settings. Holistic Nurs Pract 1(2):64–74, 1987
56. Polk GC, Brown BE: Family violence. J Psychosoc Nurs Ment Health Serv 26(2):34–37, 1988
57. Pond VE: The angry adolescent. J Psychosoc Nurs Mental Health Serv 26(12):15–17, 1988
58. Reid WH: Clinical evaluation of the violent patient. Psychiatr Clin North Am 11(4):527–537, 1988
59. Ryan JA, Poster EC: The assaulted nurse; short-term and long-term responses. Arch Psychiatr Nurs 3(6):323–331, 1989
60. Sherburne S, Utley B, McConnell S, Gannon J: Decreasing violent or aggressive theme play among preschool children with behavior disorders. Except Child 55(2):166–172, 1988
61. Stuart GW, Sundeen SJ: Principles and Practice of Psychiatric Nursing, 3rd ed. St Louis, CV Mosby, 1987
62. Tardiff K: Management of the violent patient in an emergency situation. Psychiatr Clin North Am 11(4):539–549, 1988
63. Thackrey M, Bobbitt RG: Patient aggression against clinical and nonclinical staff in a VA medical center. Hosp Community Psychiatry 41(2):195–197, 1990
64. Thomas SP: Theoretical and empirical perspectives on anger. Issues Ment Health Nurs 11:203–216, 1990
65. Turnbull J, Aitken I, Black L, Patterson B: Turn it around: short-term management for aggression and anger. J Psychosoc Nurs Ment Heath Serv 28(6):7–10, 1990
66. Westermeyer J, Wahmenholm K: Assessing the victimized psychiatric patient. Hosp Community Psychiatry 40(3):245–249, 1989
67. Winger J, Schirm V, Stewart D: Aggressive behavior in long-term care. J Psychosoc Nurs Ment Health Serv 25(4):28–33, 1987

▬ ANXIETY (MILD, MODERATE, SEVERE, EXTREME/PANIC)

── Definition[4,16,17,20,23,28,32-34,40-41]

Anxiety—an uncomfortable experience of varying intensity of an impending subjective danger for which the source of danger is unknown

── General Principles[1-41]

Normal anxiety—does not involve repressive or other defensive mechanisms

State anxiety—an emotional state of nervousness, apprehension, tension

Trait anxiety—the relatively stable anxiety-proneness of an individual

Process anxiety—a complex sequence of cognitive, behavioral, and affective responses resulting in response to stressors

- The explanation for the origins of anxiety include biological, family, genetic, behavioral, cognitive, psychoanalytic, and interpersonal models (see also Chapters 1 and 7).
- Anxiety can be experienced at conscious, preconscious, and/or unconscious levels.
- Ego defense mechanisms (e.g., displacement, identification, projection, regression, denial [see also Chapter 1]) operate to cope (generally at the unconscious levels) with anxiety but can lead to maladaptive responses, depending on the extent of reality distortion.
- The same stressor will not lead to anxiety or to the same level of anxiety in all persons.
- Response to anxiety can be constructive (task-oriented behavior) or destructive (defensive-oriented reactions).
- When the anxiety level exceeds a person's adaptive coping strategies, maladaptive patterns of behavior may result.
- Anxiety can manifest itself through physiological changes in the gastrointestinal system (lack of appetite, diarrhea, abdominal discomfort), the cardiovascular system (increased heart rate, faintness), urinary system (frequent urination), integumentary system (flushed appearance, itching, sweating), neuromuscular system (insomnia, pacing, increased reflexes), respiratory system (increased respiratory rate, shortness of breath).
- Anxiety can manifest itself through behavioral responses (accidents, withdrawal), cognitive responses (decreased concentration, lack of objectivity), and affective responses (jittery, tension).
- Anxiety can manifest itself as a predominant clinical feature in such psychiatric disorders as anxiety disorders, anxiety disorders of childhood and adolescence, or adjustment disorder with anxious mood.

— Related Factors[4,16–17,21,23,28,32–34,40–41]

Unmet needs
Terminal illness or threat of death
Threat to, or change in, health status
Threat to personal security system
Perceived or actual change in socioeconomic status
Threat to environment
Maturational or situational crises
Adverse interpersonal relationships, especially in childhood
Threat to meaningful interpersonal relationships and patterns
Threat to, or change in, role functioning
Interpersonal transmission and contagion
Perceived or actual failure of adaptive coping skills
Threat to self concept
Perceived or actual threat to goal achievement
Internal conflict
Threat to value system, ideals, or beliefs
Failure of ego defense mechanisms

— Defining Characteristics[4,16,17,21,23,28,32–34,40–41]

Mild Anxiety

Purposeful movements
Mild skeletal muscle tension
Calm voice
Good eye contact
Heightened awareness of stimuli
Increased alertness
Noises appear louder
Slight discomfort
Mild restlessness and irritability
Mild sleep disturbance
Mild attention seeking behavior
Mild idle hostility and belittling
Increased awareness, problem solving abilities
Broad perceptual field and ability to see more connections between
    events
Curiosity, repetitive questioning
Increased attention on problem situation
Enhanced ability to deal with stressor
Feelings of confidence and optimism

Moderate Anxiety

Increased blood pressure and respiratory and heart rate
Increased muscle tension
Shakiness
Mixed tension and excitement
Pupillary dilation
Moderate discomfort
Change in voice pitch
Narrowing of perceptual field, selective inattention

Moderate ability to perceive and understand connections between
    events
Increased focus of attention on specific problem situation and
    concentration on sensory data relevant to problem
Element of voluntary control; i.e., ability to be directed to
    unattended stimuli
Ability to perform well-learned skills
Potential for some learning
Moderate self doubts about ability and resources
Moderate uncertainty about positive outcomes
Mixed sense of optimism, confidence, and fear
Motivation to resolve problem
Potential for creativity and growth
Perspiration
Urinary frequency

Severe Anxiety

Tachycardia
Tense, rigid muscles
Hyperventilation
Headaches, dizziness
Pacing, purposeless activity
Immobility
Loss of appetite, nausea
Frequency, urgency
Rapid, fragmented sentences
High-pitched voice
Preoccupied expression
Clenching of jaws
Tendency to dissociate anxious feelings from self
Denial of existence of uncomfortable feelings to protect self
Somatization
Sense of impending doom
Greatly reduced range of perception
Focus on small or scattered detail
Inability to see connections between events or details
Difficulty with learning
Difficulty with and inappropriate verbalizations
Difficulty with concentration
Expectations of negative consequences

Extreme Anxiety (Panic)

Extreme gross motor agitation
Vomiting
Disorganized actions
Dizziness, faintness
Pale, weary appearance
Grimacing
High pitched, loud voice
Extreme discomfort, dread, terror
Feeling of being overwhelmed, impotent, helpless, defenseless
Feelings of anger and rage

Verbal or physical acting out
Immobility
Reliance on earlier coping patterns (curling up, shouting)
Unrealistic and severely restricted perception of situation
Distortion and enlargement of detail, disruption of perceptual field
Impervious to external stimuli
Disconnected and distorted activities
Inability to differentiate between reality and unreality
Extreme difficulty with problem solving
Feelings of personality disintegration
Preoccupation with negative outcomes

— Nursing Assessment[1-41]

- Determine level of anxiety by identifying physiological and/or psychological signs and symptoms
- Observe for stressors or threats to any of the following:
  Health status
  Stability of environment
  Personal security system
  Meaningful interpersonal relationships
  Role functioning
  Self concept
  Core or essence of personality
  Value system, ideals, and beliefs
- Observe adaptive or maladaptive behavioral responses to anxiety.
- Determine behavioral changes or physiological changes resulting from anxiety.
- Assess influence of ward milieu or interpersonal level of anxiety on patients.
- Determine what patient has done in past to reduce anxiety.
- Identify patient's current adaptive and maladaptive strategies for coping with anxiety.
- Determine available resources and patient strengths for coping with anxiety.

— Patient Outcomes and Nursing Interventions[1-41]

Patient Outcome: Experience Anxiety at a Level at which Problem-Solving Can be Effective

- Develop a positive interpersonal relationship with patient.
- Convey empathy, unconditional positive regard, and congruence.
- Do not probe for cause of behavior.
- Recognize reciprocal anxiety in oneself as care provider and develop control over own responses.
- Use short, simple sentences and a calm, firm tone in speaking with a highly anxious patient.
- Provide simple, brief, and clear information about experiences that patient might encounter during hospitalization.
- Clarify and validate information as necessary.

- Be a good listener.
- Administer anti-anxiety drugs in collaboration with psychiatrist.
- Intervene early to prevent escalation of anxiety to severe or extreme levels.
- Keep highly anxious patient in a calm milieu.
- Remove patient from stress-producing situation when anxiety level is high, until level of anxiety decreases.
- Limit contact with other anxious patients.
- Avoid requests for decision making, asking for cause of behavior, or making interpretations when patient is highly anxious.
- Avoid inadvertently contributing to or causing anxiety-provoking situations (threats, insincerity, focus on weakness, indiscriminate use of psychiatric or medical terminology, unreasonable demands, indiscriminate use of confrontation of behavior, indifference or unconcerned attitude, interference with patient's rights and goals, judgmental attitude, impatience).
- Engage patient in recreational and diversional activities aimed at reducing anxiety: group singing; volley ball; ping-pong; walking; swimming; simple, concrete tasks; simple games; routine tasks; housekeeping chores; grooming; puzzles; cards; music (see Chapter 5, *stress management*).
- Develop a mutually agreed upon daily schedule of activities, incorporating patient's preferences and strengths.
- During short-term hospitalization, offer additional support and assistance to patient in dealing with anxiety during transition points, such as on admission and upon notification of discharge.
- Permit crying.
- Encourage ventilation of feelings, considering readiness of patient; e.g., difficulties experienced with significant other.

Patient Outcome: Recognize Presence of Anxiety, Develop Insight into Cause, and Develop Adaptive Coping Strategies and Behavioral Response

- If anxiety is at low or moderate level
  - Help patient identify anxiety by asking questions such as, "Are you uncomfortable right now?" Point out your awareness of patient's discomfort by providing feedback on nonverbal behaviors that indicate presence anxiety.
  - Assist patient in discovering similarity of the immediate situation and past experiences in which comparable discomfort was experienced. Ask questions such as, "Have you, in the past, ever felt like you feel right now? What was happening then to you? What did you do to feel less anxious?"
  - Ask patient to describe what was desired, thought, or expected before becoming anxious and to discover the relationship between the state of anxiety to consequent adaptive or maladaptive behavior.
  - Explore possible reasons for anxiety with patient by helping

patient to identify misconceptions and to clarify the nature of problem realistically.

- Assist patient in developing alternative solutions and methods to reduce anxiety; have patient choose solutions for use. Role play solutions where possible and encourage patient to try out solutions. (See Chapter 5–*decision making*.)
- Evaluate results with patient. Encourage task-oriented versus self-oriented evaluation.
- Have patient explore upcoming events. Use role play to help patient cope with anxiety-provoking encounters.
- Teach patient
    - that some anxiety is part of living and that enduring mild levels of anxiety can enhance learning, problem solving, and movement towards self-actualization;
    - to observe what is happening, describe it, analyze what was expected and how expectations differ from the actual situation; to develop alternatives to solve problem or change expectations, and to validate situation with others;
    - assertive communication skills (see Chapter 5);
    - stress management techniques (see Chapter 5);
    - to reduce severe or extreme anxiety by talking to someone; walking; taking part in simple games; performing simple, concrete tasks; participating in sports; or, if anxiety is extreme, seeking professional help.
- Encourage new interests and hobbies.
- After anxiety is lowered and relationship with staff member is established
    - encourage social activities even if patient demonstrates reluctance and fears;
    - accompany patient first few times to activity and permit patient to leave if anxiety level becomes too high;
    - Gradually encourage patient's attendance independent of staff support.
- Utilize and assist patient in choosing objective environmental interventions to deal with anxiety if the patient is basically optimistic, open to experience, and flexible.
- Assist patient in developing a more optimistic and constructive world view if subjective world is deadened, closed, or distorted.
- Assist patient in reducing life-style of negative expectations.
- Allow patient freedom to work at own level and pace in solving problems.
- Reduce secondary gains patient achieves from maladaptive behavioral responses.
- Encourage participation in individual or group psychotherapy
- Involve family members or significant others in patient treatment plan.
- Actively involve patient in discharge planning (See Chapter 5— *discharge planning*.)

—— Evaluation/Outcome Criteria

- Anxiety reduced or resolved
  - Reduced or absent defining characteristics of anxiety
- Anxiety identified, analyzed, and constructive strategies used
  - Identifies presence of anxiety in self
  - Indicates beginning understanding of cause of anxiety
  - Utilizes constructive anxiety-reducing strategies
- Recognizes constructive aspects of anxiety
  - Recognizes growth potential of mild anxiety

■■ REFERENCES

1. Anxiety disorders. AAOHN Journal 34(1):42–43, 1986
2. Adams A, Dixey D: Running an anxiety management group. Health Visitor 61(12):375–376, 1988
3. Beck AT, Rush AJ: A cognitive model of anxiety formation and anxiety resolution. Issues Ment Health Nurs 7(1–4):349–365, 1985
4. Becket N: Anxiety. In McFarland G, McFarlane E: Nursing Diagnoses and Intervention: Planning for Patient Care. St Louis, CV Mosby, 1989
5. Berthot BD, Lapierre ED: What does it mean? A new scale for rating patients' behavior. J Psychosoc Nurs Ment Health Serv 27(10):25–28, 1989
6. Breznitz S: False alarms: their effects on fear and adjustment. Issues Ment Health Nurs 7(1–4):335–347, 1985
7. Chartier L, Coutu-Wakulczyk G: Families in ICU: their needs and anxiety level. Intensive Care Nurs 5:11–18, 1989
8. Dubovsky SL, Katz JL, Scherger JE, Uhde TW: Anxiolytics: when? why? which one? Patient Care 21(17):60–81, 1987
9. Epstein S: Anxiety, arousal, and the self-concept. Issues Ment Health Nurs 7(1–4):265–303, 1985
10. Evans CL: Reducing AIDS anxiety on the unit with preventive infection control. J Psychosoc Nurs Ment Health Serv 28(1):36–39, 1990
11. Eysenck HJ: A genetic model of anxiety. Issues Ment Health Nurs 7(1–4):160–199, 1985
12. Ferguson S, Campinha-Bacote J: Humor in nursing. J Psychosoc Nurs Ment Health Serv 27(4):29–34, 1989
13. Gray JA: The neuropsychology of anxiety. Issues Ment Health Nurs 7(1–4):201–227, 1985
14. Hamilton V: A cognitive model of anxiety: implications for theories of personality and motivation. Issues Ment Health Nurs 7(1–4):229–249, 1985
15. Jessell JC, Veltri FJ: Trait-anxiety among physically disabled adolescents. J Rehabil 52(1):45–49, 1986
16. Jones P, Jacob D: Anxiety revisited—from a practice perspective. In Kim M, McFarland G, McLane A (eds): Classification of Nursing Diagnoses: Proceedings of the Fifth National Conference. St Louis, CV Mosby, 1984
17. Kim M, McFarland G, McLane A: Pocket Guide to Nursing Diagnoses, 4th ed. St Louis, CV Mosby, 1991

18. Lader M: The nature of clinical anxiety in modern society. Issues Ment Health Nurs 7(1–4):309–334, 1985

19. Laraia MT, Stuart GW, Best CL: Behavioral treatment of panic-related disorders; a review. Arch Psychiatr Nurs 3(3):125–133, 1989

20. McFarland G, Bates T: Mild anxiety, moderate anxiety, severe anxiety, extreme anxiety (panic). In Kim M, McFarland G, McLane A: Pocket Guide to Nursing Diagnoses, 4th ed. St Louis, CV Mosby, 1991

21. McGinnis J, Foote K: Rapid neuroleptization. J Psychosoc Nurs Ment Health Serv 24(10):17–22, 1986

22. McReynolds P: Changing conceptions of anxiety: a historical review and a proposed integration. Issues Ment Health Nurs 7(1–4):131–157, 1985

23. Meldman M, McFarland G, Johnson E: The Problem Oriented Psychiatric Index and Treatment Plans. St Louis, CV Mosby, 1976

24. Miller LE: Modeling awareness of feelings: a needed tool in the therapeutic communication workbox. Perspect Psychiatr Care 25(2):27–29, 1989

25. Pancheri P, DeMartino V, Spiombi G, Biondi M, Mosticoni S: Life stress events and state-trait anxiety in psychiatric and psychosomatic patients. Issues Ment Health Nurs 7(1–4):367–395, 1985

26. Pasquali EA: Learning to laugh: humor as therapy. J Psychosoc Nurs Ment Health Serv 28(3):31–35, 1990

27. Pender NJ: Effects of progressive muscle relaxation training on anxiety and health locus of control among hypertensive adults. Res Nurs Health 8:67–72, 1985

28. Peplau H: A working definition of anxiety. In Burd S, Marshall M (eds): Some Clinical Approaches to Psychiatric Nursing. New York, Macmillan, 1966

29. Sarason I, Spielberger C (eds): Stress and Anxiety, Vol 7. New York, Hemisphere Publishing, 1980

30. Scavnicky-Mylant ML: The hospitalized school-age child's capacity for an appraisal of threat. West J Nurs Res 9(4):503–526, 1987

31. Smith BJ, Cantrell PJ: Distance in nurse patient encounters. J Psychosoc Nurs Ment Health Serv 26(2):22–26, 1988

32. Spielberger CD: Anxiety; state trait process. In Spielberger CD, Sarason IG (eds): Stress and Anxiety: The Series in Clinical Psychology, Vol 1. Washington DC, Hemisphere Publishing Corporation, 1975

33. Spielberger CD: Conceptual and methodological issues in research on anxiety. In Spielberger CD (ed): Anxiety: Current Trends in Theory and Research, Vol 2. New York, Academic Press, 1972

34. Spielberger CD, Sarason I, Milgram N (eds): Stress and Anxiety, Vol 8. New York, Hemisphere Publishing, 1982

35. Sullivan-Taylor L: The worried well patient. In Durham J, Hardin S: The Nurse Psychotherapist in Private Practice. New York, Springer Publishing Co, 1986

36. Tilley S: Alcohol, other drugs and tobacco use and anxiolytic effectiveness. Br J Psychiatry 151:389–392, 1987

37. Titlebaum HM: Relaxation. Holistic Nurs Pract 2(3):17–25, 1988

38. Turnbull JM, Turnbull SK: Anxiety disorders in elderly women. Physician Assistant 10(1):132–138, 1986

39. Vogelsang J: The Visual Analog Scale: an accurate and sensitive

method for self-reporting preoperative anxiety. J Post Anesthes Nurs 3(4):235–239, 1988
40. Whitley GG: Anxiety: defining the diagnosis. J Psychosoc Nurs Ment Health Serv 27(10):7–12, 1989
41. Whitley GG: Anxiety (mild, moderate, severe, extreme/panic). In McFarland GK, Thomas MD: Psychiatric Mental Health Nursing. Philadelphia, JB Lippincott 1991

■ COMMUNICATION, IMPAIRED

— Definition[21,26,27,30–32]

- *Communication*—a dynamic reciprocal process involving a sender, message, and receiver in which information is exchanged
- *Impaired communication*—a communication pattern in which the receiver often arrives at a meaning that differs from that intended by the sender

— General Principles[1–58]

- Impaired communication responses include the following:
  - *Impervious response*—outright failure to acknowledge another's attempt to communicate, suggesting that the speaker is unimportant and does not merit attention (e.g., irrelevant response, no response, interrupting).
  - *Tangential response*—response that is directed only to an incidental part of speaker's communication (e.g., shifting focus, responding with "yes" or "no," then talking about something else)
  - *Ambiguous response*—response that is confusing because more than one, often conflicting, message is contained (e.g., straddling the fence by saying both "yes" and "no," use of nonverbal communication that is incongruous with verbal communication
  - *Inadequate response*—response that is confusing because the message is lost in trivia, is incomplete, or is overqualified
  - *Projective response*—a mystifying response in which the speaker implies that what is going on inside the other person is known or that the speaker is qualified to judge the correctness of the other's feelings
  - *Crossed transaction*—the response received is not appropriate, is unexpected, and does not follow the natural order of healthy human interactions as opposed to complimentary transactions
  - *Ulterior transaction*—the transaction occurs at two levels simultaneously: the social and the psychological.
- Impaired communication patterns include the following:
  - *Games*—a well-structured series of ulterior transactions leading to a well-defined, predictable, but often painful outcome

- *Symmetrical escalation*—one person seeks to make the other conform to expectations that are met with defiance
- *Rigid complementarity*—one person is strong and overprotective of the other

— Related Factors[21,26,27,30–32]

Sensory deficit (e.g., lack of hearing)
Anatomical deficit (e.g., cleft palate)
Physical barrier (e.g., tracheostomy)
Psychiatric disorder (e.g., catatonic schizophrenia)
Emotional state (e.g., extreme anxiety)
Developmental or age-related factors
Multiple stressors
Impaired perception
Poor communication skills
Inadequate self concept
Cultural differences

— Defining Characteristics[21,26,27,30–32]

Stuttering, slurring
Lack of speech
Apparent inability to find or form words
Apparent inability to identify objects
Disorientation
Inappropriate message for context
Inconsistent verbal and nonverbal messages
Frequent misunderstandings or misinterpretations
Apparent unresponsiveness to communication
Verbosity
Loose association of ideas
Inconsistent nonverbal messages
Inappropriate feedback
Disparity of punctuation
Inappropriately timed messages
Absence of gratification
Difficulty expressing feelings
Nonassertive communication style
Inability to speak language of other culture
Inability to understand meaning of nonverbal messages of other culture

— Nursing Assessment[1–58]

- Observe for defining characteristics indicative of impaired communication.
- Note presence of sensory or anatomical deficits, physical barriers, psychiatric disorders, or developmental factors affecting communication.
- Assess for presence of stressors.
- Assess patient's description of perceptions.

- Evaluate patient's emotional state.
- Note patient's communication abilities and limitations during the interview.
- Determine the patient's perceptions about ability to communicate with others.
- Determine the perceptions of significant others regarding patient's ability to communicate.
- Observe for dysfunctional communication responses, such as tangential, ambiguous, inadequate, and projective responses in patient's interactions.
- Observe for frequency of crossed transactions, ulterior transactions, and type of games in which patient involves self.
- Evaluate effect of patient's self concept on communication.
- Evaluate patient's interaction with significant others.
- Assess presence of cultural or subcultural influences on communication patterns.

— Patient Outcomes and Nursing Interventions[1–58]

Patient Outcome: Communicate Effectively

- Use therapeutic communication techniques (see Chapter 5).
- Encourage patient to seek assistance in correcting, modifying, or preventing physical conditions or anatomical deficits that interfere with communication.
- In collaboration with psychiatrist, administer medications for psychiatric disorder or emotional state as necessary.
- In working phase of relationship, discuss discrepancies in message and the metacommunication sent and/or discrepancies in the message sent and the context within which it is sent.
- Assist patient in reviewing perceptions and assumptions.
- Help patient increase awareness of strengths and limitations when communicating with others, regarding type of message sent, timing, etc.
- Increase patient's awareness of areas in which he or she is sensitive, and discuss whether and how to share with another.
- Assist patient in examining the effect of communication skills and patterns and seeking honest feedback about the effect from others.
- Assist patient in developing plan to cope with stressors.
- Discuss how perceptions influence communication.
- Assist patient to identify and focus on relevant stimuli.
- Help patient develop insight into dynamics of relationships.
- Increase patient's awareness of the feelings of others.
- Help patient tolerate disagreement and resolve conflict.
- Help patient develop the ability to give and receive in a relationship.
- Encourage initiation of interactions and communication with others.
- Encourage participation in groups.
- Discuss communication in groups and types of messages sent and received.

- Based on individual assessment, refer patient to transactional analysis group or communication program in which understanding of transactions and games can be increased
- Encourage patient to practice reducing use of dysfunctional communication responses:
  - Reduce nagging.
  - Decrease use of generalizations.
- Teach patient communication skills such as the following:
  - Assertive communication skills (see Chapter 5—*assertiveness training*)
  - Active listening skills
  - Requesting feedback from the other person to make certain that communications are accurately understood; for example, "By telling me . . . do you mean . . . ?"
  - Giving feedback on other person's overt or covert communication, for example, "You're telling me that the whole experience makes you 'livid' "
  - Responding to other person in a manner that conveys a sincere effort to understand how that person perceives world; for example, "As you see it, I just shouldn't have purchased that fur coat without discussing it with you. You feel left out and in a way, 'put-upon' "
  - Listening actively to what the other person is saying and not focusing in own personal response to be made
  - Requesting feedback from the other person to check patient's own perception and interpretation of the other person's communication; for example, "You're giving me the impression that you're totally bored with the movie"
  - Encouraging verbalization, by verbal and nonverbal means, to help other person keep talking; for example, "Go on" "You were saying?" Nodding head
  - Providing feedback by describing some aspect of the other person's communication and its impact on the patient
  - Confronting the other person by describing discrepancies between what is said and what is actually done
- Support patient's use of communication skills.
- Increase patient's acceptance of positive and negative feedback.
- Assist patient in increasing self-esteem.
- Refer to community resources for increasing knowledge of language.
- Assist patient in coping with cultural differences.

—— Evaluation/Outcome Criteria[21,26,27,30–32]

Initiates interactions with others
Is appropriately responsive to the communication of others

Communicates clearly enough so patient can be understood by
  others
Focuses on appropriate input
Considers context when communicating
Utilizes congruent verbal and nonverbal communication
Demonstrates assertive communication skills
Experiences minimal misunderstandings or misperceptions
Gives and accepts feedback
Expresses feelings appropriately
Experiences satisfaction with communication
Demonstrates ability to consider cultural meaning when
  communicating

▬ REFERENCES

1. Berne E: Games People Play. New York, Grove Press, 1966
2. Berne E: What Do You Say After You Say Hello? New York, Bantam Books, 1973
3. Buckwalter KC, Cusack D, Beaver M, Sidles E, Wadle K: The behavioral consequences of a communication intervention on institutionalized residents with aphasia and dysarthria. Arch Psychiatr Nurs 2(5):289–295, 1988
4. Champion R et al: Clinicians' effectiveness in detecting patients' requests during an initial screening. Hosp Community Psychiatry 40(4):413–415, 1989
5. Chapman GE: Reporting therapeutic discourse in a therapeutic community. J Adv Nurs 13(2):255–264, 1988
6. DeCarlo JJ, Mann WC: The effectiveness of verbal versus activity groups in improving self-perception of interpersonal communication skills. Am J Occup Ther 39(1):20–27, 1985
7. Dowden P, Honsiager M, Beukelman D: Serving nonspeaking patients in acute care settings: an intervention approach. AAC 1:25–32, 1986
8. Earl WL, Addison S, Holmquist L: Crosstalk. J Psychosoc Nurs Ment Health Serv 27(1):20–24, 1989
9. Emrich K: Helping or hurting? Interacting in the psychiatric milieu. J Psychosoc Nurs Ment Health Serv 27(12):26–29, 1989
10. Farran CJ, Keane-Hagerty E: Communicating effectively with dementia patients. J Psychosoc Nurs Ment Health Serv 27(5):13–16, 1989
11. Farran CJ et al: Goal-related behaviors in short-term psychiatric hospitalization. Arch Psychiatr Nurs 2(3):159–164, 1988
12. Ferguson S, Campinha-Bacote J: Humor in nursing. J Psychosoc Nurs Ment Health Serv 27(4):29–34, 1989
13. Forchuk C, Brown B: Establishing a nurse-client relationship. J Psychosoc Nurs Ment Health Serv 27(2):30–34, 1989
14. Gerety EK, McKim JD, Sosnovec PA, Cowan ME: Instructor's Manual for McFarland/Thomas's Textbook of Psychiatric Mental Health Nursing: Application of the Nursing Process. Philadelphia, JB Lippincott, 1991
15. Haber J, Leach A, Schudy S, Sideau B: Comprehensive psychiatric nursing. New York, McGraw Hill, 1987
16. Hardin S, Halaris A: Nonverbal communication of patients and high

and low empathy nurses. J Psychosoc Nurs Ment Health Serv 21(1):14–19, 1983

17. Harrison TM et al: Assessing nurses' communication: a cross-sectional study. West J Nurs Res 11(1):75–91, 1989

18. Hedlund N: Therapeutic communication. In Beck CK, Rawlins RP, Williams SR (eds): Mental Health-Psychiatric Nursing, 2nd ed. St Louis, CV Mosby, 1988

19. Heineken J: Treating the disconfirmed psychiatric client. J Psychiatr Nurs Ment Health Serv 21(1):21–25, 1983

20. Kasch C: Role of strategic communication in nursing: theory and research. Adv Nurs Sci 7:56, 1984

21. Kim MJ, McFarland GK, McLane AL: Pocket Guide to Nursing Diagnoses, 4th ed. St Louis, CV Mosby, 1991

22. Kneisl CR: Communication. In Wilson HS, Kneisl CR: Psychiatric Nursing, 3rd ed. Menlo Park, Addison Wesley, 1988

23. Lane PL: Nurse-client perceptions: the double standard of touch. Issues Ment Health Nurs 10:1–13, 1989

24. Loughlin N: Symbolism as a memory tool in learning therapeutic communication techniques. Perspect Psychiatr Care 21(1):9–17, 1983

25. Mazzuca SA: How clinician communication patterns affect patients' comprehension and satisfaction. Diabetes Educ 12(4):370–373, 1986

26. McFarland GK, Naschinski CE: Impaired communication: a descriptive study. Nurs Clin North Am 20(4):775–785, 1985

27. McFarland GK, Naschinski CE: Impaired verbal communication. In Kim MJ, McFarland GK, McLane AL: Pocket Guide to Nursing Diagnoses, 4th ed. St Louis, CV Mosby, 1991

28. Miller LE: Modeling awareness of feelings: a needed tool in the therapeutic communication workbox. Perspect Psychiatr Care 25(2):27–29, 1989

29. Moccia P: Response to "women's talk and nurse-client encounters: developing criteria for assessing interpersonal skill." Scholarly Inquiry Nurs Pract 1(3):257–260, 1987

30. Naschinski CE: Communication, impaired. In McFarland GK, Thomas MD: Psychiatric Mental Health Nursing. Philadelphia, JB Lippincott, 1991

31. Naschinski CE: The communication process. In McFarland GK, Thomas MD: Psychiatric Mental Health Nursing. Philadelphia, JB Lippincott, 1991

32. Naschinski CE, McFarland GK: Impaired verbal communication. In McFarland GK, McFarlane E: Nursing Diagnosis and Intervention: Planning for Patient Care. St Louis, CV Mosby, 1989

33. Northouse P, Northouse L: Health Communication: A Handbook for Health Professionals. Englewood Cliffs, Prentice-Hall, 1985

34. Pasquali EA: Learning to laugh: humor as therapy. J Psychosoc Nurs Ment Health Serv 28(3):31–35, 1990

35. Patterson M: Nonverbal exchange: past, present and future. J Nonverbal Behav 8:350–359, 1984

36. Pavitt C, Haight L: The competent communicator as a cognitive prototype. Human Commun Res 12(2):225–241, 1985

37. Pesut D: Aim versus blame. J Psychosoc Nurs Ment Health Serv 27(5):26–30, 1989

38. Prilleltensky I, Lobel T: The experience of being understood: a phe-

nomenological-structure analysis. Multivar Exp Clin Res 8(2):221–238, 1987

39. Reakes JC: Communication. In Johnson BS: Psychiatric Mental Health Nursing: Adaptation and Growth. Philadelphia, JB Lippincott, 1989
40. Rosenberg L: Managing the group monopolist. Perspect Psychiatr Care 25(1):15–19, 1989
41. Rubin R: Communication Research: Strategies and Sources. Monterey CA, Wadsworth, 1985
42. Ruesch J: Disturbed Communication. New York, WW Norton, 1972
43. Sandman PO et al: Verbal communication and behavior during meals in five institutionalized patients with Alzheimer-type dementia. J Adv Nurs 13(5):571–580, 1988
44. Satir V: Conjoint Family Therapy. Palo Alto, CA, Science and Behavior Books, 1967
45. Satir V: People Making. Palo Alto, CA, Science & Behavior Books, 1972
46. Scott D, Oberst M, Dropkin M: A stress-coping model. Adv Nurs Sci 95(2):99–108, 1980
47. Sherman JB, Cardea JM, Gaskill SD, Tynan CM: Caring: commitment to excellence or condemnation to conformity? J Psychosoc Nurs Ment Health Serv 27(8):25–29, 1989
48. Taylor A et al: Communicating. Englewood Cliffs NJ, Prentice-Hall, 1986
49. Tedesco-Carreras P: Communicating with difficult patients. Imprint 33:36–38, 1986
50. Thomas MD: Therapeutic relationships with clients. In McFarland GK, Thomas MD: Psychiatric Mental Health Nursing. Philadelphia, JB Lippincott, 1991
51. Thompson BM: Interpersonal skills: learning the importance of listening. J Aust Nurses 16(3):45–47, 1986
52. Thorne SE: Helpful and unhelpful communications in cancer care: the patient perspective. Oncol Nurs Forum 15(2):167–172, 1988
53. Topf M: Verbal interpersonal responsiveness. J Psychosoc Nurs Ment Health Serv 26(7):8–16, 1988
54. Watzlawick P, Beavin J, Jackson D: Pragmatics of Human Communication. New York, WW Norton, 1967
55. Williams CA: Biopsychosocial elements of empathy: a multidimensional model. Issues Ment Health Nurs 11:155–174, 1990
56. Wilmot W: Dyadic Communication. New York, Random House, 1986
57. Wong SE, Woolsey JE: Re-establishing conversational skills in overtly psychotic, chronic schizophrenic patients. Behav Modif 13(4):415–430, 1989
58. Zappe C, Epstein D: Assertive training. J Psychosoc Nurs Ment Health Serv 25(8):23–25, 1987

■ COPING, DEFENSIVE (DENIAL, INEFFECTIVE DENIAL)

— Definition[5,7,13,14]

Denial—an involuntary, unconscious, protective mechanism (defense mechanism) by which the presence and impact of a threatening reality is disowned and replaced with a more pleasant or acceptable version

Ineffective denial—a degree of denial which puts the person at increased risk and danger, e.g., increased severity of illness or threat of death

— General Principles[1-20]

Denial may reflect a healthy, coordinated process of protecting the ego and can alter external or internal reality by not acknowledging awareness of the painful event or situation. It can be reversible, or may be replaced by a more mature defense mechanism in a changing process over time. Denial can serve as a temporary defense to buffer sudden, unexpected traumatic events or stressors. Denial, however, can be pathological, especially if over used. The more elements of external reality that are denied the more the person is put at risk from the resulting consequences.

- Denial can protect the ego, manage instincts, reduce or mitigate internal conflicts, keep emotions within bearable limits, allow for mastering change in the self concept, maintain the patient's sense of well-being, and preserve interpersonal relationships.
- Denial can allow for mobilization of elements of the coping repertoire and coping resources of the patient and can promote eventual awareness and acceptance of the traumatic situation.
- The process of denial can be described in four phases:
  - *Preconscious appraisal* of danger, trauma, or stressor
  - *Painful affect* and the initiation of defensive actions
  - *Cognitive arrest* in which threatening information is excluded from conscious awareness
  - *Screen behavior* in which ideas and behaviors lend credibility to the denial
- Denial serves as an attention-focusing function and occurs at different levels and in different ways.
- Denial can become ineffective depending on timing, circumstance, and pervasiveness; e.g., when it interferes with medical or psychiatric treatment and puts the patient at increased risk.
- Denial may be the hallmark of specific psychiatric disorders.

— Related Factors[5,7,13,14]

Physical illness
Compromised physical status following illness
Severe pain
Personal injury
Negative consequences of health problem
Psychiatric disorders
Substance abuse
Overwhelming stressors
Negative past experiences
Significant unexpected loss
Learned response pattern
Inadequate coping skills

Lack of ego strength
Lack of knowledge
Lack of adequate resources
Lack of social support
Threat to values or beliefs

— Defining Characteristics[5,7,13,14]

Denial

Preconscious appraisal of danger, trauma, or stressor
Disowns threatening reality
Excludes significance of threat from awareness
Distorts threatening reality
Inappropriate affect
Minimizes symptoms
Displaces source of symptoms to other organs
Inability to recognize the impact of symptoms on lifestyle
Makes dismissive comments about distressing event such as illness
Relies on self diagnosis and treatment

Ineffective Denial

Delays seeking health care to the detriment of health
Refuses health care treatment to the detriment of health
Noncompliance with treatment to the detriment of health
Inability to problem-solve
Inability to meet role expectations
Substance abuse

— Nursing Assessment[5,7,13,14]

- Maintain respect and a high degree of sensitivity to readiness of patient to discuss situation.
- What is the meaning of the experience to the patient and the underlying cause for denial? How does the patient perceive and evaluate the significance of what is happening to him or her?
- Evaluate level of feelings such as anger, anxiety.
- Evaluate degree and phase of denial. Tools to measure denial may be helpful: WOC-R (Folkman & Lazarus), Defense Mechanism Inventory (Glesner & Ihilivech), Denial Defense Scale (Haan), Denial Scale (Hackett & Cassem).
- Examine the patient's symptoms in comparison to patient's own self report and some other person's objective report.
- How has patient coped with similar stressors in the past?
- What were the patient's usual coping repertoire and resources when health problems occurred in the past?
- Evaluate the patient's current coping response repertoire and coping resources (see ineffective individual coping and situational crisis section, this chapter)
- How long has the patient denied symptoms of the health problem?
- What are the likely consequences to the patient of continued denial of the health problem?

- What treatment resources are available to the patient?
- What are the patient's social support resources to assist with health problems?
- What are the prominent cultural norms related to obtaining health care treatment? Is stigma connected with the patient's present health problem?
- Assess conflicting thoughts and feelings that may be perpetuating denial.

Patient Outcomes and Nursing Interventions[1-19]

Patient Outcome: Maintain Ego Integrity, Self-Concept, and Tolerable Emotional Level

- Try to understand the patient's experience, perceptions, and context which increase levels of anxiety and contribute to an increase in denial.
- Do not confront denial directly, especially in the initial phase of developing a therapeutic relationship with patient.
- Do not blame patient for use of denial.
- Do not try to get patient to "prove" that denial is present; i.e., don't try to get the patient to "prove" that he or she is not "lying."
- Provide supportive and predictable milieu (see Chapter 5—*milieu therapy*).
- Offer own presence as appropriate (see Chapter 5—*supportive therapy-presence*).
- Assist patient in finding ways to decrease anxiety or aggression (see Chapter 4—*anxiety, aggression*).
- Help the patient to identify areas which increase levels of discomfort.
- Delay any intervention with denial, if denial is not posing a problem to patient and/or appears to be a temporary mechanism to deal with sudden unexpected stressor.
- Use the technique of agreeing with aspect of denial that is reality based, when appropriate.

Patient Outcome: Cope with Stressful Situation in an Adaptive Problem-Solving Manner

- Do not confront denial directly.
- Support patient when distortions of reality are recognized.
- Assist the patient in developing awareness of coping response repertoire used in dealing with health problems.
- Introduce discussion related to contradictions behind reality of situation and the patient's perceptions gradually and in a carefully timed manner. Work on the least anxiety-producing aspect of the situation first.
- Enhance the patient's perceptions of strengths and coping skills.
- Examine the patient's current coping behaviors and their consequences, allowing for patient to have enough time for adequate exploration in an atmosphere free from tension.
- Explore realistic interpretations and events together with patient.

- Support the patient in reexamining and interpreting threatening situations and feelings.
- Assist the patient in acquiring new knowledge. Provide additional needed information.
- Develop mutually agreeable goals with the patient.
- Assist the patient in deployment of an adaptive coping repertoire and coping resources (see ineffective individual coping and situational crisis section, this chapter).
- Offer grief counseling, if appropriate (see Chapter 5—*supportive therapy-grief counseling*).
- Facilitate the patient's eliciting help from others.
- Assess for presence of denial in family member.
- Work through family member's support of patient's denial, if present.
- Develop a plan for working through the need for denial with other team members, the family, and other caregivers.
- Ensure that family and significant others understand that denial protects the patient from the anxiety of accepting reality.
- For ineffective denial, if situation is urgent and continued denial of reality is detrimental to patient's health and welfare, assist physician in assessment of competency to consent or refuse treatment, and get alternate consent, if appropriate.

— Evaluation/Outcome Criteria[5,7,13,14]

Experiences less anxiety and stress
Uses defense mechanism of denial appropriately
Begins to develop realistic awareness and appraisal of situation
Uses effective problem solving techniques
Meets role expectations
Seeks out needed treatment for health problems
Complies with treatment regimen for health problems

▬ REFERENCES

1. Bond M, Gardner ST, Christian J, Sigal JJ: Empirical study of self-rated defense styles. Arch Gen Psychiatry 40:333–338, 1983
2. Bond MP, Vaillant JS: Am empirical study of the relationship between diagnosis and defense style. Arch Gen Psychiatry 43:285–288, 1986
3. Breznitz S: The seven kinds of denial. In Breznitz S (ed): The Denial of Stress. New York, International University Press, 1983
4. Connor SR: Measurement of denial in the terminally ill: a critical review. Hospice J 2(4):51–68, 1986
5. Fitch MI, O'Brien-Pallas LL: Defensive coping. In McFarland GK, Thomas MD: Psychiatric Mental Health Nursing. Philadelphia, JB Lippincott, 1991
6. Folkman S, Lazarus RS: If it changes, it must be a process: study of emotion and coping during three stages of a college examination. J Pers Soc Psychol 48(1):150–170, 1985
6a. Forchuk C: Cognitive dissonance: negative self concepts and denial among alcoholic patients. Nursing Papers 16(Fall): 57–69, 1984

7. Forchuk C, Westwell J: Denial. J Psychosoc Nurs Ment Health Serv 25(6):9–13, 1987

7a. Forchuk C, Westwell J: Denial. In Baumann A, Johnson N, Atai-Otong D: Decision Making in Psychiatric and Psychosocial Nursing. Toronto, BC Decker, 1990

8. Freud A: The Ego and Mechanisms of Defense. New York, International Universities Press, 1946

9. Gleser G, Ihilivech D: An objective instrument for measuring defense mechanisms. J Consult Clin Psychol 33(1):51–60, 1969

10. Haan N: Conceptualizations of ego: processes, functions, regulations. In Monat A, Lazarus RS (eds): Stress and Coping: an Anthology. New York, Columbia University Press, 1985

11. Haan N: Coping and Defending: Processes of Self Environment Organization. New York, Academic Press, 1977

12. Hackett TP, Cassem NH: Development of a quantitative rating scale to assess denial. J Psychosom Res 18(2):93–100, 1974

13. McFarland GK, Thompson JM, Hirsch JE, Tucker SM, Bowers AC: Ineffective denial. In Thompson JM, McFarland GK, Hirsch JE, Tucker SM, Bowers AC: Mosby's Manual of Clinical Nursing. St Louis, CV Mosby, 1989

14. O'Brien-Pallas L, Graydon JE, McFarland GK: Ineffective denial. In Kim MJ, McFarland GK, McLane A: Pocket Guide to Nursing Diagnoses, 4th ed. St Louis, CV Mosby, 1991

15. Vaillant GE: Adaptation to Life. Boston, Little Brown, 1977

16. Vaillant GE: Defense mechanisms. In Nicholi AM (ed): The New Harvard Guide to Psychiatry. Cambridge, Harvard University Press, 1988

17. Vaillant GE: A 12-year follow-up of New York narcotic addicts. IV: Some characteristics and determinants of abstinence. Am J Psychiatry 123:573–584, 1966

18. Vaillant GE, Drake RE: Maturity of ego defenses in relation to DSM-III Axis II personality disorder. Arch Gen Psychiatry 42:597–601, 1985

19. Vaillant GE, Bond M, Vaillant CO: An empirically validated hierarchy of defense mechanisms. Arch Gen Psychiatry 43:786–794, 1986

20. Westwell J, Forchuk C: Denial: buffer and barrier. Can Nurse 85(9): 16–18, 1989

■ COPING, INEFFECTIVE INDIVIDUAL

— Definition

Ineffective individual coping is an inability to: (a) formulate an accurate, realistic appraisal of stressor(s), (b) develop and to use adequate response repertoire, and (c) mobilize adequate coping resources, resulting in maladaptive behaviors.[26,49,50]

— General Principles[1–51]

- Coping generally refers to the ability to deal with stressors and life demands in an adaptive manner.
- Prerequisites for effective coping include accurate appraisal of the stressor, the context, and the self; an adequate response repertoire including assertive behavior skills, problem solving

skills, communication skills; appropriate availability and deployment of coping resources; and recovery and adaptive behavior in response to the stress-coping episode.
- A positive self-concept enables a person to develop and use adequate coping responses and coping resources.

— Related Factors[26,49,50]

- Major stressors
  Physical illness (e.g., neurological disorder)
  Severe pain
  Poor physical condition (e.g., malnourishment)
  Psychiatric disorder
  Memory loss
  Sensory impairment
  Sensory overload
  Significant loss (e.g., loss of loved one)
  Multiple life changes in short time period
  Institutionalization (e.g., jail)
  Maturational crisis (e.g., career choice in adolescence)
  Multiple stressors over time
  Treatment-related stressors (e.g., disfigurement caused bysurgery)
- Inaccurate appraisal of stressors
  Inability to evaluate source of threat
  Inability to redefine or interpret source of threat
  Inability to identify own source of strengths
  Focus on previous negative experiences
  Interfering assumptions
  Unrealistic goals
  Incompatible goals
  Inability to develop personal meaning about threat
- Inadequate appraisal of the context or situation
- Impaired self-concept
- Inadequate response repertoire
  Inappropriate emotional responsiveness (e.g., emotional response too prolonged or too severe)
  Difficulty in expressing feelings
  Inappropriate use of defense mechanisms
  Defensive avoidance behaviors
  Impaired communication skills
  Impaired problem-solving or decision-making skills
  Lack of perceived control
  Helplessness
  Lack of assertive behavior
  Inability to develop alternate goals and plans
  Inability to seek out or learn new skills and the knowledge needed to resolve life demands
  Hopelessness
  Conflicting values and beliefs
- Inadequate or difficulty in deployment of coping resources
  Difficulty in using decision-making skills

Lack of ability to transfer knowledge or skills to problem
resolution
Fears about initiating action
Disruption of emotional bonds (e.g., relocation)
Dysfunctional family system
Unsatisfactory social support network
Lack of adequate treatment resources
Disruption in physical environment (e.g., natural disaster)
Cultural instability

—— Defining Characteristics[26,49,50]

Verbalization of inability to cope
Nonperformance of activities of daily living
Inability to meet basic needs
Nonproductive lifestyle
Somatic complaints
Increased illness rate
High accident rate
Substance abuse
Maladaptive behaviors (e.g., acting-out behavior, passive-aggressive
behavior)

—— Nursing Assessment

- Evaluate potential for suicidal or homicidal behavior.
- Evaluate emotional state (e.g., level of anxiety).
- Identify nature of stressor(s).
- Determine physical and emotional condition.
- Obtain information about previous coping style
- Assess cognitive abilities.
- Identify history of exposure to major stressors.
- Identify number of major life changes with past year.
- Identify how patient interprets threatening events or stressors.
- Determine degree of focus on previous negative experiences.
- Assess patient's goals.
- Evaluate patient's self concept.
- Assess patient's response repertoire.
    - Identify history of crisis resolution.
    - To what extent is patient able to express feelings?
    - Are defense mechanisms over-used? Underused?
    - Is patient using avoidance behaviors?
    - Evaluate patient's communication skills.
    - Evaluate patient's degree of perceived control in present
      situation.
    - What is patient's degree of helpless? Hopelessness?
- Evaluate patient's availability and use of coping resources.
    - Evaluate history and present degree of assertive behavior.
    - What are patient's beliefs and values regarding the current
      situation?
    - Is social withdrawal present? To what degree?
    - Assess available social support network.

- Is there evidence of unsatisfactory societal interaction?
- Is patient overdependent on significant others?
- Is patient overdependent on professional help or social institutions?
- Does patient experience an inability to perform role expectations?
- Has patient relinquished hope or spiritual values?

—— Patient Outcomes and Nursing Interventions[1–51]

Patient Outcome: Perceive Self as Able to Cope With Stressor/Threatening Event

- Convey trust in patient's ability to take action and respond to situation.
- Assist patient in lowering anxiety level or degree of aggression.
- Identify what patient has done to help self in past.
- Focus on patient's strengths.
- Allow patient time to become aware of self and reality rather than confronting with reality. Begin with a small piece of reality if confrontation is appropriate.
- Avoid interactions that focus on messages such as, "You *do* have a problem—I don't."
- Assist patient in understanding the interplay among stressor(s), perception, response repertoire, and use of coping resources.

Patient Outcome: Engage in Objective Appraisal of the Stressor

- Explore patient's assumptions and perception of the event by encouraging description.
- Provide factual information about the threatening stimulus.
- Provide preparatory information to any patient who is undergoing new procedures and experiences, especially describing the physical sensations and causes of the sensations.
- Raise questions, encourage data gathering, and promote an attitude of openness to new information.
- Avoid evaluative statements when providing information to the patient.
- Help patient work through unresolved memories of past events, using image-based reconstruction.
- Encourage patient to consult professionals in medicine, social work, and law for assistance with interpretation of stressors.
- Make referral for spiritual counseling to assist client in finding meaning in a situation.
- Give feedback about reality, especially identifying distortions of reality.
- Help the patient examine and develop realistic goals.

Patient Outcome: Develop an Awareness of Current Response Repertoire

- Provide assistance in dealing with emotional responses.
- Offer empathy to the patient's expressions of feelings and encourage acceptance of these feelings.

- Elicit from the patient what is feared and what makes the patient angry.
- Provide factual information about the responses of others to crisis (e.g., anger, depression, withdrawal, the powers of crisis resolution, and the grief-mourning process).
- Give feedback about observed behavior and the feelings expressed.
- Assist the patient in identifying feelings with names that are acceptable and understandable.
- Assist the patient in developing ideas about the relationship of emotional state, thought patterns and behaviors.
- Set limits on irrational demands.
- Assist the patient in beginning to deal with emotional reactions by examining relationships.

Patient Outcome: Achieve Increased Self-Concept

- Teach the patient to monitor self for ineffective thoughts about self or maladaptive behaviors.
- Explore past situations in which effective coping behaviors were demonstrated.
- Teach the patient to observe changes in the behavior of others as the patient changes or uses another action.

Patient Outcome: Use Adequate Coping Response Repertoire

- Help the patient reduce anxiety by using recreational and diversional activities as well as by working through feelings of anxiety.
- Foster constructive outlets for anger and hostility by teaching warning signs of outbursts, ways to gain self-control, and appropriate ways to express anger.
- Foster expression of feelings through open communication.
- Assist the patient in mobilizing others for emotional support.
- Assist the patient in identifying and making changes in health behaviors that are necessary because of the stress.
- Serve as a role model and/or social support when assisting the patient in performing activities of daily living.
- Assist the patient in identifying areas in which he or she can act and exert a reasonable amount of control and areas in which the patient has little or limited possibility of control.
- Assist the patient in working through denial or other defensive mechanisms and to understand and accept defensive mechanisms as coping responses useful at a point in time.
- Teach the patient to observe for coping responses of defensive avoidance and hypervigilance, which may impede decision-making.
- Encourage an attitude of realistic hope as a way to deal with feelings of helplessness.
- Teach the effect negative self-reflections and derogatory ideas have on emotional responses.
- Teach patient skills relevant to problem solving, decision making, assertive communication, goal setting, evaluation, study, relaxation, and help seeking (see Chapter 5).

- Assist the patient in identifying coping responses that are being used and other coping responses that are possible.
- Assist the patient in setting reasonable goals.

Patient Outcome: Develop and Use Adequate Coping Resources

- Help patient strengthen available new coping resources and develop new ones.
- Assist patient in working through remaining fears about starting an action plan to resolve difficult life demands.
- Encourage the patient to role-play the use of problem-solving and decision-making skills.
- Encourage and support the patient in trying out knowledge learned regarding dealing with the current problem situation.
- Encourage the patient to use social support resources (e.g., encourage a visit with a friend). Engage the patient in role rehearsal and mental imagery for active social role participation.
- Refer the patient for family therapy as needed.
- Engage in grief counseling (see Chapter 5—*supportive therapy; grief counseling*).
- Identify and refer the patient to treatment resources for any physical or mental disorders.

Patient Outcome: Evaluate Impact of Coping Response Repertoire and Use of Coping Resources

- Give feedback on the patient's behavior in order to make patient aware of maladaptive responses that tend to foster dependency, and manipulation of others.
- Confront the patient about impaired judgment when appropriate.
- Provide feedback to the patient and assist patient in eliciting feedback from others.
- Assist the patient in developing cues for self to indicate whether the patient is reacting automatically or objectively.
- Give the patient a conceptual model for understanding the event or treatment regimen (e.g., model of emotion, model of stress).

— Evaluation/Outcome Criteria[26,49,50]

Accurately appraises stress or threatening event and situation
Demonstrates constructive emotional and cognitive responses
Demonstrates use of problem-solving abilities
Abstains from relying on substance abuse
Uses adequate coping resources
Resolves stress-producing episode
Engages in adaptive behaviors

■ REFERENCES

1. Barnfather JS, Erickson HC: Construct validity of an aspect of the coping process: potential adaptation to stress. Issues Ment Health Nurs 10:23–40, 1989
2. Burckhardt CS: Coping strategies of the chronically ill. Nurs Clin North Am 22(3):543–550, 1987

3. Christman N, McConnell EA, Pfeiffer C, Webster KK, Schmitt M, Ries J: Res Nurs Health 11:71–82, 1988

4. Clark S: Nursing diagnosis: ineffective coping. Planning care. Heart Lung 16(6):677–684, 1987

5. Clark S: Nursing diagnosis: ineffective coping. A theoretical framework. Psychol Aspects Crit Care 16(6):670–676, 1987

6. deChesnay M, Magnuson N: How healthy families cope with stress. AAOHNJ 36(9):361–365, 1988

7. Dellasega C: Coping with caregiving. J Psychosoc Nurs Ment Health Serv 28(1):15–22, 1990

8. Gass KA: Aged widows and widowers: similarities and differences in appraisals, coping, resources, type of death, and health dysfunction. Arch Psychiatr Nurs 11(4):200–210, 1988

9. Gass KA: Coping strategies of widows. J Gerontol Nurs 13(8):29–33, 1987

10. Gass KA, Chang AS: Appraisals of bereavement, coping, resources, and psychosocial health dysfunction in widows and widowers. Nurs Res 38(1):31–36, 1989

11. Goldberger L, Breynitz S: Handbook of Stress: Theoretical and Clinical Aspects. New York, Free Press, 1982

12. Gonzales-Osler E: Coping with transition. J Psychosoc Nurs Ment Health Serv 27(6):29–33, 1989

13. Gurklis JA, Menke EM: Identification of stressors and use of coping methods in chronic hemodialysis patients. Nurs Res 37(4):236–239, 248, 1988

14. Haan N: Conceptualizations of ego: processes, functions, regulations. In Monat A, Lazaras RS (eds): Stress and Coping: An Anthology. New York, Columbia University Press, 1985

15. Haggmark C, Theorell T, Ek B: Coping and social activity patterns among relatives of cancer patients. Soc Sci Med 25(9):1021–1025, 1987

16. Harris RB: Reviewing nursing stress according to a proposed coping-adaptation framework. Adv Nurs Sci 11(2):12–28, 1989

17. Harvis KA: Dementia: helping family caregivers cope. J Psychosoc Nurs Ment Health Serv 27(5):7–8, 10–11, 1989

18. Hays JC: Patient symptoms and family coping. Cancer Nurs 9(6):317–325, 1986

19. Johnson JE, Lauver DR: Alternative explanations of coping with stressful experiences associated with physical illness. Adv Nurs Sci 11(2):39–52, 1989

20. Kadner KD: Resilience: responding to adversity. J Psychosoc Nurs Ment Health Serv 27(7):20–25, 1989

21. Korniewicz DM, O'Brien ME, Larson E: Coping with AIDS and HIV. J Psychosoc Nurs Ment Health Serv 23(3):14–21, 1990

22. LaMontagne LL: Adopting a process approach to assess children's coping. J Ped Nurs 3(3):159–163, 1987

23. Lazarus RS: The psychology of stress and coping. Issues Ment Health Nurs 7(1–4):399–418, 1985

24. Long CG: Group coping skills training for anxiety and depression: its application with chronic patients. J Adv Nurs 13(3):358–364, 1988

25. Lowery BJ: Stress research: some theoretical and methodological issues. Image: J Nurs Scholarship 19(1):42–46, 1987

26. McFarland GK, Wasli EL: Ineffective individual coping. In Kim MJ, McFarland GK, McLane A: Pocket Guide to Nursing Diagnoses, 4th ed. St Louis, CV Mosby, 1991

27. McNett SC: Social support, threat, and coping responses and effectiveness in the functionally disabled. Nurs Res 36(2):98–103, 1987

28. Meichenbaum D, Novaco R: Stress innoculation: a preventative approach. Issues Ment Health Nurs 7(1–4):419–435, 1985

29. Miller LE: Modeling awareness of feelings: a needed tool in the therapeutic communication workbox. Perspect Psychiatr Care 25(2):27–29, 1989

30. Musil CM, Abraham IL: Coping, thinking, and mental health nursing: cognitions and their application to psychosocial intervention. Issues Ment Health Nurs 8(3):191–201, 1986

31. Nyamathi A: Comprehensive health seeking and coping paradigm. J Adv Nurs 14:281–290, 1989

32. Nyamathi A, vanServellen G: Maladaptive coping in the critically ill population with acquired immunodeficiency syndrome: nursing assessment and treatment. Heart Lung 18(2):113–120, 1989

33. Nyamathi A, Dracup K, Jacoby A: Development of a spousal coping instrument. Prog Cardiovasc Nurs 3(1):1–6, 1988

34. Parkes KR: Coping in stressful episodes: the role of individual differences, environmental factors, and situational characteristics. J Personal Soc Psychol 51(6):1277–1292, 1986

35. Plante TG: Social skills training: a program to help schizophrenic clients cope. J Psychosoc Nurs Ment Health Serv 27(3):7–10, 1989

36. Poole D: Ineffective individual coping. In McFarland GK, Thomas MD: Psychiatric Mental Health Nursing, Philadelphia, JB Lippincott, 1991

37. Roberts J, Browne G, Brown B, Byrne C, Love B: Coping revisited: the relation between appraised seriousness of an event, coping responses and adjustment to illness. Nurs Papers/Perspect Nurs 19(3):45–54, 1987

38. Rundell JR, Ursano RJ, Holloway HC, Silberman EK: Psychiatric responses to trauma. Hosp Community Psychiatry 40(1):68–73, 1989

39. Ryan NM: The stress-coping process in school-age children: gaps in the knowledge needed for health promotion. Adv Nurs Sci 11(1):1–12, 1988

40. Scavnicky-Mylant ML: The process of coping among young adult children of alcoholics. Issues Ment Health Nurs 11:125–139, 1990

41. Smilkstein G: Health benefits of helping patients cope. Consultant 28(1):56–67, 1988

42. Sumners AD: Humor: coping in recovery from addiction. Issues Ment Health Nurs 9:169–179, 1988

43. Sutherland S: Burned adolescents' descriptions of their coping strategies. Heart Lung 17(2):150–157, 1988

44. Tache J, Selye H: On stress and coping mechanisms. Issues Ment Health Nurs 7(1–4):3–24, 1985

45. Titlebaum HM: Relaxation. Holistic Nurs Pract 2(3):17–25, 1988

46. vanServellen G, Nyamathi AM, Mannion W: Coping with a crisis: evaluating psychological risks of patients with AIDS. J Psychosoc Nurs Ment Health Serv 27(12):16–21, 1989

47. Vincent KG: The validation of a nursing diagnosis. Nurs Clin North Am 20(4):631–640, 1985

48. Walker CL: Stress and coping in siblings of childhood cancer patients. Nurs Res 37(4):208–212, 1988
49. Wasli EL: Ineffective individual coping. In McFarland GK, McFarland E: Nursing Diagnosis and Intervention: Planning for Patient Care. St Louis, CV Mosby, 1989
50. Wasli EL: Ineffective individual coping. In Thompson JM, McFarland GK, Hirsch JE, Tucker SM, Bowers AC: Clinical Nursing, 2nd ed. St Louis, CV Mosby, 1989
51. Webster KK, Christman NJ: Perceived uncertainty and coping post myocardial infarction. West J Nurs Res 10(4):384–400, 1988

■ CRISIS, SITUATIONAL

— Definition[2,19]

Crisis—a state of disequilibrium resulting from an imbalance between a person's perception of an event as threatening to psychological or physical well-being and available current coping mechanisms and situational supports to deal with stressor(s)
Situational Crisis—a disequilibrium resulting from an event or sequence of events evaluated as threatening, along with an inadequate coping repertoire and resources to deal with event/stressor

— General Principles[1–40]

- Crisis can occur as individual crisis, family crisis, or community crisis.
- Events or stressors may represent
  threat to integrity of self or instinctual needs;
  a real or perceived loss;
  a challenge.
- Outcomes are influenced by social support and other resources available, perception of event, and coping skills.
- Crisis offers opportunities for personal growth if successfully resolved.
- Maladaptive resolution of crisis may lead to lowered level of functioning, suicide, violence, or prolonged mental illness.
- A person is more open to suggestions, learning, and potential emotional growth during a crisis.
- A person may be aware of the stressor and state of disequilibrium and seek assistance, or may feel helpless to do anything about it.
- Crisis is self-limiting, with average duration 6 weeks. The precipitating event often occurs 10–14 days before the client comes for assistance.
- Crisis phases can include
  Denial—occurs initially but may persist throughout crisis
  Increased free-flowing anxiety—Activities of normal living are continued but with much difficulty; some hyperactivity or psychomotor retardation.

Disorganization—Activities of normal living are limited or ceased; they may include severe anxiety, fear, guilt, shame, helplessness, depression, or anger. There is preoccupation with the current hazardous event and earlier symbolically linked events.

Attempted reorganization—The patient uses a familiar coping repertoire and resources lasting several weeks, if successful; if unsuccessful, this may lead to escape mechanisms such as blaming others for difficulty or substance abuse resulting in unsuccessful crisis resolution.

Local and general reorganization—There is lower, same, or improved functioning as compared with precrisis level, usually attained in 6 weeks from onset of crisis.

— Related Factors[1–40]

Imbalance between actual/perceived resources and actual or perceived hazardous event
Unexpected, traumatic situational event
Inadequate personal resources
Physical disorder
Mental disorder
Memory loss
Sensory impairment
Major financial loss
Perceptual impairment
Impaired thought processes
Inadequate coping skills
History of maladaptive responses to stress
Lack of supportive social network
Lack of community resources

— Defining Characteristics[1–39]

Denial
Physical symptoms, e.g., headache
Difficulty with activities of daily living
Hyperactivity
Psychomotor retardation
Disorganization
Dysfunctional non-goal-directed behavior
Difficulties with communications
Severe anxiety
Extreme anxiety (panic)
Helplessness
Depression
Suicide threat
Guilt, self-blame
Blaming others
Extreme anger
Family disruption
Inappropriate deployment of coping resources

—— Nursing Assessment[1-40]

- What are the current behavioral manifestations? Are any suicidal or homicidal impulses present? What is the current level of role functioning?
- What is the nature of the crisis? Onset? Intensity and duration of precipitating factor(s) or event(s)?
- How does the patient perceive difficulties?
- What coping strategies and problem-solving skills does the patient possess?
- What coping skills have been successfully used in the past?
- Is social support available, such as family and friends? (Instruments such as the Norbeck Social Support Questionnaire[25,26] or the Personal Resource Questionnaire[39] can be used for assessing social support.)
- Does the patient's crisis affect other family members or significant others? How?
- What community resources are available?

—— Patient Outcomes and Nursing Interventions[1-40]

Patient Outcome: Achieve Lowered Level of Anxiety and Emotional State So Patient Can Function in a Goal-Directed Manner

- Provide immediate therapy in crisis to reduce disorganization and anxiety, enhance optimal resolution, and prevent psychopathology (also see anxiety, in this chapter).
- Establish rapport through warm, empathic, supportive, caring, trustworthy, nonjudgmental approach.
- Assist the patient in recognizing and expressing feelings such as anxiety, anger, and sadness.
- If relevant, support active grieving process. Provide grief counseling (see Chapter 5).
- Offer careful, simple explanations during early crisis phase.
- Reinforce coping strategies used effectively in the past by the patient to reduce tension.
- Help patient decrease the blaming of self or others.

Patient Outcome: Achieve Realistic Perception of Precipitating Event and Subsequent Experiences

- Ask the patient to describe the sequence of events in the process of adjusting to the stressor.
- Help the patient gain an understanding of the crisis by discussing the effect of the stressor(s) and the link to subsequent behaviors.
- Offer ego support.
- Convey to the patient that difficulties can be understood, that others have undergone similar problems, and that ways for solving the difficulty can be identified.
- Offer hope (see Chapter 5—*supportive therapy*).
- Focus on present, not past, difficulties.
- Outline target behaviors and goals for therapy, using patient input.

- Assist the patient in defining problem (see Chapter 5—*crisis intervention*).
- Clarify experiences by restating previously unconnected facts.
- Facilitate resourcefulness; i.e., the ability for patient to self-regulate internal responses so that the stressful event can be managed.

Patient Outcome: Utilize and Increase Repertoire of Coping Skills

- Teach how to monitor emotional state and recognize when it is interfering with problem solving.
- Encourage use of existing problem-solving skills.
- Encourage the patient to describe own accomplishments in dealing with crisis.
- Summarize positive changes during therapy.
- Promote individual responsibility for problem solving and decision making.
- Teach the patient decision-making skills (see Chapter 5).
- Teach the patient problem-solving skills by
  - Clearly defining problem;
  - Generating potential solutions;
  - Describing projected consequences of proposed solutions;
  - Choosing alternatives;
  - Testing behavior or action;
  - Evaluating results;
  - Redefining problem, if necessary
- Explore and examine alternate ways of managing stress (see Chapter 5).
- Give information and guidance as needed.
- Assist the patient to formulate plan of action that
  - Uses situational supports;
  - Identifies and mobilizes use of strengths and decision-making skills;
  - Develops a number of options for action.
- Support the patient in an emerging, more positive self-concept.

Patient Outcome: Utilize and Develop Situational Supports

- Recognize and activate social supports.
- Make home visits as needed.
- Offer information about community resources (e.g., residential housing), make referrals, or assist the patient in contacting agencies.
- Provide easy access to the therapist, within limits.
- Encourage the patient's use of the phone as a communication link.
- Encourage the patient's use of, and reliance on, community supports, social service agencies, or significant others.
- Monitor the patient's dependency on the therapist and reduce dependency, if appropriate.
- Seek input from the patient in developing a treatment plan.
- Assist the patient in increasing his or her social sphere.
- Explore resources known by the patient.

- Use the preventive technique of anticipatory planning, tailored to the patient's unique circumstances; have patient describe potential future crises and possible coping strategies.

—— Evaluation/Outcome Criteria

Demonstrates pre-crisis level of functioning.
Demonstrates improvement over pre-crisis level of functioning.

■ REFERENCES

1. Adams A, Dixey D: Running an anxiety management group. Health Visitor 61(12):375–376, 1988
2. Aguilera D, Messick J: Crisis Intervention, Theory and Methodology, 6th ed. St Louis, CV Mosby, 1989
3. Barnfather JS, Swain MA, Erickson HC: Construct validity of an aspect of the coping process: potential adaptation to stress. Issues Ment Health Nurs 10:23–40, 1989
4. Bennett G: Stress, social support, and self-esteem of young alcoholics in recovery. Issues Ment Health Nurs 9:151–167, 1988
5. Breznitz S: False alarms: their effects on fear and adjustment. Issues Ment Health Nurs 7(1–4):335–347, 1985
6. Buckwalter KC, Abraham IL: Alleviating the discharge crisis: the effects of a cognitive-behavioral nursing intervention for depressed patients and their families. Arch Psychiatr Nurs 1(5):350–358, 1987
7. Burstein A: Post-traumatic stress disorder in victims of motor vehicle accidents. Hosp Community Psychiatry 40(3):295–297, 1989
8. Caplan G: Principles of Preventive Psychiatry. New York, Basic Books, 1964
9. Cervantes RC, deSnyder V, Padilla AM: Post-traumatic stress in immigrants form Central America and Mexico. Hosp Community Psychiatry 40(6):615–619, 1989
10. Cohen S: Cognitive processes as determinants of environmental stress. Issues Ment Health Nurs 7(1–4):65–81, 1985
11. Dellasega C: Coping with caregiving: stress management for caregivers of the elderly. J Psychosoc Nurs Ment Health Serv 28(1):15–22, 1990
12. Dohrenwend BS: Social status and responsibility for stressful life event. Issues Ment Health Nurs 7(1–4):105–127, 1985
13. Ellison JM, Hughes DH, White KA: An emergency psychiatry update. Hosp Community Psychiatry 40(3):250–259, 1989
14. Ferguson S, Campinha-Bacote J: Humor in nursing. J Psychosoc Nurs Ment Health Serv 27(4):29–34, 1989
15. Fisher HL: Psychiatric crises: making the most of an emergency room visit. J Psychosoc Nurs Ment Health Nurs 27(11):4–8, 1989
16. Gonzales-Osler E: Coping with transition. J Psychosoc Nurs Ment Health Serv 27(6):29–33, 1989
17. Kadner KD: Resilience: responding to adversity. J Psychosoc Nurs Ment Health Serv 27(7):20–25, 1989

18. Karl GT: Survival skills for psychic trauma. J Psychosoc Nurs Ment Health Serv 27(4):15–19, 1989
19. Leichman SS: Crisis, maturational and situational. In McFarland G, Thomas M: Psychiatric Mental Health Nursing. Philadelphia, Lippincott, 1991
20. Levy S, Guttman L: Worry, fear, and concern differentiated. Issues Ment Health Nurs 7(1–4):251–263, 1985
21. McDougle CJ, Southwick SM: Emergence of an alternate personality in combat-related post-traumatic stress disorder. Hosp Community Psychiatry 41(5):554–555, 1990
22. McGinnis J, Foote K: Rapid neuroleptization. J Psychosoc Nurs Ment Health Serv 24(10):17–22, 1986
23. Meichenbaum D, Novaco R: Stress inoculation: a preventative approach. Issues Ment Health Nurs 7(1–4):419–435, 1985
24. Miller LE: Modeling awareness of feelings: a needed tool in the therapeutic communication workbox. Perspect Psychiatr Care 25(2):27–29, 1989
25. Norbeck JS, Lindsey AM, Carrieri VL: The development of an instrument to measure social support. Nurs Res 30(5):264–269, 1981
26. Norbeck JS, Lindsey AM, Carrieri VL: Further development of the Norbeck Social Support Questionnaire: normative data and validity testing. Nurs Res 32(1):4–9, 1983
27. Pancheri P, DeMartino V, Spiombi G, Biondi M, Mosticoni S: Life stress events and state-trait anxiety in psychiatric and psychosomatic patients. Issues Ment Health Nurs 7(1–4):367–395, 1985
28. Robinson JW: Stress and wellness. Champaign, IL, Well Way Publishers, 1985
29. Rundell JR, Ursano RJ, Holloway HC, Silberman EK: Psychiatric responses to trauma. Hosp Community Psychiatry 40(1):68–73, 1989
30. Singer JE: Traditions of stress research: integrative comments. Issues Ment Health Nurs 7(1–4):25–33, 1985
31. Stanley SR: When the disaster is over: helping the healers to mend. J Psychosoc Nurs Ment Health Serv 28(5):12–16, 1990
32. Stelzer J, Elliott CA: A continuous-care model of crisis intervention for children and adolescents. Hosp Community Psychiatry 41(5):562–564, 1990
33. Stokols D: A congruence analysis of human stress. Issues Ment Health Nurs 7(1–4):35–57, 1985
34. Suedfeld P: Stressful levels of environmental stimulation. Issues Ment Health Nurs 7(1–4):83–103, 1985
35. Tache J, Selye H: On stress and coping mechanisms. Issues Ment Health Nurs 7(1–4):3–23, 1985
36. Titlebaum HM: Relaxation. Holistic Nurs Pract 2(3):17–25, 1988
37. Sullivan-Taylor: The worried-well patient. In Durham J, Hardin S (eds): The Nurse Psychotherapist in Private Practice. New York, Springer Publishing Co, 1986
38. Weinert C: A social support measure: PRQ85. Nurs Res 36:273–277, 1987
39. Wheeler BR: Crisis intervention. AORN J 47(5):1242–1246, 1988
40. Wright LK: Life-threatening illness. J Psychosoc Nurs Ment Health Serv 23(9):7–11, 1985

▬ DECISIONAL CONFLICT (SPECIFY)

▬ Definition

Decisional conflict is uncertainty about taking a specific action when the choice involves selecting among competing alternative that can involve a personal risk, loss, or challenge to personal values.[14,25-27,34]

▬ General Principles[1-35]

- Personal values affect decision making and reflect a person's preference for the perceived outcomes of an alternative.
- Personal goals and beliefs affect the decision-making process because they reflect a person's beliefs about the likelihood of an outcome of a particular action.
- In the decision-making process, actions that are perceived as familiar, less risky, or as resulting in desirable outcomes are generally selected.
- A conflicted decision results when alternative actions will probably produce both positive and negative consequences for the person, and one specific alternative cannot meet the person's personal goals and values.
- The behavioral, cognitive, and emotional response to a conflicted decision varies, depending on the level of conflict in the decision. While a low level of conflict may be stimulating and enhance decision making, a moderate level of conflict may result in defensiveness, and a high degree of conflict may result in hypervigilence and an extreme level of distress.

▬ Related Factors[14,25-27,34]

Mental disorder
Impaired cognitive function
Anxiety (moderate, severe, extreme/panic)
Unrealistic goals or beliefs
Lack of skills in decision making
Conflicting information about alternatives and consequences
Insufficient or conflicting information about alternatives and
    consequences
Anticipated outcome having both negative and positive
    consequences
Lack of social resources
Interference from others in the decision-making process
Threatened value system
Unclear personal values

▬ Defining Characteristics[14,25-27,34]

Moderate distress, tension
Severe distress, tension
Hypervigilence
Self-focused

Defensiveness
Verbalization of moderate to extreme uncertainty about alternative
  choices available
Verbalization of distress from recognition of undesired consequences
Vacillation among alternative choices
Delayed or passive decision making
Vacillation in beliefs or values

—— Nursing Assessment[1-35]

- Assess patient's cognitive functioning and level of anxiety.
- Does the patient have a mental disorder? How is functioning affected?
- Assess the patient's goals, beliefs, and values in relation to the focus of decision making.
- Does patient have skills and experience in decision making?
- What information does the patient possess related to the area in which decision-making is necessary?
- Are there social supports or interferences for the patient engaging in decision making?
- Is the patient experiencing uncertainty (and at what level) about alternative choices?
- Is the patient verbalizing or manifesting distress on recognition of a degree of undesirable consequences regarding all the choices available?
- Does the patient vacillate among alternative choices?
- Does the patient delay decision making?

—— Patient Outcomes and Nursing Interventions[1-35]

Patient Outcome: Engage in Effective and Timely Decision Making

- Assess and, if necessary, reduce level of anxiety.
- Do not force decision making when cognitive functioning is impaired.
- Assist patient to deal with feelings generated by decisions to be made.
- Assist the patient in dealing with behavioral, cognitive, and emotional aspects of a mental disorder to a level where the patient can engage in decision making.
- Assist the patient in overcoming any procrastination, and work on the decision when he or she is well rested and least distracted.
- Encourage the patient to explore and develop an understanding of the conflicting decision situation.
- Identify knowledge gaps and provide needed information.
- Assist the patient in exploring and clarifying goals and expectations.
- Assist the patient, if necessary, in developing goals that are aligned with reality.
- Assist the patient in exploring and clarifying own values.

- Help the patient identify and examine available alternative choices and the consequences of each choice. Teach the patient different techniques to identify creative alternatives (e.g., brainstorming) and to look at problems from different perspectives. (See Chapter 5—*decision making.*)
- Assist the patient in developing an understanding of the potential outcomes of each alternative.
- Assist the patient in realigning unrealistic goals and outcomes.
- Help the patient become fully aware of conflicts inherent in the decision.
- Assist the patient in identifying alternatives that are congruent with his or her values and that result in the most positive outcomes.
- Provide appropriate assistance in implementing action. Use role playing when possible.
- Discuss situations with patient that have a potential for decisional conflict.
- Encourage and assist the patient as necessary in evaluating outcome; e.g., recognizing presence of decisional conflict.

— Evaluation/Outcome Criteria[14,25–27,34]

Verbalizes awareness of goals and beliefs
Identifies available alternatives
Identifies realistic outcomes
Engages in selecting actions consistent with own values
Implements action
Evaluates outcome of actual decision made

■ REFERENCES

1. Alvino D: A caring concept: providing information to make decisions. Top Clin Nurs 8(2):70–76, 1986
2. Barros A: The process of effective decision making. J Med Technol 3; 10:525–528, 1986
3. Bennett J: Helping people with AIDS live well at home. Nurs Clin North Am 23(4):731–748, 1988
4. Bille DA: Locus of decision making in patient and family education: its effect on promoting wellness. Nurs Admin Quart 11(3):62–65, 1987
5. Brown KC: Effective decision making. AAOHN J 38(3):139–140, 1990
6. Busch D: Ethical decision-making in paradoxical intervention. J Child Adolesc Psychiatr Ment Health Nurs 1(2):58–65, 1988
7. Doudera AE: Decision making and patients' rights. Am Health Care Assoc J 11(3):5–8, 1985
8. Ericksen J: Steps to ethical reasoning. Can Nurse 85(7):23–24, 1989
9. Fuchs J: Use of decisional control to combat powerlessness. ANNAJ 14(1):11–13, 56, 1987
10. Grainger RD: Making better decisions. Am J Nurs 90(6):15–16, 1990
11. Hammond KR, McClelland GH, Mumpower J: Human Judgment and Decision Making. New York, Praeger Publishing, 1980
12. Harris T: Assessing decision-making skills. J Psychosoc Nurs Ment Health Serv 28(5):23–26, 1990

13. Harrison H: Neonatal intensive care: parents' role in ethical decision making. Birth 13(3):165–175, 1986
14. Hiltunen E: Nursing diagnosis: decisional conflict (specify). In Carroll-Johnson RM (ed): Classification of Nursing Diagnoses: Proceedings of the Eighth Conference. Philadelphia, JB Lippincott, 1989
15. Huckabay LM, Daderian AD: Effect of choices on breathing exercises post-open heart surgery. Dimens Crit Care Nurs 9(4):190–201, 1990
16. Janis IL, Mann L: Decision Making. New York, Free Press, 1977
17. Kaczorowski JM: Sustaining treatment. J Psychosoc Nurs Ment Health Serv 26(3):9–12, 1988
18. Keeney RL: Decision analysis: an overview. Operations Res 30:803–838, 1982
19. Kelly KM, Sautter F, Tugrul K, Weaver MD: Fostering self-help on an inpatient unit. Arch Psychiatr Nurs 4(3):161–165, 1990
20. Lachman VD: Nine ways to make better decisions. Nurs 16(6):73–74, 1986
21. McConnell EA: Decision making. AORNJ 49(5):1382–1385, 1989
22. Nettleman MD: Practical applications of decision analysis. Infect Control Hosp Epidemiol 9(5):214–218, 1988
23. O'Connor AM: Effects of framing and level of probability on patient's preferences for cancer chemotherapy. J Clin Epidemiol 42:119–126, 1989
24. O'Connor AM, Boyd NF, Tritchler DL, Kriukov Y, Sutherland H, Till J: Eliciting preferences for alternative cancer drug treatments: the influence of framing, medium, and rater variables. Med Decis Making 5:453–463, 1985
25. O'Connor AM, D'Amico JM: Decisional conflict. In McFarland GK, Thomas MD: Psychiatric Mental Health Nursing. Philadelphia, JB Lippincott, 1991
26. O'Connor AM, McFarland GK: Decisional conflict (about seeking antenatal genetic counseling and testing). In Kim MJ, McFarland GK, McLane AL: Pocket Guide to Nursing Diagnoses, 4th ed. St Louis, CV Mosby, 1991
27. O'Connor AM, O'Brien-Pallas LL: Decisional conflict (specify). In McFarland GK, McFarlane EA: Nursing Diagnosis and Intervention: Planning for Patient Care. St Louis, CV Mosby, 1989
28. Pender NJ: Health promotion in nursing practice. Norwalk, Appleton & Lange, 1987
29. Porter-Tibbetts S: A compliance protocol: psychiatric emergency services and brief encounters. Issues Ment Health Nurs 8:223–236, 1986
30. Rothert ML, Talarczyk GJ: Patient compliance and the decision-making process of clinicians and patients. J Compliance Health Care 2:55–71, 1987
31. Shewchuk RM, Francis KT: Principles of clinical decision making—an introduction to decision analysis. Phys Ther 68(3):357–359, 1988
32. Slimmer LW, Brown RT: Parents' decision-making process in medication administration for control of hyperactivity. J Sch Health 55:221–225, 1985
33. Taylor SG, Pickens JM, Geden EA: Interactional styles of nurse practitioners and physicians regarding patient decision making. Nurs Res 38(1):50–55, 1989
34. Thompson JM, McFarland GK, Hirsch JE, Tucker SM, Bowers AC:

Decisional conflict (specify). In Thompson JM, McFarland GK, Hirsch JE, Tucker SM, Bowers AC: Mosby's Manual of Clinical Nursing. 2nd ed. St Louis, CV Mosby, 1989

35. Walker RA, Bibeau DL: Health decisions and evidence. Health Ed 17(4):18–21, 1986

▬ DEPRESSION

—— Definition

Depression is an emotional state, ranging in severity from mild to severe, characterized by discouragement, sadness, worthlessness, psychomotor retardation or agitation, and varying degrees of inability to care for self[14]

—— General Principles[1–47]

- A number of theories, models, and explanations shed light on an understanding of depression: psychoanalytic, interpersonal, cognitive, behavioral, genetic, and psychophysiological.
- Genetic factors play a potential role for depression in the multidimensional systems model, while childhood experiences can serve as predisposing factors. Stressors, various buffers, and the meaning the person attaches to the event then interact, resulting in the precipitating factors.
- Risk factors for depression may include age (the elderly have a higher incidence), socioeconomic status (higher levels of depression are associated with lower social class status), gender (women are more likely to report depressive symptomatology), unemployment (higher levels of depressive symptomatology are associated with unemployment), level of social participation and social support (social participation and social support appear to have a positive effect on mental health).
- Depression is reversible and in later life is no more likely to become chronic than at any other life period, especially if properly diagnosed and treated.
- A major depressive syndrome occurs secondary to schizophrenia in 20–30% of patients and may be associated with an increased suicide risk, increased rate of relapse, and poor psychosocial functioning.
- Because one fourth to one third of patients with Alzheimer's-type dementia develop depression, observation is extremely important in order to detect the presence of depression.
- The depressed patient's low self-esteem can be modified and improved by the caring attitude of the nurse, by helping the patient become aware of negative feelings, by assisting the patient to develop decision-making and coping skills.
- A caring supportive approach will help the patient feel better about self and less likely to ruminate on suicidal thoughts.
- Vegetative signs such as lack of appetite or constipation will lessen as the patient begins to perceive hope, works through feelings, and becomes physically involved in activities.

— Related Factors[1-47]

Genetic factors
Hormonal imbalances or changes
Neurotransmitter dysfunction
Physical illness
Mental illness
Medication side effects
Psychological factors
 Fear of failing
 Guilt
 Loss of feeling of control
 Anger
 Negative thoughts
 Internal conflict
Cognitive errors
 Negative idea of self
 Negative idea of world and future
Crisis, especially involving separation, death, loss
Catastrophic financial loss
Unemployment
Social factors
 Role loss
 Cultural change
 Alienation from group
 Lack of social support

— Defining Characteristics[1-47]

Physical complaints
Sleep disturbance
Change in appetite or weight
Constipation
Poor personal hygiene
Lack of energy, fatigue
Psychomotor retardation
Agitation
Loss of interest in sex
Difficulties in carrying out activities of daily living
General lack of motivation
Flat affect; sad, gloomy mood
Verbalization of feelings of worthlessness
Hopelessness
Helplessness
Inappropriate guilt
Frequent crying spells
Suicidal ideation
Suicide attempts
Confusion, disorientation
Difficulty concentrating
Complaints of memory impairment
Poor problem-solving skills

Decrease in social activities
Limited interactions
Lack of meaning in life.

— Nursing Assessment[1-47]

- Determine suicide potential. Be especially observant as patient becomes agitated or experiences loss of significant person.
- Determine homicidal potential and be especially observant if patient becomes agitated.
- Ascertain whether there has been a recent loss of significant other, an insult to self-esteem, a major change such as socioeconomic status, or any other major stressor.
- List physical complaints and identify actions taken by patient to cope with them.
- Note changes in physical complaints and determine their relationship to the level of anxiety.
- Determine patient's current sleep pattern and inquire what might help to correct the sleep pattern, if irregular.
- Observe current eating pattern and potential for weight loss.
- Note verbal indications of appetite.
- Assess change in bowel patterns as potential constipation.
- Note recurring thought content and verbalizations; e.g., thoughts about self-worth, fear, worries, expressions of worthlessness, hopelessness, helplessness.
- Observe for increased complaining, hypercritical behavior, or skepticism.
- Identify which activities the patient does for self.
- Determine extent of withdrawal from family and friends.
- Identify person with whom the patient feels comfortable in talking.
- Observe changes in coping strategies or ability to plan activities for the day.

— Patient Outcomes and Nursing Interventions[1-47]

Patient Outcome: Gain a Positive Attitude Toward Self and Experience Less Worthlessness, Hopelessness, Helplessness

- Establish therapeutic relationship (see Chapter 2).
- In collaboration with psychiatrist, administer antidepressant medications.
- Set limits on physical abuse of self or others.
- Assist patient as needed in areas of self-care deficits, such as personal hygiene.
- Encourage physical activity.
- Help patient focus on a here-and-now activity rather than on a physical complaint
- Set realistic limits on behavior.
- Assist patient in setting small goals and experiencing success.
- Support and give positive feedback for small decisions made.
- Use firmness when patient hesitates to do things for self.
- Confront irrational demands.

- Assist in constructive expression of anger or anxiety.
- When patient begins ruminating, redirect to other activities or ask for further information about a part of the story.
- Spend time with patient even when nothing is being said.
- Respond to expressions of feelings; for example, if patient states, "I'm no good," or "There is nothing to live for," respond with "I understand you feel worthless."
- Begin to question the statement "I am no good" by responding with "In what area?"
- Avoid arguments or making moral judgments.
- Prevent isolation from others.
- Assist patient in redefining ideas or self or the situation.
- Assist patient to expand coping response repertoire and coping resources.
- Teach patient:
  - To recognize tension in self;
  - To be alert to sad feelings that may be disguised as anger;
  - To recognize other symptoms of depression;
  - To identify the thoughts that occur just before feelings of hopelessness or sadness;
  - To choose a behavior that will help reduce such feelings;
  - To identify potentially stressful situations;
  - When to seek professional help;
  - The importance of doing activities;
  - To reward self;
  - To recognize the beneficial effects of exercise on self-esteem;
  - To focus on accomplishments instead of the things not done;
  - Information about medications.

— Evaluation/Outcome Criteria

Makes positive statements about self
Has normal mood pattern
Performs activities of daily living
Uses problem-solving skills
Meets role expectations
Makes plans that reflect desire to live

■ REFERENCES

1. Alger I: Manic-depression, depression, and adolescent suicide. Hosp Community Psychiatry 40(4):347–349, 1989
2. Badger TA, Cardea JM, Biocca LJ, Mishel MH: Assessment and management of depression: an imperative for community-based practice. Arch Psychiatr Nurs 4(4):235–241, 1990
3. Baier M: The "Holiday Blues" as a stress reaction. Perspect Psychiatr Care 24(2):64–68, 1987/88
4. Becker RE: Depression in schizophrenia. Hosp Community Psychiatry 39(12):1269–1275, 1988
5. Beeber LS: Enacting corrective interpersonal experiences with the de-

pressed client: an intervention model. Arch Psychiatr Nurs 3(4):211–217, 1989

6. Blazer D: Major depression in later life. Hosp Pract 24(9A):69–79, 1989

7. Browning MA: Depression. In Hogstel MO (ed): Geropsychiatric Nursing. St Louis, CV Mosby, 1990

8. Bruss CR: Nursing diagnosis of hopelessness. J Psychosoc Nurs Ment Health Serv 26(3):28–31, 1988

9. Buckwalter KC, Abraham IL: Alleviating the discharge crisis: the effects of a cognitive-behavioral nursing intervention for depressed patients and their families. Arch Psychiatr Nurs 1(5):350–358, 1987

10. Buckwalter KC, Kerfoot KM, Stolley JM: Children of affectively ill parents. J Psychosoc Nurs Ment Health Serv 26(10):8–14, 1988

11. Campbell L: Hopelessness. J Psychosoc Nurs Ment Health Serv 25(2):18–22, 1987

12. Condon EH: Dementia and depression: a devastating pair. Geriatr Nurs 10(1):26–27, 1989

13. Dean PR, MacDonald CC: The dysthymic patient. Perspect Psychiatr Care 24(2):69–73, 1987/88

14. Dunne-Maxim K: Survivors of suicide. J Psychosoc Nurs 24(12):31–35, 1986

15. Farill MM, Klopfenstein CB: Depression. In McFarland GK, Thomas MD: Psychiatric Mental Health Nursing. Philadelphia, JB Lippincott, 1991

16. Farran CJ, Popovich JM: Hope: a relevant concept for geriatric psychiatry. Arch Psychiatr Nurs 4(2):124–130, 1990

17. Fellin P: Perspectives on depression among black Americans. Health Soc Work 14(4):245–25, 1989

18. Fopma-Loy J: The prevalence and phenomenology of depression in elderly women: a review of the literature. Arch Psychiatr Nurs 2(2):74–80, 1988

19. Ganzini L, McFarland BH: Prevalence of mental disorders after catastrophic financial loss. J Nerv Ment Dis 178(11):680–685, 1990

20. Goldwyn RM: Educating the patient and family about depression. Med Clin North Am 72(4):887–896, 1988

21. Gordon VC, Gordon EM: Short-term group treatment of depressed women: a replication study in Great Britain. Arch Psychiatr Nurs 1(2):111–124, 1987

22. Grainger RD: Depression. AJN 90(5):13–14, 1990

23. Greydanus DE, Porter J, Rypma CB, Heuer T, Granberg A, Ruch R: The behavioral medicine unit: a community hospital model for inpatient treatment of adolescent depression. Semin Adolesc Med 2(4):311–319, 1986

24. Hinds PS: The relationship of nurses' caring behaviors with hopefulness and health care outcomes in adolescents. Arch Psychiatr Nurs 2(1):21–29, 1988

25. Hughes DY: Alzheimer's disease and psychiatric nursing: treating the depression. Perspect Psychiatr Care 24(1):5–8, 1987/1988

26. Kerr NJ: Signs and symptoms of depression and principles of nursing intervention. Perspect Psychiatr Care 24(2):48–63, 1987/88

27. Knowles RD: The depressed patient. In Durham J, Hardin S (eds): The

Nurse Psychotherapist in Private Practice. New York, Springer Publishing Co, 1986

28. LaGodna GE: Aging women and depression: unresolved conceptual, etiologic, and epidemiologic issues. Issues Ment Health Nurs 9:285–298, 1988

29. Long CG, Bluteau P: Group coping skills training for anxiety and depression: its application with chronic patients. J Adv Nurs 13(3):358–364, 1988

30. Lum TL: An integrated approach to aging and depression. Arch Psychiatr Nurs 2(4):211–217, 1988

31. Macey JC: Depression: it happened to me! Perspect Psychiatr Care 24(1):25–31, 1987

32. Miller LE: Modeling awareness of feelings: a needed tool in the therapeutic communication workbox. Perspect Psychiatr Care 25(2):27–29, 1989

33. Morofka V: Mental health. In Thompson JM, McFarland GK, Hirsch JE, Tucker SM, Bowers AC, 2nd ed.: Mosby's Manual of Clinical Nursing. St Louis, CV Mosby, 1989

34. Nelson PB: Social support, self-esteem, and depression in the institutionalized elderly. Issues Ment Health Nurs 10:55–68, 1989

35. O'Connell RA, Mayo JA: The role of social factors in affective disorders: a review. Hosp Community Psychiatry 39(8):842–849, 1988

36. Parker SD: Accident or suicide? J Psychosoc Nurs Ment Health Serv 26(6):15–33, 1988

37. Pollack LE: Improving relationships; groups for inpatients with bipolar disorder. J Psychosoc Nurs Ment Health Serv 28(5):17–22, 1990

38. Rubin EH, Zorumski CF, Burke WJ: Overlapping symptoms of geriatric depression and Alzheimer-type dementia. Hosp Community Psychiatry 39(10):1074–1079, 1988

39. Simmons-Alling S: New approaches to managing affective disorders. Arch Psychiatr Nurs 1(4):219–224, 1987

40. Simon JM: Therapeutic humor. J Psychosoc Nurs Ment Health Serv 26(4):8–12, 1988

41. Slimmer LW, Lopez M, LeSage J, et al: Perceptions of learned helplessness. J Gerontol Nurs 13(5):33–37, 1987

42. Stuart GW, Laraia MT, Ballenger JC, Lydiard RB: Early family experiences of women with bulimia and depression. Arch Psychiatr Nurs 4(1):43–52, 1990

43. Swanson B, Cronin-Stubbs D, Colletti MA: Dementia and depression in persons with AIDS: causes and care. J Psychosoc Nursing Ment Health Serv 28(10):33–39, 1990

44. Thomas MD, Sanger E, Whitney JD: Nursing diagnosis of depression. J Psychosoc Nurs Ment Health Serv 24(8):6–12, 1986

45. Thomas SP, Wilt D, Noffsinger AR: Pathophysiology of depressive illness: review of the literature and case example. Issues Ment Health Nurs 9:271–284, 1988

46. Valente SM, Saunders JM: Dealing with serious depression in cancer patients. Nursing 19(2):44–47, 1989

47. Wright LK: Mental health in older spouses: the dynamic interplay of resources, depression, quality of the marital relationship, and social participation. Issues Ment Health Nurs 11:49–70, 1990

▬ FAMILY PROCESSES, ALTERED

── Definition

An altered family process is the state in which a family that normally functions effectively experiences a disruption in the structure and functioning of its system and is unable to meet the developmental or sustenance needs of one or more of its members.[7,41]

── General Principles[1-62]

- Characteristics of healthy and normally functioning families include engaging in behaviors which enhance member growth and development; meeting member sustenance, physical, and emotional needs; demonstrating ability to remain flexible; engaging in effective, shared decision making and problem solving; demonstrating open, trusting communication; showing mutual respect and support for each other; respecting each other's autonomy yet sharing affection and closeness.
- Families are multicultural as well as multidimensional; e.g., cultural differences are reflected in the manner in which families communicate—how directly family members communicate with each other, for example.
- Families evolve through a series of developmental stages and transitions.
- Changes in individual behavior affect the entire family system, while changes in family processes affect individual behaviors.

── Related Factors[7,8,17,41]

Unsuccessful achievement of previous development stage(s)
Intrapsychic conflicts in family member(s)
Developmental transitions and/or crisis
    Gain of family member
    Loss of family member
    Major role changes
    Hospitalization of family member
    Retirement
Situational transition and/or crisis
    Physical illness of member
    Mental illness of member
    Treatment demands
        Unusually time-consuming treatment
        Very expensive treatment
        High-energy-consuming treatment
        Multiple side effects from treatment
    Moral deviance of family member
    Unemployment
    Financial problems
    Natural disaster
    War

Lack of skills conducive to family functioning
    Lack of ability to negotiate roles
    Faulty communication techniques
    Inability to adapt to varying demands
    Inadequate conflict negotiation skills
    Inadequate coping skills
    Learned maladaptive behavioral patterns
Cultural factors
    Conflicting values or beliefs
    Excessive demands from customs

— Defining Characteristics[7,8,17,26,41]

Inability to meet member needs; e.g., developmental/growth needs, physical needs, emotional needs, security needs
Anxiety
Inability to deal with stressors that affect family
Inability to adapt to changing circumstances
Ineffective communication patterns
    Poorly communicated rules, rituals, symbols
Difficulty in expressing and accepting feelings
Ineffective family decision making
Lack of shared decision making
Decreased ability to problem solve as a family unit
Severe difficulty in conflict resolution
Role disturbances
    Rigid inflexible roles
    Inability to give or receive help from each other
    Role reversals
    Severe sense of being separate
    Overly close relationships, with disrespect for autonomy
    Disrespect or distrust among family members
Minimum socialization with persons outside family
Isolation from community activities
Inappropriate boundary maintenance of family with nonfamily members

— Nursing Assessment[7,8,17,26,41]

- Observe and interview the entire family, if possible.
- Obtain a family history that includes birth, death, marriage, work, education, major moves, and illness of members.
- Listen carefully to descriptions by individual family members of the current situation; e.g., presence of conflict, presence of crisis.
- Observe the family system for role reversals, rules, secrets, methods of decision making, scapegoating.
- Observe the family communication patterns; e.g., are members openly able to say to others what they really think and mean? are children able to discuss problems with parents?
- Observe the family for presence or absence of mutual support; e.g., are "put-downs" or sarcastic comments frequently expressed? Are family members hostile towards each other?

- Observe the family's ability to solve problems and make decisions.
- Note the level of closeness or separateness among family members.

Family Outcomes and Nursing Interventions[1-62]

Family Outcome: Develop Open Communication

- Help the family identify strengths and maximize use of them.
- Teach family members to say what is really meant in a way that is understood by all.
- Point out when a family member is trying to "read" another's mind.
- Act as mediator, being careful not to take sides.
- Encourage differing points of view.
- Serve as a role model in being clear, seeking clarification, showing respect, listening to expression of feelings, giving suggestions, expressing opinions, setting limits, making clear statements.
- Discuss the role of anxiety in disrupting communication and in developing triangles.
- Act as consultant as members work at discovering how to improve communication.

Family Outcome: Achieve Effective Problem-Solving and Decision-Making Skills

- Assist the family in clarifying the issue that needs to be resolved, describing what is occurring as specifically as possible.
- Assist members in identifying problems appropriate for the family to discuss and resolve as a group versus focusing on problems appropriate for the individual to work on.
- Help the family to redefine the whole situation in favorable terms; e.g., perceive the situation as changeable.
- Assist members in stating alternatives to resolve problems.
- Teach the family steps in problem-solving and decision-making processes (see Chapter 5).
- Provide information about family dynamics that will facilitate the problem-solving process.
- Teach the recognition of emotional factors in the process of problem solving, especially the effects of anxiety.
- Assist the family in developing an appropriate level of flexibility in rules and regulations that allows for maximum functioning for entire family.
- Assist the family in recognizing changes in the environment and adapting to them.

Family Outcome: Experience Mutual Support, Nurturance, and Growth Among All Members

- Assist family members in identifying ways they can be supportive to each other.
- Encourage family members to express mutual support to each other.

- Point out family strengths and encourage the use of them.
- Give positive feedback when family members are supportive to each other.
- Assist family members in recognizing the need for closeness and affection.
- Assist family members to recognize and accept differences.
- Refer for family therapy as needed.

—— Evaluation/Outcome Criteria

Basic needs of family met
Maintains growth of family members
Demonstrates clear communication
Demonstrates constructive interactions and role differentiation
Engages in problem solving and decision making
Maintains contact with community

REFERENCES

1. Allen DG: Critical social theory as a model for analyzing ethical issues in family and community health. Fam Commun Health 10(1):63–72, 1987
2. Amundson MJ: Family crisis care: a home-based intervention program for child abuse. Issues Ment Health Nurs 10:285–296, 1989
3. Baird SF: Helping the family through a crisis. Nursing 17(6):66–67, 1987
4. Baker HM: Behavioral issues: some thoughts on helping grieving families. J Emergency Nurs 13(6):359–362, 1987
5. Bishop SM: The primacy of the family in child psychiatric and mental health nursing. J Child Adol Psychiatr Ment Health Nurs 1(2):45, 1988
6. Bluhm J: Helping families in crisis hold on. Nursing 17(10):44–46, 1987
7. Bowers JE: Family processes, dysfunctional. In McFarland GK, Thomas MD: Psychiatric Mental Health Nursing. Philadelphia, JB Lippincott, 1991
8. Bowers JE: Family therapy. In McFarland GK, Thomas MD: Psychiatric Mental Health Nursing. JB Lippincott, 1991
9. Bright MA: Therapeutic ritual: helping families grow. J Psychosoc Nurs Ment Health Serv 28(12):24–29, 1990
10. Buckwalter KC, Kerfoot KM, Stolley JM: Children of affectively ill parents. J Psychosoc Nurs Ment Health Serv 26(10):8–14, 1988
11. Bulow BV, Sweeney JA, Shear MK, Friedman R, Plowe C: Family satisfaction with psychiatric evaluations. Health Soc Work 290–295, 1987
12. Carter EA, McGoldrick M: The Family Life Cycle: A Framework for Family Therapy. New York, Gardner Press, 1980
13. Chafetz L, Barnes LE: Issues in psychiatric care giving. Arch Psychiatr Nurs 3(2):61–68, 1989
14. Choi T, Josten L, Christensen ML: Health-specific Family Coping Index for Noninstitutional Care. NLN Pub No. 21-2194, 161–167. New York, 1987

15. Collison CR, Miller SL: The role of family re-enactment in group psychotherapy. Perspect Psychiatr Care 23(2):74–78, 1985
16. Cuff-Carney D: Holistic family therapy: individuals or families? A therapist's perspective. Holistic Nurs Pract 2(1):45–51, 1987
17. deChesnay M, Magnuson N: How healthy families cope with stress. AAOHN J 36(9):361–365, 1988
18. Dellasega C: Coping with caregiving: stress management for caregivers of the elderly. J Psychosoc Nurs Ment Health Serv 28(1):15–22, 1990
19. Duffy ME: Health promotion in the family: current findings and directives for nursing research. J Adv Nurs 13:109–117, 1988
20. Flannery D, Link I: A model comprehensive family program for relatives of adult schizophrenics. Psychosoc Rehab J 9(3):15–24, 1986
21. Forisha B, Grothaus K, Luscombe R: Dinner conversation: meal therapy to differentiate eating behavior from family process. J Psychosoc Nurs Ment Health Serv 28(11):12–16, 1990
22. Francell CG, Conn VS, Gray DP: Families' perceptions of burden of care for chronic mentally ill relatives. Hosp Community Psychiatry 39(12):1296–1300, 1988
23. Friedemann ML: Closing the gap between grand theory and mental health practice with families. Part 1: the framework of systemic organization for nursing of families and family members. Arch Psychiatr Nurs 3(1):10–19, 1989
24. Friedemann ML: Closing the gap between grand theory and mental health practice with families. Part 2: the control-congruence model for mental health nursing of families. Arch Psychiatr Nurs 111(1):20–28, 1989
25. Gantt AB, Green RS: Telling the diagnosis: implications for social work practice. Soc Work Health Care 11(2):101–110, 1986
26. Garver PM: Altered family processes. In McFarland GK, McFarlane EA: Nursing Diagnosis and Intervention. St. Louis, CV Mosby, 1989
27. Geiser R, Hoche L, King J: Respite care for mentally ill patients and their families. Hosp Community Psychiatry 39(3):291–295, 1988
28. Greenberg L, Fine SB, Cohen CC, Larson K, Michaelson-Baily A et al.: An interdisciplinary psychoeducation program for schizophrenic patients and their families in an acute care setting. Hosp Community Psychiatry 39(3):277–282, 1988
29. Gross D: At risk: children of the mentally ill. J Psychosoc Nurs Ment Health Serv 27(8):14–19, 1989
30. Grunebaum H, Friedman H: Building collaborative relationships with families of the mentally ill. Hosp Community Psychiatry 39(11):1183–1187, 1988
31. Haber J: A family systems model for divorce and the loss of self. Arch Psychiatric Nurs 4(4):228–234, 1990
32. Harter L: Multi-family meetings on the psychiatric unit. J Psychosoc Nurs Ment Health Serv 26(8):18–22, 1988
33. Hays A: Family care: the critical variable in community-based long-term care. Home Health Care Nurse 6(1):26–31, 1988
34. Hays JC: Patient symptoms and family coping: predictors of hospice utilization patterns. Cancer Nurs 9(6):317–325, 1986
35. Heiney SP: Assessing and intervening with dysfunctional families. Oncology Nurs Forum 15(5):585–590, 1988
36. Herrick CA, Goodykoontz L: Neumann's systems model for nursing

practice as a conceptual framework for a family assessment. J Child Adolesc Psychiatr Ment Health Nurs 2(2):61–67, 1989

37. Hughes L, Joyce B, Staley D: Does the family make a difference? J Psychosoc Nurs Ment Health Serv 25(8):8–13, 1987
38. Jones SL: Family, marital, and couples therapy: a comparison. Arch Psychiatric Nurs 4(3):145–146, 1990
39. Kane CF: Family social support: toward a conceptual model. Adv Nurs Sci 10(2):18–25, 1988
40. Kiehne AM: Children in the addicted family: an overview. Holistic Nurs Pract 2(4):14–19, 1988
41. Kim MJ, McFarland GK, McLane AM: Pocket guide to nursing diagnoses, 4th ed. St Louis, CV Mosby, 1991
42. King J, McSwain K, Reid S: A nursing family assessment program. Psychiatr Nurses July:12–14, 1986
43. Kuipers L, Bebbington P: Relatives as a resource in the management of functional illness. Br J Psychiatry 147:465–470, 1985
44. LaChance R: Schizophrenic family processes. C J Psychiatr Nurs 28(4):9–14, 1987
45. Landenburger K: A process of entrapment in and recovery from an abusive relationship. Issues Ment Health Nurs 10:209–277, 1989
46. Maurin JT, Boyd CB: Burden of mental illness on the family: a critical review. Arch Psychiatr Nurs 4(2):99–107, 1990
47. Mays RM: Family stress and adaptation. Nurs Pract 13(8):53–56, 1988
48. Miller TW: Group sociotherapy: a psychoeducative model for schizophrenic patients and their families. Perspect Psychiatr Care 25(1):5–9, 1989
49. Moller MD, Wer JE: Simultaneous patient/family education regarding schizophrenia: the Nebraska model. Arch Psychiatr Nurs 3(6):332–337, 1989
50. Noh S, Turner RJ: Living with psychiatric patients: implications for the mental health of family members. Soc Sci Med 25(3):263–271, 1987
51. Nubel AS, Solomon LZ: Addicted adolescent girls: familial interpersonal relationships. J Psychosoc Nurs Ment Health Serv 26(1):32–35, 1988
52. Nyamathi A, Dracup K, Jacoby A: Development of a spousal coping instrument. Prog Cardiovasc Nurs 3(1):1–6, 1988
53. Polk GC, Brown BE: Family violence: development of a master's level specialty track in family abuse. J Psychosoc Nurs 26(2):34–37, 1988
54. Rose L, Finestone K, Bass J: Group support for the families of psychiatric patients. J Psychosoc Nurs Ment Health Serv 23(12):24–29, 1985
55. Seymour RJ, Dawson NJ: The schizophrenic at home. J Psychosoc Nurs Ment Health Serv 24(1):28–30, 1986
56. Solomon P, Beck S, Gordon B: Family members' perspectives on psychiatric hospitalization and discharge. Commun Ment Health J 24(2):108–117, 1988
57. Stockdale S, Hutzenbiler T: How you can comfort a grieving family. Nurs Life 6(3):23–26, 1986
58. Walker CL: Stress and coping in siblings of childhood cancer patients. Nurs Res 37(4):208–212, 1988
59. Weinstein RK: The patient experiencing marital conflict. In Durham

J, Hardin S (eds): The Nurse Psychotherapist in Private Practice. New York, Springer Publishing Co, 1986

60. Wilk J: Family environments and the young chronically mentally ill. J Psychosoc Nurs Ment Health Serv 26(10):15–20, 1988
61. Youssef FA: Discharge planning for psychiatric patients: the effects of a family-patient teaching programme. J Adv Nurs 12:611–616, 1987
62. Zimmerman RS, Connor C: Health promotion in context: the effects of significant others on health behavior change. Health Ed Q 16(1):57–75, 1989

▬ GRIEVING, ANTICIPATORY

— Definition

Anticipatory grieving is the process taking place prior to and in preparation for a significant actual or potential loss.

— General Principles[1–48]

- The significant losses can include such losses as, for example, a limb through planned surgery, loss of a friend who is planning to move abroad, or the potential death of a significant person who is terminally ill.
- Behaviors and feelings exhibited and experienced during anticipatory grieving are very similar to those that are experienced during normal grieving.
- There may be differences between anticipatory grieving and the normal grieving process that follows a significant loss in terms of end-point, hope, acceleration, and ambivalence.
- Anticipatory grieving can be influenced by interpersonal, sociocultural, and psychological variables.
- Anticipatory grieving can help a person adjust to the actual loss and lighten the burden of grieving after the loss.
- Anticipatory grieving can also result in negative consequences, such as depression following actual loss.
- Depending on the experience of anticipatory grieving and the responses of significant others in the environment, anticipatory grieving can be either functional or dysfunctional.

— Related Factors[15–17,25,31–34,40]

Perceived potential loss of body part
Perceived potential loss of body function(s)
Perceived impending death of self
Perceived potential loss of physiopsychosocial well-being
Perceived potential loss of prized material possession
Perceived potential loss of pet animal
Perceived potential loss of social role
Perceived potential loss of significant person

— Defining Characteristics[15-17,25,31-34]

Normal grieving upon anticipation of loss
Denial of potential loss
    Disbelief
    Avoidance of focus on loss
Physiological symptoms
    Emptiness in stomach
    Choking sensations
    Exhaustion
    Decreased appetite
Preoccupation with self
Disinterest in daily living
Anger
Guilt
Weeping
Sadness
Difficulty in concentration
Sense of unreality
Social withdrawal
Ambivalence
Altered communication patterns
Altered activity levels
Hope for preventing loss

— Nursing Assessment[15-17,25,31-34]

- What is the significance of the impending loss to the person?
- What characteristics of normal grieving are present?
- Are characteristics of dysfunctional grieving present?
- How do significant others respond to the person who is experiencing anticipatory grieving?
- To what extent can the person carry out self care, social, and occupational responsibilities?
- Identify cultural factors that influence grieving process.

— Patient Outcomes and Nursing Interventions[1-48]

Patient Outcome: Engage in constructive anticipatory grieving

- Encourage good health habits.
- Be accepting, supportive, and reassuring.
- Assist the person in working through denial.
- Assist in working through feelings of anger.
- Provide support during bargaining and depression phases.
- Assist patient to accept reality of potential loss. Offer realistic hope.
- Discuss what to expect in the expected loss.
- Assist patient to adapt to role changes.
- Teach use of problem-solving skills.
- Support and assist patient in coping with impending loss.
- Encourage use of support network including family, self-help groups, and spiritual counselors

- Assess for risk factors related to dysfunctional grieving and provide patient with extra assistance as needed during anticipatory grieving process.

(See also goal for dysfunctional grieving—engage in normal grieving.)

—— Evaluation/Outcome Criteria

Engages in constructive anticipatory grief work
Meets self-care requirements
Meets social and occupational responsibilities

—— GRIEVING, DYSFUNCTIONAL

—— Definition[1-47]

- *Grieving*—a normal process by which a person adaptively adjusts to a significant loss; this process includes
  - Emotional emancipation from significant loss of object, person, or other established patterns of life;
  - Readjustment to environment;
  - Development of new relationships, emotional investment in new objects in order to restructure new life and achieve personal reorganization.
- *Dysfunctional grieving*—Normal grieving process becoming stuck in one phase of grieving, with presence of excessive emotional reactions or excessive length of time in a phase.

—— General Principles[1-48]

- Normal grieving unaccompanied by mental problems does not usually require psychiatric referral but is facilitated by skilled interpersonal intervention to prevent the occurrence of dysfunctional grieving.
- Physical symptoms that do not last long and frequently appear immediately after loss can include
  - Sighing respirations;
  - Choking sensation;
  - Empty feelings in stomach, digestive upsets;
  - Physical distress;
  - Shortness of breath.
- The exact nature of the normal grief reaction may vary from person to person. Behaviors can include the following:
  - *Denial*—patient avoids acceptance of loss, thereby developing a buffer against reality; acts as if deceased is still present or loss has not occurred; searching behavior
  - *Anger*—channeled toward lost object or person, toward self, or displaced toward other object or person; may place blame on health professionals or may misinterpret what is said by them

- *Bargaining*—last attempt to postpone realization of loss, which may include bargaining with a deity; attempts to negotiate for change in reality
- *Realization of loss*—full awareness of loss, including meaning and value of person or object to self, awareness of lost or changed roles, realization of new responsibilities and roles; preoccupation with loss.
- *Acceptance and reintegration*—problem-solving behavior initiated relative to loss and concomitant problems and change; restructuring and reordering of life.
- Dysfunctional grieving can include prolonged, excessive denial; prolonged depression; and, can lead to mental illness, especially clinical depression.

— Related Factors[15–17,25,31–34]

Perceived or actual loss of body function, part, or physiopsychosocial well-being
Perceived or actual loss of significant person, animal, or prized possession
Perceived or actual loss of, or change in, social role(s)
Unexpected or sudden death of significant other
Multiple overlapping losses with unresolved grief
Stressful and prolonged anticipatory loss
Inadequate social supports
Secondary gains from grieving
Overidentification or unfinished business with deceased
Inability to attend to grieving because of other tasks
Dysfunctional grieving of parents (if loss is a child)
Unconscious maneuvers of family members to control fate or alleviate guilt (if loss is a child)

— Defining Characteristics[15–17,25,31–34]

Excessive time in any stage of normal grieving
Excessive or distorted emotional reactions
    Prolonged or excessive denial
    Prolonged social isolation or withdrawal
    Behavior suggesting that loss occurred yesterday
    Developmental regression
    Extremely low self-esteem
    Severe feelings of identity loss
    Unabated searching behavior for lost person or object
    Excessive idealization of dead person
    Excessive guilt and self-blame
    Extreme/prolonged hostility toward dead person
    Suicidal ideation
    Severe hopelessness
    Prolonged panic attacks
    Prolonged depression

Somatic complaints
Engaging in self-detrimental activities
Delayed emotional reaction(s)

—— Nursing Assessment[15-17,25,31-34]

- What is the degree of depression? Are there suicidal tendencies?
- Are defining characteristics of dysfunctional grieving present?
- What stage of grieving and behavioral manifestations does the patient currently present?
- What is the patient's behavior between actual occurrence of loss and present?
- What is the nature of the loss? When did it occur?
- How did the patient perceive the loss? Special meaning/value? Significance of loss in relation to patient's perceived and real abilities to meet own needs?
- How has patient coped with loss in the past? What strengths were demonstrated in coping with loss?
- Is the patient at high risk for dysfunctional grieving? Examples of such patients at high risk are those with
  - Ambivalent relationship with person prior to death;
  - Social isolation or poor social network;
  - Divorce or separation
  - History of multiple past losses and use of maladaptive coping strategies;
  - Presentation of a brave, stoic front.
- What is the nature of the social network present?
- What are significant others' reactions to patient's response to loss?
- Identify cultural factors that may influence perception of loss or grieving process.

—— Patient Outcomes and Nursing Interventions[1-48]

Patient Outcome: Engage in Normal Grieving

- Help patient to understand the physical symptoms.
- Recognize that while the patient may have worked through denial or anger or bargaining, there is still the possibility of the periodic reoccurrence of these emotions.
- Assist the patient in working through denial. (also see *defensive coping* in this chapter).
  - Help the patient understand that others respond similarly when mourning a loss.
  - Be genuine, honest, and realistic about loss.
  - Permit visual and tactile contact with body of dead when possible.
  - Use caring tone of voice.
- Assist the patient in working through feelings of anger (also see *aggression* in this chapter).
  - Demonstrate tolerance, patience, and empathy.
  - Permit open expression of feelings. Do not become defensive.

- Assist the patient in understanding reasons for feelings.
- If the patient has difficulty in expressing anger, place with patients who can express feelings openly.
- Reassure the patient that feelings of guilt are part of the normal grieving process; assist in working through feelings of guilt.
- Encourage the patient to work out conflicting aspect of relationship with the deceased; work through any ambivalence.

- Assist the patient in working through bargaining.
  - Acknowledge the patient's need to talk about loss through active listening.
  - Permit expression of feelings and thoughts; gently point out reality.
- Assist through realization of loss.
  - Be physically present; offer support and enhance self-esteem.
  - Offer presence (see Chapter 5—*supportive therapy*).
  - Offer acceptance and unconditional positive regard.
  - Correct misinformation about cause of loss.
  - Reinforce past and present strengths in dealing with difficulty.
  - Through sympathetic understanding show that crying is acceptable.
  - Encourage support for patient from family members and friends.
  - Observe for and monitor depression.
  - Facilitate review of positive and negative aspects of lost person, object, or life pattern.
  - Clarify and offer missing factual information.
  - Use touch to offer support, if appropriate.
- Assist through acceptance of loss.
  - Explore nature of problems encountered that are linked to loss with patient.
  - Raise questions regarding next steps in coping.
  - Assist in thinking through adaptive coping strategies.
  - Assist or coordinate resources to develop new skills, to make readjustments in lifestyle, and to make new emotional investments.
  - Support the patient as new coping strategies are tried. Use role playing techniques when possible.
- Avoid suppression of symptoms of grieving with drugs such as benzodiazepines; use supportive intervention (see Chapter 5— *supportive therapy; grief counseling*).
- Answer questions directly and tactfully.
- Orient the patient to new aspects of environment in a simple, clear way.
- Foster an environment in which loss can be placed in spiritual context by engaging the patient in religious and spiritual rituals and practices as desired.
- Be cognizant of the possibility of different stages of grieving occurring among family members. Help the patient and family members communicate with each other.

- Offer extensive support and guidance in performing activities of living during bewilderment experienced immediately after loss.
- Demonstrate caring and concern, especially immediately after the loss.
- Encourage the patient to seek help and not be "too proud."
- Use role play as a way to help work through feelings.
- Do not abandon the patient during the experience of loss.
- Provide anticipatory guidance and support anticipatory grieving to avoid development of dysfunctional grieving.
  - Assist the patient in coping with expected and impending loss.
  - Encourage open discussion of the impending loss and expression of feelings.
  - Teach use of problem-solving skills:
    - Define potential life changes and problems anticipated from the loss.
    - Develop alternative potential strategies to deal with problems.
    - Map out possible consequences of each strategy.
    - Prioritize strategies in terms of usefulness for potential problem resolution.
- Offer extra assistance in process of grieving to those at high risk for dysfunctional grieving, such as
  - Those who had a traumatic, difficult or ambivalent relationship with person who is now deceased;
  - Those who present cheerful, brave, and stoic behavior;
  - Those who are socially isolated or who have a poorly developed social network;
  - Those who have a history of multiple past losses and have used maladaptive coping strategies;
  - Those who perceive their social network as nonsupportive;
  - Those with very traumatic circumstances surrounding the death of a spouse—anger- or guilt-provoking death, unexpected or untimely death.
  - Those with concurrent life crises.
- Provide psychological intervention to the person during bereavement, to reduce potential for dysfunctional grieving (see also Chapter 5—*grief counseling*).

Patient Outcome: Resolve dysfunctional grieving

- Apply interventions outlined for normal grieving.
- Assist the patient in getting through the phase in which the patient is stuck.
  - Assess present stage of grieving and the current objects or facts that patient still links to the loss.
  - Encourage use of relaxation techniques (See Chapter 5).
  - Use genogram to assist in identification of unresolved losses.
  - Consider need for referral to brief psychotherapy.
  - Determine need for evaluation for antidepressant therapy.

(See also Chapter 5—*supportive therapy; grief counseling*.)

— Evaluation/Outcome Criteria

Engages in normal grief work
Works through phases of normal grieving
Recognizes reality of loss
Demonstrates emotional reactions congruent with cultural and
personal expectations.
Restructures and reorders life constructively
Develops new relationships and emotional investments.

■ REFERENCES

1. Aldrich C: Some dynamics of anticipatory grief. In Schoenberg B, Carr A, Peretz D, Kutscher A (eds): Psychological Aspects of Terminal Care. New York, Columbia University Press, 1974
2. Allan JD, Hall BA: Between diagnosis and death: the case for studying grief before death. Arch Psychiatr Nurs 2(1):30–34, 1988
3. Assimacopoulos L: Realizing empathy in loss. J Psychosoc Nurs Ment Health Serv 25(11):26–29, 1987
4. Bower F (ed): Nursing and the Concept of Loss. New York, John Wiley & Sons, 1980
5. Burnard P: Existentialism as a theoretical basis for counselling in psychiatric nursing. Arch Psychiatr Nurs 3(3):142–147, 1989
6. Collison C, Miller S: Using images of the future in grief work. Image 19(1):9–11, 1987
7. Dugan DO: Death and dying. J Psychosoc Nurs Ment Health Serv 25(7):21–29, 1987
8. Engel G: Grief and grieving. AJN 64(9):93–98, 1964
9. Farnham R: Grief work with mothers of retarded children in a group setting. Issues Ment Health Nurs 9:73–82, 1988
10. Fulton R, Gottesman D: Anticipatory grief. Br J Psychiatry 139:79–80, 1981
11. Fulton R, Gottesman D: Anticipatory grief: a psychosocial concept reconsidered. Br J Psychiatry 137:45–54, 1980
12. Garrett JE: Multiple losses in older adults. J Gerontol Nurs 13(8):8–12, 1987
13. Gass KA: Aged widows and widowers: similarities and differences in appraisal, coping, resources, type of death, and health dysfunction. Arch Psychiatr Nurs 2(4):200–210, 1988
14. Gass KA: Coping strategies of widows. J Gerontol Nurs 13(8):29–36, 1987
15. Gerety EK: Grieving, anticipatory grieving, dysfunctional grieving. In McFarland GK, Thomas MD: Psychiatric Mental Health Nursing. Philadelphia, JB Lippincott, 1991
16. Gerety EK, McFarland GK: Anticipatory grieving. In McFarland GK, McFarlane EA: Nursing Diagnosis and Intervention: Planning for Patient Care. St Louis, CV Mosby, 1989
17. Gerety EK, McFarland GK: Dysfunctional grieving. In McFarland GK, McFarlane EA: Nursing Diagnosis and Intervention: Planning for Patient Care. St Louis, CV Mosby, 1989
18. Glaser B, Strauss A: Awareness of Dying. Chicago, Aldine Publishing, 1968

19. Glaser B, Strauss A: Time for Dying. Chicago, Aldine Publishing, 1968
20. Hartz GW: Adult grief and its interface with mood disorder: proposal of a new diagnosis of complicated bereavement. Compr Psychiatry 27(1):60–64, 1986
21. Henderson KJ: Dying, God, and anger. J Psychosoc Nurs Ment Health Serv 27(5):17–20, 1989
22. Houseman C, Pheifer WG: Potential for unresolved grief in survivors of persons with AIDS. Arch Psychiatr Nurs 2(5):296–301, 1988
23. Humphrey MA: Effects of anticipatory grief for the patient, family member, and caregiver. In Rando TA (ed): Loss and Anticipatory Grief. Lexington, MA: Lexington Books, 1986
24. Johnson S: The grieving patient. In Durham J, Hardin S (eds): The Nurse Psychotherapist in Private Practice. New York, Springer Publishing Co, 1986
25. Kim MJ, McFarland GK, McLane AM: Pocket Guide to Nursing Diagnosis, 4th ed. St Louis, CV Mosby, 1991
26. Kirschling JM, Austin JK: Assessing support—the recently widowed. Arch Psychiatr Nurs 2(2):81–86, 1988
27. Kovarsky RS: Loneliness and disturbed grief: a comparison of parents who lost a child to suicide or accidental death. Arch Psychiatr Nurs 3(2):86–96, 1989
28. Kubler-Ross E: On Death and Dying. New York, Macmillan, 1969
29. Lindemann E: Symptomatology and management of acute grief. Am J Psychiatry 101(2):141–148, 1944
30. Martocchio BC: Grief and bereavement. Nurs Clin North Am 20(2):327–341, 1985
31. McFarland GK, Gerety EK: Anticipatory grieving. In Kim MJ, McFarland GK, McLane AM: Pocket Guide to Nursing Diagnoses, 4th ed. St Louis, CV Mosby, 1991
32. McFarland GK, Gerety EK: Anticipatory grieving. In Thompson JM, McFarland GK, Hirsch JE, Tucker SM, Bowers AC: Mosby's Manual of Clinical Nursing, 2nd ed. St Louis, CV Mosby, 1989
33. McFarland GK, Gerety EK: Dysfunctional grieving. In Kim MJ, McFarland GK, McLane AM: Pocket Guide to Nursing Diagnoses, 4th ed. St Louis, CV Mosby, 1991
34. McFarland GK, Gerety EK: Dysfunctional grieving. In Thompson JM, McFarland GK, Hirsch JE, Tucker SM, Bowers AC: Mosby's Manual of Clinical Nursing, 2nd ed. St Louis, CV Mosby, 1989
35. Morrow BR, Maier GJ, Kelley W: Dying with dignity: hospice care on the unit. J Psychosoc Nurs Ment Health Serv 27(11):10–13, 1989
36. Parkes C: Anticipatory grief. Br J Psychiatry 138:183, 1981
37. Pheifer WG, Houseman C: Bereavement and AIDS. J Psychosoc Nurs Ment Health Serv 26(10):21–25, 1988
38. Pollock GH: The mourning-liberation process in health and disease. Psychiatr Clin North Am 10(3):345–354, 1987
39. Poncar PJ: The elderly widow: easing her role transition. J Psychosoc Nurs Ment Health Serv 27(2):6–11, 1989
40. Rando T: A comprehensive analysis of anticipatory grief: perspectives, processes, promises, and problems. In Rando T (ed): Loss and Anticipatory Grief. Lexington, MA: Lexington Press, 1986
41. Rando T: Understanding and facilitating anticipatory grief in the loved

ones of the dying. In Rando T (ed): Loss and Anticipatory Grief. Lexington, MA: Lexington Press, 1986

42. Ruetz E: Help for the grieving. Health Prog 70(4):74–77, 1989
43. Rynearson EK: Psychotherapy of pathologic grief. Psychiatr Clin North Am 10(3):487–499, 1987
44. Stockdale L, Hutzenbiler T: How you can comfort a grieving family. Nurs Life 6(3):23–27, 1986
45. Sweeting HN, Gilhooly MLM: Anticipatory grief: a review. Soc Sci Med 30(10):1073–1080, 1990
46. Vachon ML: Unresolved grief in persons with cancer referred for psychotherapy. Psychiatr Clin North Am 10(3):467–486, 1987
47. Warner SL: A comparative study of widows' and widowers' perceived social support during the first year of bereavement. Arch Psychiatr Nurs (4):241–250, 1987
48. York CR, Stichler JF: Cultural grief expressions following infant death. Dimens Crit Care Nurs 4(2):120–127, 1985

■ MANIPULATION

— Definition

Manipulation is a mode of interaction in which other people are controlled, exploited, or used to meet immediate needs and desires or to avoid discomfort frequently experienced in a manner in which the other person's needs, goals, and feelings are disregarded, and the other person feels dehumanized and treated as an object.[4,5,9,11,12]

— General Principles[1–13]

- As one among a large repertoire of behaviors, and used occasionally, manipulation can be a purposeful, directed way of getting needs met and does not necessarily have harmful consequences.
- When demands and needs are not fulfilled by another person, manipulation serves to maneuver the reluctant-other into behaviors to satisfy such demands and needs.
- Manipulation used as a primary mode of meeting personal needs is self-defeating in that interpersonal relationships are negatively affected.
- Interpersonal relationships are maintained at a superficial level by such behaviors as establishing pseudo-intimate rapport using flattery, antagonistic behaviors such as aggressive touching, or playing one staff member against another.
- Interpersonal closeness and spontaneity, as well as self-knowledge, self-disclosure, and personal growth are jeopardized for the person who relies on manipulation as a primary mode of meeting needs.
- Manipulative behaviors may increase if the nurse attempts to avoid the patient.
- Self-awareness is essential for the nurse, including his or her own areas of vulnerability and unmet needs.

—— Related Factors[1-13]

Psychiatric disorder (e.g., borderline personality disorder,
    psychoactive substance use disorder)
Developmental factors
Anxiety
Fear
Low frustration tolerance
Crisis
Feelings of lack of control
Need for power
Unmet dependency needs
Alienation
Family communication factors
Decreased family stability
Parental/significant other use of manipulation as primary mode of
    behavior
Lack of parental role model
Social network support for use of manipulation
Conflicted milieu
Low self-esteem

—— Defining Characteristics[1-13]

Multiple suicidal gestures
Controlling behaviors
Power struggles
Deliberate "forgetting"
Tearfulness
Use of aliases
Uncooperative behavior
Difficulty accepting controls, limits, rules
Defiance of authority
Dehumanizing use of others
Deception, dishonesty
Demanding
Exploiting weaknesses of others
Intimidation
Overinvolvement in other's problems while ignoring own
Overuse of flattery, charm
Attempts to get special treatment
Frequent attention-seeking behaviors
Use of seductive behaviors
Pseudo-intimate relationships
Superficial relationships
Aggressive touching
Playing one person against another
Intense, unstable relationships
Overly dependent relationships
Ambivalent relationships
Lack of trust in a relationship
Lack of motivation to change

Underachievement
Distorted beliefs
Lack of personal growth

—— Nursing Assessment[1-13]

- Identify the range of manipulative behaviors being used by the patient.
- Note what or who becomes the major focus of manipulative behaviors.
- Determine what problems the patient is avoiding or what needs he or she is trying to meet.
- Observe for situational factors that tend to increase the manipulation.
- Note what or who becomes the major focus of manipulative behaviors.
- Assess level of anxiety, aggression.
- Assess for increase in patient's ability to identify own feelings and wants.
- Describe type of interpersonal relationships patient has developed with family and significant others and is developing with health team members.
- Evaluate family member/significant other's response to patient's use of manipulative behaviors.
- Describe rewards patient receives for engaging in manipulative behavior.
- Examine own feelings about and response to patient's manipulation.
- Collect data from team members about cause, nature, and patterns of patient's manipulative behaviors.

—— Patient Outcomes and Nursing Interventions[1-13]

Patient Outcome: Experience Trust and Security in Interpersonal Relationship

- Encourage patient to anticipate needs and when possible, meet these needs, so that manipulative behaviors are not necessary.
- Gently help patient to explore distancing behaviors.
- Demonstrate concern and respect for other, modeling behaviors that can be imitated.
- Initially set limits in areas where there is need to protect others or patient.
- Establish realistic, enforceable consequences for breaking and keeping rules.
- Carefully explain community rules and consequences for breaking or keeping them.
- Clarify reasons for limit setting and the consequences of breaking or keeping to the limits.
- Enforce limits consistently. A coordinated team effort is needed.
- Evaluate the effects of the limits and means for enforcing them.
- Ensure documentation of nursing care plan in order to foster a

coordinated and consistent effort among all health team members.
- Demonstrate a willingness to admit to mistakes.
- Assign to the patient a designated staff member to answer questions and respond to requests in order to avoid reinforcing manipulative behavior.
- Offer the patient constructive opportunities for exerting control or influence (e.g., mutual goal setting and development of treatment plan, use of contracting).
- Provide opportunities to use strengths and skills constructively.

Patient Outcome: Experience Increased Self-Worth and a Reduced Need to Engage in Manipulative Behaviors

- Teach patient
    - Responsibilities for self (i.e., make requests clearly and to one member of team; attend therapies);
    - Relaxation techniques to deal with feelings or stress (see Chapter 5—*stress management*);
    - To outline activities of the day and to concentrate on accomplishing these;
    - How to approach others in order to meet needs;
    - To recognize when own needs or requests have been met and the interactions in which consideration and respect was experienced;
    - To identify family rules and how to participate in their formulation and abide by them;
    - To set limits on self;
    - To recognize signs of anxiety and how to relieve this feeling;
    - How to identify positive behaviors and to reward self.
- Set realistic, rational limits.
- Allow for testing of interpersonal limits.
- Assist the patient in changing view of self as a victim by having patient define and clarify rights.
- Help the patient clarify own personal wishes and desires as opposed to doing something because another demands it.
- Be nonjudgmental as patient examines manipulative behaviors.
- Give feedback of effects of manipulative attempts on others.
- Seek regular times to interact with the patient that are not contingent on patient behavior or demands.
- Avoid rejective and retaliatory behaviors and power struggles, because those behaviors decrease self-esteem.
- Help patient to delay the immediate satisfaction of every wish or need.
- Frequently ask the patient to describe perceptions of "here and now" and to describe recognition of feelings in current situation.
- Discuss alternative ways of dealing with people, particularly those of authority.
- Use behavioral rehearsal to try out alternative behaviors.

— Evaluation/Outcome Criteria

Decreases use of negative manipulation
Verbalizes positive ideas about self

Shows acceptance of responsibility for self
Develops satisfying interpersonal relationships.

■ REFERENCES

1. Bockle F: The Manipulated Man. New York, Herder & Herder, 1971
2. Chitty K, Maynard C: Managing manipulation. J Psychosoc Nurs Ment Health Serv 24(6):9–13, 1986
3. Earl WL, Addison S, Holmquist L: Crosstalk. J Psychosoc Nurs Ment Health Serv 27(1):20–25, 1989
4. Ellis N: Manipulation. In Beck C, Rawlins R, Williams S (eds): Mental Health-Psychiatric Nursing, 2nd ed. St Louis, CV Mosby, 1988
5. Haber J, Hoskins P, Leach A, Sideleau B: Comprehensive Psychiatric Nursing, 3rd ed. New York, McGraw-Hill, 1987
6. Johnson G, Werstlein P: Reframing: a strategy to improve care of manipulative patients. Issues Ment Health Nurs 11:237–241, 1990
7. Kumler FR: An interpersonal interpretation of manipulation. In Burd S, Marshall B (eds): Some Clinical Approaches to Psychiatric Nursing. New York, MacMillan Publishing, 1963
8. McMorrow ME: The manipulative patient. AJN 81(6):188–190, 1981
9. Meldman M, McFarland GK, Johnson E: The problem-oriented psychiatric index and treatment plan. St Louis, CV Mosby, 1976
10. Richardson J: The manipulative patient spells trouble. Nursing 11:48–52, 1981
11. Sengstacken JK: Manipulation. In McFarland GK, Thomas MD: Psychiatric Mental Health Nursing. Philadelphia, JB Lippincott, 1991
12. Stuart G, Sundeen S: Principles and Practice of Psychiatric Nursing, 3rd ed. St Louis, CV Mosby, 1987
13. Vogel CH, Nihart MA, Buckwalter KC, Stolley J: Exploring the concept of manipulation in psychiatric settings. Arch Psychiatr Nurs 1(6):429–435, 1987

■ POWERLESSNESS

— Definition

Powerlessness is the perceived lack of control over a current situation or happening and the perception that one's own actions are not able to significantly affect the outcome.[4,12,14,16,17]

— General Principles[1–23]

- Everyone has a desire for control.
- There are different reactions to a loss of control.
- Five bases for personal social power are[9]
    - Power based on punishment;
    - Power based on reward;
    - Power based on one's legitimate role in an organization;
    - Power based on knowledge;
    - Power based on personal characteristics.
- Locus of control influences how a person views a given situation:

- Those high in external locus of control perceive situations to be controlled by external factors (e.g., fate).
- Those high in internal locus of control view themselves to be more in control of what happens in any given situation.
- Powerlessness can have an impact on the desire to learn.
- Two types of powerlessness are trait (refers to person's general affect and lifestyle) and situational (refers to person's perceived lack of control in a circumscribed situation).
- Loss of power in one aspect of a person's life can be counterbalanced by an increase in another source of power in another aspect of life or with the introduction of a new source of power.

— Related Factors[4,12,15-17]

Acute physical illness
Chronic, progressively debilitating illness
Threat to physical integrity (e.g., disfigurement)
Mental illness
Loss of control
Sensory deficits
Weak identity
Perception of locus of control
Major losses
Difficulty in accomplishing developmental tasks
Maturational factors (e.g., career pressures)
Lack of knowledge
Lifestyle of helplessness
Repeated interpersonal problems or failures
Inability to perform role responsibilities
Lack of available social resources
Insufficient finances
Hospitalization
Institutional limitations (non-growth-promoting health care
    environment)
    Removal of personal possessions
    Invasion of privacy
    Lack of individualization
    Abuse of authority
    Lack of explanation from caregivers
    Inability to participate in decision making
    Staff monopoly of important resources
    Isolation from significant others
    Staff misuse of rewards and negative reinforcers

— Defining Characteristics[4,12,15-17]

Severe
    Verbal expressions of having no control or influence over
        situation
    Verbal expressions of having no control or influence over
        outcome

Verbal expressions of having no control over self-care
Depression over physical deterioration that occurs despite patient
   compliance with regimen
Apathy
Resignation
Withdrawal
Severe level of emotions such as violence, panic, or depression
Moderate
Nonparticipation in self-care or decision-making when
   opportunities are provided
Expressions of dissatisfaction and frustration over inability to
   perform previous tasks and/or activities
Failure to monitor progress
Expression of doubt regarding role performance
Reluctance to express true feelings, fearing alienation from
   caregivers
Inability to seek information regarding self-care
Failure to learn
Dependence on others that may result in irritability, resentment,
   anger, and guilt
Failure to defend self-care practices when challenged
Passivity
Moderate level of emotional feelings; e.g., moderate anxiety
Low
Increasing passivity
Expressions of uncertainty about fluctuating energy levels
Mild depression, or anxiety, or aggression

—— Nursing Assessment[1-23]

- Evaluate for current contributing factors
- Observe for signs and symptoms indicating presence and level of
  depression.
- Evaluate presence and level of feelings such as anxiety, fear, and
  aggression.
- Evaluate ability to perform activities of daily living.
- Assess patient's perceptions about situation and outcome.
- Note areas that the patient believes cannot be changed.
- Determine the control the patient perceives to have over present
  health problem.
- Identify internal versus external locus of control.
- How much control does the patient perceive to have over the
  present health problem or situation?
- Evaluate resistance to change in order to determine whether the
  patient is afraid of change or is trying to maintain some control
  over life.
- Note pattern and involvement in decision-making.
- Observe for indications of increase in the patient's passivity.
- Note the ability to express feelings.
- Does the patient actively seek out information about the health
  problem or situation?
- Observe for strengths and limitations in role performance.

- How has the patient coped with previous stressors?
- Note presence of interpersonal difficulties related to powerlessness.
- Note increase in complaints, demands, and refusal to go along with treatment program.
- Watch for increasing isolation, resistance, and rejection.
- Note the degree of dependency on others.
- Evaluate the caregiver's support of patient's need for control and assumption of as much responsibility for self-care as possible.

— Patient Outcomes and Nursing Interventions[1-23]

Patient Outcome: Experience Ability to Control Activities and Outcomes and Feel Less Powerless

- Intervene to decrease extreme or moderate level of feelings so that the patient is more comfortable and functional (see *aggression, anxiety, depression* in this chapter).
- Allow for expression of feelings.
- Provide for basic needs with acceptance of dependence but with encouragement of individual freedom, choice, and an increase in self-care.
- Assist the patient in identifying feelings of powerlessness.
- Encourage the patient to explore factors that contribute to feelings of powerlessness.
- Encourage identification and use of strengths and potential. (See Chapter 5—*advocacy*.)
- Help the patient identify personal values.
- Help the patient set realistic goals for self.
- Help the patient differentiate those situations that can be changed from those that cannot.
- Help identify areas that the patient can control.
- Develop a therapeutic milieu in which the patient can regain a sense of control.
    - Refrain from labeling the patient.
    - Call the patient by full name or name chosen by patient.
    - Maximize the use of personal possessions within limits of safety.
    - Protect personal privacy.
    - Provide time for the patient to be alone.
    - Encourage the patient to structure own immediate surroundings, e.g., include family pictures or other familiar objects.
    - Encourage patient to participate in patient council and/or therapeutic community meetings.
    - Respond to make environmental changes suggested by patients.
    - Individualize care as much as possible (e.g., time for grooming).
    - Encourage the patient to participate in setting goals and determining the treatment plan as much as possible.
    - Encourage decision making in developing and planning the day's activities.

- Offer realistic options in the treatment plan.
- Provide opportunities for social interaction and visits from significant others.
- Maintain the patient's interest and participation in the treatment regimen.
- Encourage questions about the treatment regimen.
- Show willingness to change rules to increase the independence of the patient in the hospital.
- Encourage the patient to participate in creating a pleasant environment.
- Minimize rules within the limits of safety, permitting maximum opportunity for the patient to exert own control.
- Convey recognition of patient for active participation in own care.
- Provide recognition for progress in taking a more active role in self care.
- Teach the patient the following:
  - Needed information about illness, treatment, and expected results
    - For patients with external locus of control, provide written information and directions and encourage patient to keep own records.
    - For patients with internal locus of control, provide as detailed and explicit information as desired.
  - Five bases of personal social power (see p. 127) and the consequences of their use.
  - Problem solving skills
  - Assertive communication skills.
- Structure opportunities in which the patient can succeed.
- Provide increased opportunities for the patient to control decisions, including negotiations with health care team.
- Assist in redefining relationships.
- Increase the number of community activities in which the patient participates.
- Identify available self-help groups and refer the patient to them.
- Convey the expectation that the patient will seek help with problems experienced in the future.

— Evaluation/Outcome Criteria

Perceives self as having control over current situation
Perceives own actions as able to influence outcomes
Participates actively in situations that are important to self

■ REFERENCES

1. Arakelian M: An assessment and nursing application of the concept of locus of control. ANS 3(1):25–42, 1980
2. Blau P: Exchange and Power in Social Life. New York, John Wiley & Sons, 1964

3. Boeing MH et al: Powerlessness in critical care patients. Dimens Crit Care Nurs 8(5):274–279, 1989
4. Butcher HK, Kirkpatrick H: Powerlessness. In McFarland GK, Thomas MD: Psychiatric Mental Health Nursing. Philadelphia, JB Lippincott, 1991
5. Byalin K: Parent empowerment: a treatment strategy for hospitalized adolescents. Hosp Community Psychiatry 41(1):89–90, 1990
6. Carpenito LJ: Nursing Diagnosis: Application to Clinical Practice, 3rd ed. Philadelphia, JB Lippincott, 1989
7. Donahue MP: Advocacy. In Bulechek GM, McCloskey JC (eds): Nursing Interventions: Treatments for Nursing Diagnoses. Philadelphia, JB Lippincott, 1985
8. Drew BL: Differentiation of hopelessness, helplessness, and powerlessness using Erik Erikson's "Roots of Virtue." Arch Psychiatr Nurs 4(5):332–337, 1990
9. French J, Raven B: The bases of social power. In Cartwright D (ed): Studies in Social Power. Ann Arbor, The University of Michigan, 1959
10. Glass C, Levy L: Perceived psychophysiological control: the effects of power versus powerlessness. Cog Ther Res 6(1):91–103, 1982
11. Hardin SB, Callahan RJ, Fierman CF, et al: Power in client and nurse-therapist relationships. Perspect Psychiatr Care 23(3):91–98, 1985
12. Kim M, McFarland G, McLane A: Pocket Guide to Nursing Diagnoses, 4th ed. St Louis, CV Mosby, 1991
13. Krouse HJ et al: Nurse-patient interactive styles: power, control, and satisfaction. West J Nurs Res 11(6):717–725, 1989
14. Markert ME: Powerlessness. In McFarland GK, McFarlane EA: Nursing diagnosis and intervention: Planning for patient care. St Louis, CV Mosby, 1989
15. McFarland GK: Powerlessness. In Thompson JM, McFarland GK, Hirsch JE, Tucker SM, Bowers AC: Mosby's Manual of Clinical Nursing, 2nd ed. St Louis, CV Mosby, 1989
16. McFarland GK, Leonard HS, Morris MM: Nursing Leadership and Management: Contemporary Strategies. New York, John Wiley & Sons, 1984
17. McFarland GK, Markert ME: Powerlessness. In Kim MJ, McFarland GK, McLane AM: Pocket Guide to Nursing Diagnoses, 4th ed. St Louis, CV Mosby, 1991
18. Meldman M, McFarland G, Johnson E: The Problem-Oriented Psychiatric Index and Treatment Plans. St Louis, CV Mosby, 1976
19. Miller J: Coping With Chronic Illness: Overcoming Powerlessness. Philadelphia, FA Davis, 1983
20. Pratt CW et al: Sharing research knowledge to empower people who are chronically mentally ill. Psychosoc Rehabil J 13(3):75–79, 1990
21. Rotter J: Generalized expectancies for internal versus external control of reinforcement. Psychol Monogr Gen Appl (Whole no. 609) 80(1):1–28, 1966
22. Shaw RJ: Powerlessness in the nursing home population. In McLane AM (ed): Classification of Nursing Diagnoses: Proceedings of the Seventh Conference. St Louis, CV Mosby, 1987
23. Sheppard K: Powerlessness: a nursing diagnosis. Dimens Oncol Nurs 1(2):17–20, 1986

■ RITUALISTIC BEHAVIOR

—— Definition

Ritualistic behavior is repetitive, uncontrollable thoughts or behaviors performed in an attempt to manage anxiety and internal conflicts.[17]

—— General Principles[1-17]

- Compulsive acts or thoughts are usually an attempt to control primary impulses and deal with related anxiety.
- Obsessive-compulsive traits, such as orderliness, cautiousness, rationality, tidiness, and precision, are useful in many aspects of life.
- Anxiety results when the person does not perform but tries to otherwise control a compulsive act or obsessive thought.
- Persons with compulsions or obsessions are characterized by a high need to control.
- Severe obsessions and compulsions can interfere with the performance of activities of daily living and role expectations.
- The person generally recognizes the obsession or compulsion as irrational.

—— Related Factors[1-17]

Physiological factors
Obsessive-compulsive disorder
Psychodynamic factors
    Conflict among id, ego, superego
    Developmental stage fixation
    Unacceptable impulses
    Unacceptable feelings about self
Anxiety
Learned behavioral response

—— Defining Characteristics[1-17]

Repetitive uncontrollable thought (obsession)
    Repetitive morbid thoughts
    Repetitive fearful thoughts
    Repetitive anxiety-provoking thoughts
    Repetitive ridiculous thoughts
Repetitive uncontrollable acts
    Repetitive handwashing
    Rigid repetitive adherence to work schedule
    Repetitive housecleaning
Increased anxiety when ritualistic behavior is interrupted
High need to control self, others, or environment
Overabundant attention to detail with little feeling
Inflexibility
Severe cautiousness, deliberateness
Problems in completing activities of daily living

—— Nursing Assessment[1-17]

- Describe the patient's current lifestyle and degree of dysfunctional behavior.
- Identify level of anxiety and any means used to channel anxiety.
- Note situations that tend to increase anxiety and lead to obsessive thoughts or compulsive acts.
- Observe for the expression of feelings of distress associated with ritual.
- Identify changes in the patient's view of self.
- Identify the patient's view of the repetitive thought or act as being alien to self.
- Collect data on relief from urgency of repetitive act or thought provided by various activities.
- Identify effect of current behavior on performance of activities of daily living, including effects on job performance requirements.
- Identify specific interpersonal relationships and health routines being adversely affected by repetitive thoughts or acts.

—— Patient Outcomes and Nursing Interventions[1-17]

Patient Outcome: Experience Reduced Anxiety and Need for Ritualistic Behavior

- Administer clomipramine (Anafranil) as ordered.
- Use calm, quiet, caring approach.
- Avoid judgmental attitude or disapproval of patient's behavior.
- Avoid confrontation of ritualistic behavior.
- Do not exert pressure for change of ritualistic behavior.
- Allow for performance of ritual without making demeaning remarks or attempting to stop behavior.
- Plan for additional time to complete rituals.
- Assist patient in making schedule of daily activities and engaging in constructive activities.
- Avoid introducing too much change into daily routine.
- Provide patient support in completing activities, particularly any new ones.
- Reassure and assist the patient in engaging in small periods of relaxation and pleasure.
- Provide opportunities to express feelings.
- Assist the patient in identifying ways of dealing with anxiety and resulting obsessive thoughts.
- Teach the patient ways of dealing with anxiety, such as identifying the feeling, controlling thoughts, exercise.
- Be aware of and take action to decrease the anxiety level aroused in staff.
- Be consistent and time-conscious when making contacts and appointments or giving specific care.
- Give feedback about expressions of obsession and assist the patient in saying directly what is meant.
- Teach ways of dealing with consequences of ritualistic behavior.
- Assist the patient in increasing the range of strategies to decrease anxiety.

- Model the desired social skill when possible.
- Have the patient rehearse the social skill that has resulted in anxiety.
- Teach the patient decision-making skills (see Chapter 5—*decision making*).
- Teach the patient the thought-stopping technique in which the patient commands self to "stop" unwanted thought.
- Teach the patient to reward self for behavior that is not ritualistic.
- Encourage participation in psychotherapy.

Evaluation/Outcome Criteria

Demonstrates less ritualistic behavior
Demonstrates more confined ritualistic behavior
Uses other effective anxiety-reducing techniques
Makes positive statements about self

REFERENCES

1. Baier M, Robinson M, DeShay E, Snider K: Issues in the nursing management of patients with water intoxication. Arch Psychiatr Nurs 3:338–343, 1989
2. Calarco MM: Managing Myra's madness. AJN 89(3):346–349, 1989
3. Delaney P: Trapped by a vacuum. Nurs Times 84(13):55–56, 1988
4. Fan CS: Obsessive compulsive neurosis. Hong Kong Nurs J 42:66–76, 1987
5. Fox H: Patterns of avoidant anxiety. In Haber J, Hoskins PP, Leach AM, Sideleau BF (eds): Comprehensive Psychiatric Nursing, 3rd ed. New York, McGraw-Hill Book Co, 1987
6. Gerety EK, McKim JD, Sosnovec PA, Cowan ME: Instructor's Manual to Accompany McFarland and Thomas's Psychiatric Mental Health Nursing. St Louis, CV Mosby, 1991
7. Grant E: The exercise fix. Psychol Today 22:24–28, 1988
8. Hagerty BK: Obsessive-compulsive behavior: an overview of four psychological frameworks. J Psychosoc Nurs Ment Health Serv 19(1):37–39, 1981
9. Lieberman J: Evidence for a biological hypothesis of obsessive compulsive disorder. Neuropsychobiology 11:14–21, 1984
10. Miller TW, Feibelman ND: Obsessional thought disturbance in a gainfully employed PTSD patient. AAOHN J 35(2):69–73, 1987
11. Petit M: Clients with anxiety, somatoform and dissociative disorders. In Wilson HS, Kneisl CR: Psychiatric Nursing, 3rd ed. Menlo Park, Addison-Wesley Publishing Co, 1988
12. Rapoport JL: The boy who couldn't stop washing: the experience and treatment of obsessive-compulsive disorder. New York, EP Dutton, 1989
13. Roy-Byrne PP, Katon W: An update on treatment of anxiety disorders. Hosp Commun Psychiatry 38:835, 1987
14. Shultz C: Flexibility-rigidity. In Beck CK, Rawlins RP, Williams SR: Mental Health-Psychiatric Nursing, 2nd ed. St Louis, CV Mosby, 1988
15. Silverman WH: Client-therapist cooperation in the treatment of com-

pulsive handwashing behavior. J Behav Ther Exp Psychiatry 17:39–42, 1986

16. Weissman MM: The epidemiology of anxiety and panic disorders: an update. J Clin Psychiatry 47:11–17, 1986
17. Whitley G: Ritualistic behavior. In McFarland GK, Thomas MD: Psychiatric Mental Health Nursing. Philadelphia, JB Lippincott, 1991

■ SELF-ESTEEM DISTURBANCE

— Definition

Self-esteem disturbances involve negative self-evaluation or feelings about oneself, including one's self-worth, self-approval, self-confidence, self-respect, and self-capabilities which may be directly or indirectly expressed.[15,20]

— General Principles

- Self-esteem is a component of the concept of self. Self-esteem disturbance can be situational (in response to a traumatic event) or chronic (long-standing negative evaluation).
- Persons with a high self-esteem are confident about their abilities, appraise themselves realistically, and feel worthwhile and significant. Goals are consistent with capabilities and can change, based on circumstances. The person appreciates self as well as others.
- Persons who have low self-esteem lack confidence, feel worthless and insignificant, and are more sensitive to negative information.
- A person's self-esteem develops over time and is influenced by the positive experiences encountered.

— Related Factors[1–42]

Gap between ideal and real self
Conflicting cognitions/perceptions
Perception of repeated negative experiences (e.g., globalizing negative events) or traumatic events
Ineffective coping skills (e.g., assertion and communication skills)
Learned helplessness
Perceived negative change in body structure or function
Unrealistic demands on self or significant others
Internalizing criticism of others
Reliance on others for self-appraisal
Difficult role transitions
Abusive relationship(s)
Dysfunctional family relationships
Conflicting cultural expectations
Poverty
Deteriorating neighborhood (e.g., high incidence of drug abuse)
Restrictive environment (e.g., hospital setting)

—— Defining Characteristics[15,20]

Devaluation of self through criticism
Low sense of self-worth
Fears or worries, especially of failure
Feelings of disappointment and helplessness
Feelings of fragility and inadequacy
Minimization of own real strengths and abilities
Sense of self-defeat
Inability to accept self
Sensitive to negative information
Denial of self-pleasure
Hesitancy to offer own viewpoints
Preoccupation with real or imagined past failures
Ambivalency and procrastination
Self-destructive behavior
Failure to achieve goals and be successful
Poor interpersonal relationships
Inability to respect own opinion and opinions of others
Difficulty in accepting positive reinforcement
Seeking secondary gains from self-criticisms
Lack of follow-through
Failure to take responsibility for self-care
Expecting the worst outcome for self

—— Nursing Assessment[1-42]

- What is the patient's present perception of self?
- What is the patient's perception of the ideal self?
- What are the patient's goals and how realistic are they?
- Identify patient's specific perceptions and cognitions related to negative self-appraisal
- What standards does the patient set for self? Are they realistic?
- Encourage the patient to assess strengths and potentials. In what ways has the patient been successful in the past? What coping strategies are used?
- Describe the patient's interpersonal relationships. Is there a social network with meaningful others with whom the patient relates well?
- Observe for manifestations of depression.

—— Patient Outcomes and Nursing Interventions[1-42]
Patient Outcome: Experience Improved Self-Esteem

- Use a constructive approach with patient that enhances patient's self-esteem.
  - Avoid judgmental attitude.
  - Do not reject patient for expressing negative feelings.
  - Convey empathy. (See Chapter 2.)
  - Demonstrate unconditional positive regard.
  - Accept the patient as a person regardless of past failures.
  - Be congruent and genuine.

- Focus on the patient's strengths and potential.
  - Encourage the patient to identify and list strengths and potentials.
  - Discourage emphasis on failure.
  - Assist the patient in developing the attitude of not always having to be perfect.
  - Encourage participation in rewarding and satisfying experiences.
  - Encourage developing new skills and activities in which success can be experienced.
  - Find ways to use strengths.
  - Encourage the patient to formulate own opinion of self and decrease reliance on opinions of others.
- Assist the patient in becoming aware when discounting own opinions.
- Assist the patient to examine own perceptions.
- Assist the patient to identify incongruent cognitions.
- Assist the patient to focus on specific events rather than globalizing.
- Provide opportunities for the patient to work through feelings of disappointment.
- Give recognition on neat appearance, activities well done, and other strengths.
- Encourage the patient to
  - Develop positive reinforcers for actual achievements;
  - Minimize encounters in which false praise is used.
- Teach the patient to use problem solving and to seek constructive resolution of current and future problems.
  - Have the patient list negative qualities and develop plans to change them.
  - Assist the patient in developing solutions to problems and in setting realistic goals and plans.
  - Help the patient plan for action to meet goals.
  - Encourage the patient to explore feelings, thoughts, and behavior and to examine own behavior critically.
  - Encourage the patient to accept responsibility for own opinions and behavior and to evaluate outcomes.
- Teach the patient to give self positive reinforcement; e.g., treat self to dinner after completing something successfully.
- Discourage use of expressions indicative of poor self-esteem for secondary gains.
- Encourage good grooming habits and personal appearance.
- Assists the patient in developing defenses against attacks on self-concept.
- Encourage the patient to accept responsibility for own opinions and behavior and to evaluate outcomes in relation to the options available.
- Spend time with the patient in groups and in a one-to-one nurse-patient relationship.
- Encourage the patient to participate in group therapy in which the emphasis is to provide support and to help the patient

recognize that there are others experiencing similar fears and failures.
- Teach the patient characteristics of assertive behavior and communication skills: (see Chapter 5—*Assertive training and social skills training.*)
    - Sensitivity to others' feelings
    - Use of "I" messages
    - Respect for behaviors, opinions, and rights of others
    - Consistency of posture, facial expression, tone of voice with verbal communication
    - Clear communication of own expectations to others
    - Recognition of negotiation as viable tactic
    - Firm but gentle expression of opinions and wishes, unyielding where appropriate, without use of threats
    - Based on own human rights
    - Emphasis on learning and competence
- Teach patients components of assertive behavior and communication skills: (see Chapter 5.)
    - Set goals and express to others honest thoughts and feelings.
    - Act on set goals in clear, consistent way.
    - Accept personal responsibility for consequences of actions.
    - Remain sensitive to rights and feelings of others.
- Encourage the patient to join appropriate self-help groups, neighborhood improvement group.
- Encourage the patient to use problem-solving skills to deal with environmental stresses.
    - Review problems identified and action plan with patient.
    - Help patient prepare for action plan; e.g., use of role playing.
    - Assist the patient in evaluating the action plan.

Evaluation/Outcome Criteria

Demonstrates positive self-esteem
Sets and achieves realistic and meaningful goals
Engages in and recognizes benefit of treatment modalities
Uses assertive behaviors and communication skills
Feels competent
Expresses own opinions in confident manner
Values own contributions
Engages in constructive behavior
Has constructive social network
Defining characteristics are eliminated, reduced, or modified.

▬ REFERENCES

1. Adams S: The relationship of clothing to self-esteem in elderly patients. Nurs Times 83:42–45, 1987
2. Antonucci T et al: Physical health and self-esteem. Fam Commun Health 6:1–9, 1983
3. Austin JK, Champion VL, Tzeng O: Cross-cultural relationships be-

tween self-concept and body image in high school-age boys. Arch Psychiatr Nurs 3:234–240, 1989

4. Barron CR: Women's causal explanations of divorce: relationships to self-esteem and emotional distress. Res Nurs Health 10:345–353, 1987
5. Bennett G: Stress, social support, and self-esteem of young alcoholics in recovery. Issues Ment Health Nurs 9:151–167, 1988
6. Bonham P, Cheney A: Concept of self: a framework for nursing assessment. In Chinn P (ed): Advances in Nursing Theory Development. Rockville, MD, Aspen Systems, 1983
7. Clark C: Assertive skills for nurses. Wakefield, Contemporary Publishing, 1978
8. Crouch M et al: Enhancement of self-esteem in adults. Fam Commun Health 6:65–78, 1983
9. Fitts W: The Self Concept and Performance. Nashville, Dede Wallace Center, 1972
10. Fitts W: The Self Concept and Psychopathology. Nashville, Dede Wallace Center, 1972
11. Forchuk C: Cognitive dissonance: denial, self-concepts, and the alcoholic stereotype. Nurs Papers 16(3):57–69, 1984
12. Gilberts R: The evaluation of self-esteem. Fam Commun Health 6:29–49, 1983
13. Hirst S, Straub V: Promoting self-esteem. J Gerontol Nurs 10:72–77, 1984
14. Hubbard JT, Romero DH, Thomas SB: A guide to photography in educational and counseling settings. Perspect Psychiatr Care 24:20–24, 1987
15. Kim MJ, McFarland GK, McLane AL: Pocket Guide to Nursing Diagnoses, 4th ed. St Louis, CV Mosby, 1991
16. Koniak-Griffin D: The relationship between social support, self-esteem, and maternal-fetal attachment in adolescents. Res Nurs Health 11:269–278, 1988
17. Lamarine RJ: Self-esteem, health locus of control, and health attitudes among native American children. J Sch Health 57:371–374, 1987
18. Lego S: The development of the self. Arch Psychiatr Nurs 1:318–321, 1987
19. Long KA, Hamlin CM: Use of the Piers-Harris Self-Concept Scale with Indian children: cultural considerations. Nurs Res 37:42–46, 1988
20. McFarland GK, von Schilling K, McCann J: Self-concept-self-perception pattern. In Thompson J, McFarland G, Hirsch J, Tucker S, Bowers A: Mosby's Clinical Nursing, 2nd ed. St Louis, CV Mosby, 1989
21. McGlashan R: Strategies for rebuilding self-esteem for the cardiac patient. Dimens Crit Care Nurs 7:28–38, 1988
22. McGonigle D: Making self-talk positive. AJN 88:725–726, 1988
23. Meldman M, McFarland G, Johnson E: The Problem-oriented Psychiatric Index and Treatment Plans. St Louis, CV Mosby, 1976
24. Miller SA: Promoting self-esteem in the hospitalized adolescent: clinical interventions. Issues Compreh Pediatr Nurs 10:187–194, 1987
25. Muhlenkamp AF, Sayles JA: Self-esteem, social support, and positive health practices. Nurs Res 35:335–338, 1986
26. Nelson PB: Social support, self-esteem, and depression in the institutionalized elderly. Issues Ment Health Nurs 10:55–68, 1989
27. Norris J, Kunes-Connell M: A multimodal approach to validation and

refinement of an existing nursing diagnosis. Arch Psychiatr Nurs 2:103–109, 1988

28. Norris J, Kunes-Connell M: Self-esteem disturbance. Nurs Clin North Am 20:745–761, 1985
29. Petersen-Martin J, Cottrell RR: Self-concept, values, and health behavior. Health Educ 18:6–9, 1987
30. Reasoner R: Enhancement of self-esteem in children and adolescents. Fam Commun Health 6:51–64, 1983
31. Rice MA, Szopa TJ: Group intervention for reinforcing self-worth following mastectomy. Oncol Nurs Forum 15:33–37, 1988
32. Roy DJ: Caring for the self-esteem of the cosmetic patient. Plast Surg Nurs 6:138–141, 1986
33. Stanwyck D: Self-esteem through the life span. Fam Commun Health 6:11–28, 1983
34. Swanson B, Cronin-Stubbs D, Sheldon JA: The impact of psychosocial factors on adapting to physical disability: a review of the research literature. Rehab Nurs 14:64–69, 1989
35. Taft LB: Self-esteem in later life: a nursing perspective. Adv Nurs Sci 8:77–84, 1985
36. Taylor M: The need for self-esteem. In Yura H, Walsh M (eds): Human Needs and the Nursing Process. Norwalk, Appleton-Century-Crofts, 1982
37. Thomas BL: Self-esteem and life satisfaction. J Gerontol Nurs 14:25–36, 1988
38. Thompson EH: Variation in the self-concept of young adult chronic patients: chronicity reconsidered. Hosp Community Psychiatry 39:771–775, 1988
39. Watson WL, Bell JM: Who are we? Low self esteem and marital identity. J Psychosoc Nurs Ment Health Serv 28(4):15–20, 1990
40. Weisberg J, Haberman MR: Enhancing self-esteem of the young through grandchildren's day in a home for the aged. Nurs Homes 36:38–40, 1987
41. Whall AL: Self-esteem and the mental health of older adults. J Gerontol Nurs 13:41–43, 1987
42. Wylie R: The Self Concept. Lincoln, University of Nebraska Press, 1974

■ SEXUAL DYSFUNCTION

— Definition

Sexual dysfunction is the state in which an individual experiences a change in sexual function that is viewed by the individual as unsatisfying, unrewarding, inadequate, or is socially inappropriate.[5,22]

— General Principles[1–22]

- Sexuality is dynamic, intrinsic to one's identity, and involves all aspects of being male or female: It is not limited to sexual intercourse.
- Sexually well-functioning persons are aware of and accept sexual feelings, accept as normal and have an understanding of

sexual functioning, have a positive body image, respect the rights of others, and are tolerant of mistakes.[27]

- Sexual functioning can be affected by disease processes, health status, pain, emotional disorders, feelings, stress or sexually traumatic experiences, interpersonal relationships, environmental conditions, cultural norms, and religious beliefs.
- Sexual dysfunction can be experienced in any aspect of being male or female.
- Sexual dysfunction can be experienced during any phase of the sexual experience; i.e., desire phase, excitement phase, orgasm/ejaculation phase.
- A person's response to any one or combination of related factors is influenced by numerous variables; e.g., previous sexual history, the nature and cause of the difficulty, meaning of current situation for person, coping repertoire and resources of the person, available professional health care, and actual use of available professional sexual counseling and assistance.

—— Related Factors[1,5,9,15–17,19,22,23,32]

Altered body structure or function
    Congenital anomalies
    Genetic factors
    Disease process
    Altered hormonal functioning
    Treatment-related factors
        Surgery
        Radiation
        Medications
Pain due to organic cause
Pain due to psychogenic cause
Fatigue
Physical abuse
Pregnancy
Childbirth
Aging
Psychiatric disorders; e.g., organic mental disorder, mood disorders
Psychosocial factors
    Psychosocial abuse
    Sexual trauma; e.g., rape, incest
    Maturational crisis
    Situational crisis
    Negative body image
    Ambivalence about sexual behavior
    Overly critical self-appraisal of sexual functioning
    Performance anxiety
    Fear of pregnancy
    Fear of AIDS or other sexually transmitted disease
    Avoidance of erotic stimulation or fantasies
    Fear of intimacy
Lack of privacy
Misinformation

Inadequate sexual techniques
Ineffective role models
Poor communication skills
Lack of significant other
Relationship problems with significant others
Partner pressure
Family norms
Unrealistic expectations
Values conflict
Spiritual factors
Religious beliefs
Cultural factors

— Defining Characteristics[5,9,15-17,19,22,23,32]

Altered/perceived limitation of sexual functioning imposed by
   disease
Altered/perceived limitation of sexual functioning imposed by
   treatment
General concern about sexual functioning
   Verbalization of problems regarding sexual functioning
   Questioning of sexual practices
   Confusion about expression of sexual desires
Sex role conflict or dissatisfaction
Negative attitude toward sexuality
Difficulty discussing sexual matters
Altered interpersonal relationships; e.g., isolating behavior
Disrupted orgasm/ejaculation phase
   Premature or retarded ejaculation
   Inhibited orgasm
Disrupted excitement phase
   Reduced sexual pleasure/satisfaction
   Lack of sexual pleasure/satisfaction
   Impotence
   Painful coitus
Disrupted desire phase
   Absence of desire
   Diminished sexual desire for significant other
Pre-orgasm/ejaculatory phase pain
Post-orgasm/ejaculatory phase pain
Dyspareunia
Phobic avoidance of sexual behavior
Disregard for welfare of other person
   Aggression
   Potential for violence
   Sex with minor
   Sex with others unable to give understood consent; e.g., the
      mentally ill, developmentally handicapped
   Use of coercion
   Use of physical force
   Inflicting injury
   Psychological degradation of other

—— Nursing Assessment[1-42]

- Assess sexual history.
- Does the patient experience altered body functions or structures that can effect sexual functioning?
- Does the patient experience mental disorder; e.g., psychoactive substance abuse, that can effect sexual functioning?
- Assess for any psychosocial factors that can effect sexual functioning; e.g., maturational crisis.
- Assess for spiritual and cultural influences that can effect sexual functioning.
- Assess for presence of stressors.
- Assess for vulnerability to sexual aggression from others; e.g., sexual rape.
- Has the patient experienced any sexual trauma in the past?
- Does the patient or partner express concern about sexual functioning?
- Have the patient describe nature and importance of sexual problem.
- Assess learning needs regarding sexual needs.
- Assess maturational stage.
- Does the patient experience difficulties in orgasm/ejaculation phase, excitement phase, desire phase? What is the nature and extent of difficulties? How important are they to the patient and/or partner?
- How comfortable is the patient in discussing sexual matters?
- Ascertain meaning of sexual behavior.
- Assess the patient's understanding of normal sexual functioning and effects of medical illness, psychiatric disorder, stressor, and/or treatment-related factors.
- Does the patient experience pre- or post-orgasm/ejaculation phase pain? Is dyspareunia present?
- What are the patient's attitudes and beliefs concerning sexuality? Evaluate level of anxiety or fear.
- Assess the patient's attitude and general respect to welfare toward sexual partner.

—— Patient Outcomes and Nursing Interventions[1-42]

Patient Outcome: Experience Personally Satisfying Sexual Functioning While Considering Rights of Others

- Be aware of and resolve own personal conflicts regarding sexual matters.
- Avoid being judgmental or biased.
- Foster atmosphere of safety and protection conducive to open discussion and expression of feelings.
- Encourage the patient to express thoughts and discuss sexual concerns openly.
- Help the patient get in touch with repressed emotions regarding sexual trauma.
- Explore with the patient roots of sexual dysfunction.
- Openly discuss meaning of sexual behaviors and desire for change.

- Assist the patient in identifying appropriate ways and/or alternatives for meeting sexual needs.
- Assist the patient in exploring means of intensifying sexual sensations.
- Assist the patient in identifying and dealing with stressors and crisis (see Chapter 5—*crisis intervention*).
- Identify and discuss sexually provocative or inappropriate behaviors.
- Assist the patient in becoming aware of and examining consequences of socially inappropriate or risk-laden sexual behaviors.
- Assist the patient in developing a more positive body image.
  - Provide information about corrective devices.
  - Refer patient to self-help group.
- Enhance self-esteem (see *self-esteem disturbance* in this chapter).
  - Assist the patient in developing more realistic expectations of self or other regarding sexual performance.
- Provide needed and accurate information about healthy sexual functioning characterized by acceptance of sexual feelings, sexual fantasies, positive body image, respect for rights and feelings of others, and tolerance of mistakes.
- Provide needed and accurate information about sexual techniques (e.g., talk about techniques for safe sex) or refer to sex counselor.
- Provide information about major structure and function of reproductive system, including birth control and safe sexual practices, and the effects of physical illness, psychiatric disorder, medication or other treatment.
- Ensure access to appropriate sexual expression in inpatient settings.
- Teach the patient the need for compliance with treatment for disease process.
- Assist the patient to improve social interaction.
- Teach the patient social skills (see Chapter 5—*social skills training*).
- Teach the patient stress management techniques (see Chapter 5—*stress management*).
- Teach the patient assertive communication techniques (see Chapter 5—*assertiveness training*).
- Discuss values, conflicting values, and spiritual beliefs, and refer for pastoral counseling as needed.
- Discuss any cultural conflict present.
- Make appropriate referrals; e.g., grief counseling, family therapy or couples therapy, sex counseling or therapy, treatment for physical illness.
- Involve partner in care decisions.
- Refer to relevant community resources and groups.

—— Evaluation/Outcome Criteria

Has minimal concerns about sexual functioning
Experiences satisfactory orgasm/ejaculation phase

Experiences sexual pleasure in excitement phase
Experiences sexual desire
Reduced or absence of pain in pre- or post-orgasm/ejaculation phase
Reduced or absence of dyspareunia
Engages in socially appropriate behaviors to meet sexual needs
Demonstrates concern for welfare of other while meeting sexual
　　needs

▪ REFERENCES

1. Arcangelo V: Sexual dysfunction. In Carpenito LJ: Nursing Diagnosis, 2nd ed. Philadelphia, JB Lippincott, 1987
2. Burgess AW, Hartman CR, Kelley SJ: Assessing child abuse: the TRI-ADS checklist. J Psychosoc Nurs Ment Health Serv 28(4):6–14, 1990
3. Burgess AW, Hartman CR, Wolbert WA, Grant CA: Child molestation: assessing impact in multiple victims (Part I). Arch Psychiatr Nurs 1(1):33–39, 1987
4. Burgess EJ: Sexually abused children and their drawings. Arch Psychiatr Nurs 2(2):65–73, 1988
5. Carroll-Johnson RM: Sexual dysfunction. In Carroll-Johnson RM (ed): Classification of Nursing Diagnoses: Proceedings of the Eighth Conference. Philadelphia, JB Lippincott, 1989
6. Coker LS: A therapeutic recovery model for the female adult incest survivor. Issues Ment Health Nurs 11:109–123, 1990
7. Cornman BJ: Group treatment for female adolescent sexual abuse victims. Issues Ment Health Nurs 10:261–271, 1989
8. Covington CH: Incest: the psychological problem and the biological contradiction. Issues Ment Health Nurs 10:69–87, 1989
9. Dickman GL, Livingston CA: Sexual dysfunction. In McFarland GK, Thomas MD: Psychiatric Mental Health Nursing. Philadelphia, JB Lippincott, 1991
10. Frank DI, Lang AR: Disturbances in sexual role performance of chronic alcoholics: an analysis using Roy's adaptation model. Issues Ment Health Nurs 11:243–254, 1990
11. Gilbert CM: Psychosomatic symptoms: implications for child sexual abuse. Issues Ment Health Nurs 9(4):399–408, 1988
12. Gilbert CM: Sexual abuse and group therapy. J Psychosoc Nurs Ment Health Serv 26(5):19–23, 1988
13. Glover J: Human Sexuality in Nursing Care. London, Croom Helm, 1985
14. Greenfeld M: Disclosing incest: the Relationships That Make it Possible. J Psychosoc Nurs Ment Health Serv 28(7):20–23, 1990
15. Hartman CR, Burgess AW: Altered sexuality patterns. In Thompson JM, McFarland GK, Hirsch JE, Tucker SM, Bowers AC: Mosby's Manual of Clinical Nursing, 2nd ed. St Louis, CV Mosby, 1989
16. Hartman CR, Burgess AW: Rape-trauma syndrome. In Thompson JM, McFarland GK, Hirsch JE, Tucker SM, Bowers AC: Mosby's Manual of Clinical Nursing, 2nd ed. St Louis, CV Mosby, 1989
17. Hartman CR, Burgess AW: Sexual dysfunction. In Thompson JM, McFarland GK, Hirsch JE, Tucker SM, Bowers AC: Mosby's Manual of Clinical Nursing, 2nd ed. St Louis, CV Mosby, 1989

18. Higgins L, Hawkins J: Human Sexuality Across the Life Span. Monterey, Wadsworth Health Sciences Division, 1984
19. Hinds SD: Rape-trauma syndrome (compound reaction and silent reaction). In McFarland GK, McFarlane EA: Nursing Diagnosis and Intervention: Planning for Patient Care. St Louis, CV Mosby, 1989
20. Hogan RM: Human Sexuality: A Nursing Perspective, 2nd ed. Norwalk, Appleton-Century-Crofts, 1985
21. Holbrook T: Policing sexuality in a modern state hospital. Hosp Commun Psychiatry 40(1):75–79, 1989
22. Kim MJ, McFarland GK, McLane AM: Pocket Guide to Nursing Diagnoses, 4th ed. St Louis, CV Mosby, 1991
23. Korb CS, Kupperberg C: Sexual dysfunction; altered sexuality patterns. In McFarland GK, McFarland EA: Nursing Diagnosis and Intervention: Planing for Patient Care. St Louis, CV Mosby, 1989
24. Krach P, Zens D: Incest: Nursing interventions for group therapy. J Psychosoc Nurs Ment Health Serv 26(10):32–34, 1988
25. Ledray LE: Counseling rape victims: the nursing challenge. Perspect Psychiatr Care 26(2):21–27, 1990
26. Limandri BJ: Disclosure of stigmatizing conditions: the discloser's perspective. Arch Psychiatr Nurs 3(2):69–78, 1989
27. Lion E: Human Sexuality in Nursing Process. New York, John Wiley & Sons, 1982
28. Lowery M: Adult survivors of childhood incest. J Psychosoc Nurs Ment Health Serv 25(1):27–31, 1987
29. Masters W, Johnson V: Human Sexuality. Boston, Little, Brown & Co, 1984
30. Mayr S, Price JL: The Io syndrome: symptom formation in victims of sexual abuse. Perspect Psychiatr Care 25(3,4):36–39, 1989
31. McArthur MJ: Reality therapy with rape victims. Arch Psychiatr Nurs 4(6):360–365, 1990
32. McFarland GK, Scipio-Skinner K: Sexual dysfunction. In Kim MJ, McFarland GK, McLane A: Pocket Guide to Nursing Diagnoses, 4th ed. St Louis, CV Mosby, 1991
33. Minden P: The victim care service: a program for victims of sexual assault. Arch Psychiatr Nurs 3(1):41–46, 1989
34. Rew L: Childhood sexual abuse: toward a self-care framework for nursing intervention and research. Arch Psychiatr Nurs 4(3):147–153, 1990
35. Rew L: Childhood sexual exploitation: long-term effects among a group of nursing students. Issues Ment Health Nurs 10:181–191, 1989
36. Rew L: Long-term effects of childhood sexual exploitation. Issues Ment Health Nurs 10:229–244, 1989
37. Spratlen LP: Sexual harassment counseling. J Psychosoc Nurs Ment Health Serv 26(2):28–32, 1988
38. Urbancic JC: Resolving incest experiences through inpatient group therapy. J Psychosoc Nurs Ment Health Serv 27(9):4–10, 1989
39. Webb C: Sexuality, Nursing, and Health. New York, John Wiley & Sons, 1985
40. Woods N: Human Sexuality in Health and Illness. St Louis, CV Mosby, 1984
41. Young EW: Sexual needs of psychiatric clients. J Psychosoc Nurs Ment Health Serv 25(7):30–32, 1987

42. Zimmerman ML, Wolbert WA, Burgess AW, Hartman CR: Art and group work: interventions for multiple victims of child molestation (Part II). Arch Psychiatr Nurs 1(1):40–46, 1987

▬ SOCIAL INTERACTION, IMPAIRED

— Definition

Impaired social interaction is the state in which an individual participates in an insufficient or excessive quantity or ineffective quality of social exchange.[9,13]

— General Principles[1–22]

- Social interaction consists of a dynamic pattern of social exchange occurring within a context involving at least two persons.
- Different levels of awareness operate continually in social interactions; e.g., awareness of external appearance.
- Cognitive abilities, reality testing, maturational state, and coping repertoire are important for effective social interaction.
- Environmental factors can have an impact on and impair social interaction.
- Individuals with chronic mental illness may experience impaired social interaction as a result of a number of factors; e.g., impaired reality testing, severe aggression, loss of interpersonal skills, poor impulse control, manipulation.
- Individuals with chronic mental illness often have few friends and often experience impaired social interactions.

— Related Factors[3,9,14,21,22]

Limited physical mobility
Sensory deficits
Speech impediment
Severe pain
Debilitating physical illness; e.g., terminal cancer
Developmental handicaps
Mental disorder
Poor impulse control
Impaired reality testing
Severe aggression
Substance abuse
Treatment-related factors; e.g., surgery
Extreme emotions; e.g., panic
Altered thought processes
Inadequate social and communication skills
Absence of available significant others
Lack of opportunity to interact with others

Maturational crisis
Cultural barriers
Language barriers
Environmental barriers; e.g., restrictive long-term care facilities
Self-concept disturbance

— Defining Characteristics[3,9,14,21,22]

Discomfort in social interaction
Feelings of loneliness or rejection
Frequently feeling misunderstood
Reports of inability to establish positive supportive relationships
Reports of inability to maintain supportive relationships
Active avoidance of others
Isolation from others
Failure to respond to other's attempts at interactions
Ineffective social behaviors
Excessive social change
Lack of close interdependent relationships
Superficial relationships
Dissatisfaction with social network
Family report of problematic patterns of interaction
Interpersonal difficulties at work

— Nursing Assessment[2,3,9,12–14,21,22]

- Assess social history and identify when change in social behavior occurred.
- Assess physical, emotional, environmental barriers to establishing effective and supportive interpersonal relationships; e.g., limited physical mobility, extreme anxiety, lack of opportunity to interact with others.
- What is the patient's perception of social interaction?
- Observe for level of discomfort in interactions.
- Ask patient to describe nature and level of satisfaction with social interactions. Use of Malone Social Network Inventory may be helpful.
- Are feelings of loneliness or rejection present?
- Is patient grieving?
- To what extent does patient initiate interactions and respond to others' attempts at interaction?
- What are the characteristics of patient's interactions with family members, friends, and co-workers?
- Is patient able to live cooperatively with others?
- Is patient able to participate with others in recreational activities?
- Are family, friends, and acquaintances available to patient?
- How do others react to patient's interpersonal difficulties?
- Assess patient's actual social and communication skills.

—— Patient Outcomes and Nursing Interventions[1-22]

Patient Outcome: Maintain Interaction with Others in Process of Daily Living with Minimal Anxiety and Engage in Satisfying Social Interactions to the Extent Possible

- Reduce barriers to establishing effective and satisfying social interactions; e.g., reduce anxiety; provide grief counseling (see Chapter 5—*supportive therapy*); provide opportunities for social interactions.
- Offer opportunities to express feelings in an acceptable manner.
- Explore with the patient his or her subjective experience of a specific social exchange.
- Improve self-esteem (see *self esteem disturbance* in this chapter).
- Encourage the patient to express perception of the difficulty.
- Assist the patient in identifying presence of discomfort and dissatisfaction.
- Provide safe atmosphere in which feelings such as rejection can easily be expressed.
- Establish therapeutic milieu that promotes social interaction (see Chapter 5), and allows for practice of new behaviors, as well as allows for social solitude.
- Help the patient identify behaviors or situations in which others are alienated.
- Discuss with patient what is conveyed through silence.
- Use nonverbal communication to encourage interaction when appropriate. (See Chapter 5—*communication techniques*.)
- Base extent of initial interaction with the patient on observed levels of tolerance.
  - Start with short but frequent encounters.
  - Discuss neutral topics of interest to the patient.
  - Keep conversation reality based.
  - Focus on what is occurring now.
  - Engage in meaningful tasks.
- Explore and support patient's strengths.
- Capitalizing on patient strengths, encourage interaction with a peer with whom the patient feels comfortable; e.g., initiate card game between the patient and peer.
- Use role-playing techniques to practice aspects of social interaction. (See Chapter 5—*social skills training*)
  - How to initiate a conversation
  - How to continue a conversation
  - How to terminate a conversation
  - How to refuse a request
  - How to ask for something
  - How to interview for a job
  - How to ask someone to participate in an activity; e.g., going to the movies
- After successful interaction in a one-to-one interaction with staff, peer, friend, and/or family member, encourage the patient to participate in small group activities.
- Encourage increasing involvement in community groups related to the patient's interests; e.g., music group.
- Teach the patient relevant skills; e.g., social skills;

communication techniques; assertive communication skills (see also Chapter 5); job interviewing skills.
- Help the patient to identify new opportunities for social interaction and encourage participation in activities with others.
- Give positive feedback for improvement in social interaction.
- Teach the family information about the patient's mental illness, related behavior, and treatment.
- Provide family guidance on interacting with patient.

— Evaluation/Outcome Criteria[3,9,14,21−22]

Verbalizes satisfaction with one-to-one interactions
Verbalizes satisfaction with group interactions
Maintains mutually supportive social network
Spends time interacting with others
Demonstrates ability to cope with new and complex social situations

■ REFERENCES

1. Copel LC: Loneliness. J Psychosoc Nurs Ment Health Serv 26(1):14–19, 1988
2. Doenges ME, Moorhouse MF: Nurse's Pocket Guide: Nursing Diagnoses with Interventions. Philadelphia, FA Davis, 1988
3. Fischer K, Schwartz M: Impaired social interaction. In Thompson JM, McFarland GK, Hirsch JE, Tucker SM, Bowers AC: Mosby's Manual of Clinical Nursing, 2nd ed. St Louis, CV Mosby, 1989
4. Forchuk C, Brown B: Establishing a nurse-client relationship. J Psychosoc Nurs Ment Health Serv 27(2):30–34, 1989
5. Foxall MJ, Ekberg JY: Loneliness of chronically ill adults and their spouses. Issues Ment Health Nurs 10:149–167, 1989
6. Harris JL: Self-care actions of chronic schizophrenics associated with meeting solitude and social interaction requisites. Arch Psychiatr Nurs 4(5):298–307, 1990
7. Hoeffer B: A causal model of loneliness among older single women. Arch Psychiatr Nurs 1(5):366–373, 1987
8. Johnson ML: Use of play group therapy in promoting social skills. Issues Ment Health Nurs 9:105–112, 1988
9. Kim MJ, McFarland GK, McLane A: Pocket Guide to Nursing Diagnoses, 4th ed. St Louis, CV Mosby, 1991
10. Kovarsky RS: Loneliness and disturbed grief: a comparison of parents who lost a child to suicide or accidental death. Arch Psychiatr Nurs 3(2):86–96, 1989
11. Lane PL: Nurse-client perceptions: the double standard of touch. Issues Ment Health Nurs 10:1–13, 1989
12. Malone J: The social support social dissupport continuum. J Psychosoc Nurs Ment Health Serv 26(12):18–22, 1988
13. Markert ME, McFarland GK: Impaired social interaction. In Kim MJ, McFarland GK, McLane A: Pocket Guide to Nursing Diagnoses, 4th ed. St Louis, CV Mosby, 1991
14. Maroni J: Impaired social interaction. In McFarland GK, McFarlane EA: Nursing Diagnosis and Intervention: Planning for Patient Care. St Louis, CV Mosby, 1989

15. Nighorn S: Narcissistic deficits in drug abusers: a self psychological approach. J Psychosoc Nurs Ment Health Serv 26(9):22–26, 1988
16. Nokes KM, Kendrew J: Loneliness in veterans with AIDS and its relationship to the development of infections. Arch Psychiatr Nurs 4(4):271–277, 1990
17. Plante TG: Social skills training. J Psychosoc Nurs Ment Health Serv 27(3):7–10, 1989
18. Rokach A: Surviving and coping with loneliness. J Psychol 124(1):39–54, 1990
19. Topf M: Verbal interpersonal responsiveness. J Psychosoc Nurs Ment Health Serv 26(7):8–16, 1988
20. Welt SR: The developmental roots of loneliness. Arch Psychiatr Nurs 1(1):25–32, 1987
21. Westwell J, Martin ML: Impaired social interaction. In McFarland GK, Thomas MD: Psychiatric Mental Health Nursing. Philadelphia, JB Lippincott, 1991
22. Willard AE: Impaired social interactions. In Carpenito LJ: Nursing Diagnosis, 2nd ed. Philadelphia, JB Lippincott, 1987

■ SUICIDE, POTENTIAL

— Definition

There is a potential for suicide when a possibility exists that the patient will kill his- or herself voluntarily and intentionally.

— General Principles[1–39]

- Theories of suicide include: (a) psychodynamic—conflict between the life and death instincts, with the death wish predominating; aggression turned inward resulting in self-destructive behavior; (b) sociological perspective—alienation from society with a difficult struggle to function without clear norms and roles. This struggle is too painful to the person and can lead to suicide; (c) cognitive—hopelessness, including extreme negative self-appraisal and anticipation of poor outcomes, can lead to suicide; (d) psychophysiologic—some biochemical alterations are being identified in research on suicide victims.
- About 80% of persons who commit suicide give some type of clue indicative of the suicide. All talk of suicide is of concern.
- Clues include the following:
    - Direct verbal clues such as, "I would like to kill myself."
    - Indirect verbal clues such as, "You'd be better off without me."
    - Coded verbalizations such as, "How can I give my body to the medical school?"
    - Behavioral clues such as suicide attempts or sudden improved affect in the depressed person.
    - Situational clues such as notification that cancer has been diagnosed or significant loss.

- A specific high-lethality suicide plan (e.g., shooting, hanging, poisoning) of recent origin in which the person has the resources available increases the potential of suicide.
- Other indications of high risk for suicide are depression (especially changing levels); major recent loss; family history of suicide; "putting house in order," i.e., giving away prized possessions; hopelessness, with few plans or goals for future; unwillingness to make a "no suicide" contract.
- Repression has been found to be highly correlated with the risk of suicide and may be a mechanism by which aggression is focused inward.
- Suicide may be prevented because persons with the potential for suicide do experience ambivalence sometime prior to actual suicide.
- More suicides occur during the period of improvement following severe depression than during the period of severe depression itself.
- A person who experiences hallucinations may respond, for example, to voices that command the patient to kill self.
- Suicide ranks among the leading cause of death in 15- to 23-year-olds.
- Suicide is the ninth leading cause of death among the elderly.
- White males over 65 are at highest risk.
- Males outnumber females in actual suicide, while females outnumber males in actual suicide attempts.

— Related Factors[1-39]

Reaction to physical illness; e.g., AIDS, cancer
Delirium
Acute or chronic pain
Psychiatric disorder
    Schizophrenia
    Mood disorder
    Psychoactive substance use disorder
    Organic mental disorder
    Adjustment disorder with depressed mood
    Personality disorder
Disturbed thought processes/perceptions
    Hallucinations
    Delusions
    Phobias
    Disorientation
    Impaired judgment
Severe stress
Developmental crisis
Threat of extreme deprivation; e.g., institutionalization
Severely impaired self-concept
Inadequate coping skills
Past history of dealing with stressors by suicide attempts
Inadequate or stressful social network
Pathological interpersonal relationship

Alienation
Suicide contagion
Family dysfunction
Child abuse or incest
Low socioeconomic status
Cultural factors
Spiritual stress

—— Risk Factors[1-39]

Directly verbalizing desire to kill self
Indirectly verbalizing desire to kill self
Verbalizing coded desire to kill self
History of previous suicide attempts
Putting unusual things in order before going on a long trip
Making a will under extraordinary circumstances
Buying a casket for self at funeral of significant other
Giving away prized possessions
Psychologically overacting when stressed
Feeling agitated
Anger
Repression of aggression
Sadness, flat affect
Specific high-lethality plan to kill self
Obtaining resources that can be used to kill self
Lacking future plans
Hopelessness
Unwillingness to agree to "no suicide or self-harm" contract
Expressing agitated concern over controlling own fate
Having unclear awareness of consequences of suicide attempt
Experiencing difficulty with problem solving
Desperate search for help, attention, reassurance
Withdrawing
Social isolation

—— Nursing Assessment

- Assess severity of intent, wish to die, and lethality, objective danger to life.
- Explore patient's present situation.
- What is the nature of the patient's suicidal behavior that lead to admission? Method? Clarity of plan? Place? Proximity of other people? Physical results? Actions to reverse physical results or obtain help?
- Does patient verbalize desire to die (e.g., "I'm tired. It's no use. No one would care if I died," or "Death would solve everything.")?
    - Ask patient the following questions:
        Have you thought of committing suicide?
        Are you thinking of committing suicide now?
        How long have you thought about it?
        What is the frequency and duration of such thoughts?

How would you go about doing it?
Do you have the means?
Have you ever attempted to commit suicide?
Has anyone in your family ever committed suicide?
What is the likelihood that you will?
How do you see your future?

- Observe patient's nonverbal behaviors: isolating self, collecting harmful objects, giving away prized possessions.
- Does patient have a history of suicidal behavior?
- Assess the significance of inadequate pain control and any associated suicidal ideation.
- Observe for signs of depression: lack of interest in activities of daily living, insomnia, lack of appetite, sadness, physical complaints, hopelessness.
- Does patient exhibit impaired judgment that may result from substance abuse?
- Has patient experienced delusions or auditory hallucinations?
- Has patient experienced disorientation, memory impairment, acute or chronic confusion?
- Has patient made any attempts at suicide in the past? Method used? Place? Proximity of other people? Physical results?
- Does patient show *changes* in level of depression?
- Are any physical illnesses present that may be masked by other behaviors?
- Assess quality of social network.
- Utilize established scales for assessing suicide potential (e.g., The Los Angeles Suicide Prevention Center Scale for Assessing Suicidal Potential).
- In evaluating suicide *potential*, consider the following variables.
  - Verbalizations of wish to die with definite plan
  - Highly lethal plan with availability of resources
  - Previous suicide attempts or self-destructive behavior
  - Perception of suicide as a release or escape
  - Recent loss of significant person, possession, or role
  - Physical pain or illness
  - Alcohol or drug abuse
  - History of or current mental illness
  - Age and sex
  - Domestic difficulties, separation, divorce
  - Occupational status, unemployment
  - Retirement
  - Financial stress
  - Lack of religious beliefs

— Patient Outcomes and Interventions[1-39]

Patient Outcome: Remain Safe and Will Not Harm Self

- In community mental health setting, if risk is high, arrange for hospitalization immediately unless patient can be safely maintained and observed.
- Create flexible, therapeutic milieu which recognizes individual as

well as group needs and promotes constructive behavior (see Chapter 5—*milieu therapy*).
- Provide safe environment, which includes freedom from sharp objects and other harmful items, so the patient will not harm self (see Chapter 5—*protective interventions-observation for suicide prevention*).
    - Discuss with team members and decide what personal items to remove from the patient and what specific environmental hazards to eliminate.
- Evaluate with team members the necessity for close observation, area restriction procedures, or one-to-one observations for suicide prevention.
- Observe the patient closely
    - Put the patient on an observation level consistent with degree of risk, e.g., constant observation every 15 minutes or every 30 minutes (see Chapter 5—*protective interventions-observation for suicide prevention*).
    - Gradually reduce level of observation as patient risk improves.
    - Consider having the patient take on responsibility by "checking in" at assigned periods with staff.
    - For patients not on constant observation, use "no suicide or self-harm" contracts for intervening periods.
    - Emphasize protective, not punitive, attitude.
- Offer support against self-destructive impulses and suggest alternative behaviors.
- Set limits in relation to destructive behavior toward self or others.
- Permit expression of anger and hostility within these limits.
- Prevent isolation; seek out patient.
- Assess impact of patient's behavior on staff or other patients.

Patient Outcome: Perform Activities of Daily Living
- Reflect a caring, concerned attitude.
- Accept the patient as a worthwhile person while conveying that self-destructive behavior is not acceptable.
- Assist the patient in meeting activities of daily living, permitting as much independence as possible and keeping within the boundaries of patient's capabilities.
- Encourage simple decision making according to patient's limitations.

Patient Outcome: Develop Adaptive Methods to Cope with Stress and Decrease Potential for Suicide
- Offer hope (see Chapter 5—*supportive therapy: offering hope*). Point out that other ways are available to cope with what is happening. Communicate opportunity to reevaluate the situation when patient is not overwhelmed by desire to die.
- Help the patient look at positive aspects of living that can be anticipated in the future. Explore possible religious/spiritual beliefs that may assist the patient in avoiding suicide.

- Identify what the patient believes will be helpful.
- Assist the patient in identifying anxiety.
- Seek ways to lower anxiety in the patient.
- Teach the patient strategies for maintaining control (e.g., walking, or resting in bed) when emotional stress increases and to seek professional help when needed.
- Help the patient identify times when angry, sources of anger, and ways to channel anger.
- Avoid interpreting remarks such as "I'll kill myself before I do that" as attention-seeking behaviors.
- Listen with sensitivity to expressions of unworthiness, without insisting that words are false.
- Convey message that having bad thoughts and making mistakes does not mean one is a "bad person."
- Avoid imposing own feelings, values, and moral judgments.
- Assist the patient in developing realistic personal goals.
- Do not use a jubilant, cheerful approach.
- Encourage the patient to interact with others.
- Teach the patient decision-making and coping skills to prevent future suicidal threats, attempts, or actual suicides. Assist patient to use the following strategies: (See Chapter 5—*decision making*).
  - Explore the present situation.
  - Establish realistic goals. Master daily activities and rely on self as much as possible.
  - Minimize distraction from immediate desires and self-indulgence by recognizing each day as an opportunity to increase self-confidence and movement toward realistic goals.
  - Identify potential solutions to problem.
  - Evaluate consequences of different alternatives; encourage the patient to change alternatives when necessary.
  - Role-play options when possible.
  - Evaluate impact of actions.
  - Demonstrate courage, persistence, and self-possession to minimize negative feedback from others.
  - Use personal goals as an overall frame of focus in order to put complex situations into perspective.
  - Be assertive so that other people's opinions do not prevent one from accomplishing new or original activities or meeting personal goals. (See Chapter 5—*assertiveness training*).
  - Develop relationships through shared activities. Resist compromising self-identity or trying to remold others in case of differences.
  - Focus on positive, not negative, thoughts.
  - Avoid feeling obligated to reveal self to others continually.
  - Find solitude to gain strength and focus on personal direction.
  - Recognize that in future stressful situations, feelings of suicide may occur and that talking to someone is an important aspect of prevention.
  - List crisis line phone number and other numbers that may be useful in an emergency.

- Collaborate with the patient to set a daily schedule, allowing for flexibility, but making the most out of each part of the day.
- Encourage the patient to avoid substance abuse, becoming exhausted, or taking sedatives.
- Stress the importance of taking medications as ordered, especially after discharge from inpatient setting.

—— Evaluation/Outcome Criteria

- Suicide potential eliminated
- Demonstrates adequate coping skills in dealing with stressors
- Exhibits appropriate mood
- Verbalizes hope for own future
- Demonstrates positive self-concept
- Establishes meaningful relationships with others
- Demonstrates adequate role functioning
- Expresses feelings appropriately

■■ REFERENCES

1. Alger I: Manic-depression depression, and adolescent suicide. Hosp Community Psychiatry 40(4):347–349, 1989
2. Apter A, Plutchik R, Sevy S, Korn M, Brown S, van Praag H: Defense mechanisms in risk of suicide and risk of violence. Am J Psychiatry 146(8):1027–1031, 1989
3. Assey JL: The suicide prevention contract. Perspect Psychiatr Care 23(3):99–103, 1985
4. Barrett TW, Scott TB: Development of the grief experience questionnaire. Suicide Life Threat Behav 19(2):201–215, 1989
5. Bassuk EL: The prevention of suicide. Physician Assist 13(2):63–72, 1989
6. Blythe MM, Pearlmutter DR: The suicide watch. Perspect Psychiatr Care 21(3):90–93, 1983
7. Boxwell AO: Geriatric suicide: the preventable death. Nurse Pract 13(6):10–19, 1988
8. Bruss CR: Nursing diagnosis of hopelessness. J Psychosoc Nurs Ment Health Serv 26(3):28–31, 1988
9. Campbell L: Hopelessness; a concept analysis. J Psychosoc Nurs Ment Health Serv 25(2):18–22, 1989
10. Clark BA: Suicide threat. Nurs 85 15(6):47, 1985
11. Curran D: Adolescent suicidal behavior. Issues Ment Health Nurs 8(4):275–277, 1986
12. Demi AS, Miles MS: Suicide bereaved parents: emotional distress and physical health problems. Death Stud 12(4):297–307, 1988
13. Dunne-Maxim K: Survivors of suicide. J Psychosoc Nurs Ment Health Serv 24(12):31–35, 1986
14. Emrich K: Helping or hurting? Interacting in the psychiatric milieu. J Psychosoc Nurs Ment Health Serv 27(12):26–29, 1989
15. Favazza AR: Why patients multilate themselves. Hosp Community Psychiatry 49(2):127–145, 1989
16. Fischer K, Schwartz M: Potential for violence: self-directed or directed

at others. In Thompson JM, McFarland GK, Hirsch JE, Tucker SM, Bowers AC: Mosby's Manual of Clinical Nursing, 2nd ed. St Louis, CV Mosby, 1989

17. Frances A, Miller LJ: Coordinating inpatient and outpatient treatment for a chronically suicidal woman. Hosp Community Psychiatry 40(5):468–470, 1989

18. Gemma PB: Coping with suicidal behavior. MCN 14(2):101–103, 1989

19. Gilead MP, Mulaik JS: Adolescent suicide: a response to developmental crisis. Perspect Psychiatr Care 21(3):94–101, 1983

20. Hall JM, Stevens PE: AIDS: a guide to suicide assessment. Arch Psychiatr Nurs 1(2):115–120, 1988

21. Harsch HH, Holt RE: Use of antidepressants in attempted suicide. Hosp Community Psychiatry 39(9):990–992, 1988

22. Hogarty SS, Rodaitis CM: A suicide precautions policy for the general hospital. J Nurs Admin 17(10):36–44, 1987

23. Hradek EA: Crisis intervention and suicide. J Psychosoc Nurs Ment Health Serv 26(5):24–27, 1988

24. Kerr NJ: Signs and symptoms of depression and principles of nursing intervention. Perspect Psychiatr Care 24(2):48–63, 1987/88

25. Kibbee P: The suicidal patient: an issue for quality assurance and risk management. J Nurs Qual Assur 3(1):63–71, 1988

26. Kovarsky RS: Loneliness and disturbed grief: a comparison of parents who lost a child to suicide or accidental death. Arch Psychiatr Nurs 3(2):86–96, 1989

27. Landeen JJ: Patient suicide: its impact on the therapeutic milieu of a psychiatric unit. Perspect Psychiatr Care 24(2):74–78, 1987/88

28. Larson LA: Potential for violence: self-directed or directed at others. In McFarland GK, McFarlane EA: Nursing Diagnosis and Intervention: Planning for Patient Care. St Louis, CV Mosby, 1989

29. Lion JR: Violence and suicide within the hospital. In Lion JR, Adler WN, Webb WL: Modern Hospital Psychiatry. New York, WW Norton & Co, 1988

30. Long KA: Suicide intervention and prevention with Indian adolescent populations. Issues Ment Health Nurs 8:247–253, 1986

31. Mullis MR, Hyers PH: Social support in suicidal inpatients. J Psychosoc Nurs Ment Health Serv 25(4):16–19, 1987

32. Nkongho NO: Suicide in the elderly: a beginning investigation. J National Black Nurses 2(2):47–57, 1988

33. Pallikkathayil L, Morgan SA: Emergency department nurses' encounters with suicide attempters: a qualitative investigation. Schol Inq Nurs Pract 2(3):237–253, 1988

34. Parker SD: Accident or suicide: do life change events lead to adolescent suicide? J Psychosoc Nurs Ment Health Serv 26(6):15–19, 1988

35. Saunders JM, Buckingham SL: When the depression turns deadly. Nurs 18(7):59–64, 1988

36. Spillers GM: Suicide potential. In McFarland GK, Thomas MD: Psychiatric Mental Health Nursing. Philadelphia, JB Lippincott, 1991

37. Thompson J, Brooks S: When a colleague commits suicide: how the staff reacts. J Psychosoc Nurs Ment Health Serv 28(10):6–11, 1990

38. Valente SM: Assessing suicide risk in the school-age child. J Pediatr Health Care 1(1):14–20, 1987

39. vanDongen CJ: The legacy of suicide. J Psychosoc Nurs Ment Health Serv 26(1):9–13, 1988

■ THOUGHT PROCESSES, ALTERED (ACUTE CONFUSION)

— Definition

Altered thought processes (acute confusion) is the abrupt onset of a cluster of transient changes and disturbances in attention, cognition, perception, psychomotor activity, and/or sleep patterns.[8,14]

— General Principles[1-22]

- The condition can become life-threatening if underlying causes are not treated.
- The patient is not necessarily disoriented in all spheres; disorientation to time occurs first, with disorientation to person last.
- Patients who have chronic confusion can also have periods of acute confusion.
- The assumption should *not* be made that disorientation is a natural consequence of aging.
- The assumption should *not* be made that disorientation is an expected natural course of changes in physiological status.
- Although mental status changes are of relatively brief duration; e.g., hours to several weeks, they are usually very frightening to the patient and family.
- Reduced level of consciousness (not always present) results in impaired awareness of self and surroundings.
- Fluctuations, waxing and waning, of mental impairment may occur from hour to hour or from day to day.
- Changes and disturbances are usually self-limiting, once the underlying cause is identified and dealt with.
- Pharmacologic management focuses on minimal use of benzodiazepines and antidepressants because of their potentiating effects on confusion (alcohol withdrawal, however, can be treated with benzodiazepines).

— Related Factors[1-22]

Vascular disorder, e.g., migraine, transient ischemic attacks, congestive heart failure, pulmonary embolism
Hematopoietic system disorders, e.g., severe anemia
Neurological conditions; e.g., head trauma, seizures, intracranial neoplasm
Metabolic encephalopathies; e.g., hypoglycemia, hyperinsulinism, dehydration, water intoxication, hypervitaminosis, vitamin deficiency
Addictive inhalants; e.g., glue, ether, nitrites, nitrous oxide

Poisons; e.g., industrial, mushrooms
Infectious processes
Injury by physical agents; e.g., heat stroke, hypothermia due to
  exposure to cold
Intoxication from alcohol, nonprescription, or recreational (street)
  drugs
Intoxication from prescription drugs, e.g., antipsychotics,
  antiparkinsonian agents, benzodiazepines, antihypertensive
  drugs, lithium, narcotic and non-narcotic analgesics, disulfiram
  (Antabuse)
Withdrawal from alcohol, sedatives, or hypnotics
Sleep deprivation
Sensory deprivation or sensory overload
High psychological stress associated with a severe physical illness
  and threat of death
Severe psychosocial stress, e.g., bereavement and relocation in the
  elderly
Social isolation

— Defining Characteristics[1-22]

Elevated blood pressure
Tachycardia
Perspiring
Dilated pupils
Flushed face
Abnormal psychomotor activity, hypoactivity or hyperactivity
Altered sleep-wake cycle; e.g., daytime drowsiness and napping
  and/or insomnia at night
Acute onset of mental status changes
Disorientation for time, place, and person with greater variation in
  disorientation to time
Unpredictable fluctuations in levels of alertness and ability to
  concentrate
Impaired attention; easily distracted
Disorganized thinking
Impaired memory
Rambling, irrelevant, or incoherent speech
Confabulation
Fragmentation in conversation
Perseveration
Inconsistent fluctuations in mood and emotional responses, e.g.,
  anger, fear, apathy, depression, euphoria
Illusions, misinterpretations of stimuli and environment
Vivid visual hallucinations (most commonly) and/or auditory
  hallucinations, tactile hallucinations
Transient, shifting and poorly organized delusions, usually of
  persecutory nature
Delusions that hallucinations are real
Lack of motivation to initiate and to successfully sustain goal-
  directed purposeful actions.

— Nursing Assessment[1-22]

- Obtain the following information from patient, family, and staff:
  - When did the confusion begin? Was there a sudden onset of mental status changes? Was there a sudden change in usual behavioral patterns, activities of daily living (ADL)?
  - Has the patient ever experienced anything of this nature before?
  - Is the patient easily distracted or having difficulty focusing attention?
  - Are there changes in short-term and/or long-term memory?
  - Observe for disorganized thinking; e.g., rambling, irrelevant conversation, abrupt shifting from one topic to another.
  - Assess level of consciousness; e.g., alert, hyperalert, drowsy, easily aroused, stuporous, coma.
  - Check for evidence of disorientation; are there fluctuations in orientation ability?
  - Assess the patient's sleep-wakefulness patterns; e.g., drowsiness during day and awake at night.
  - Observe for behaviors indicative of delusional thinking or hallucinations, particularly visual hallucinations.
  - Is the patient experiencing illusions or misinterpretations?
  - What is the patient's activity pattern? Observe for evidence of psychomotor activity or psychomotor retardation.
- What are the patient's vital signs?
- Review the patient's current prescription as well as over-the-counter medication history; has a new medication been introduced?
- Is there evidence of infection; e.g., pulmonary, urinary tract?
- Review laboratory work for variations from normal limits; e.g., electrolytes, thyroid functioning, BUN, WBC, hemoglobin, hematocrit.
- Does the patient use street drugs, alcohol?
- What is the state of the patient's overall health, including current medical problems for which the patient is receiving treatment?
- Has the patient experienced recent psychosocial stressors?
- What is the patient's current living situation and social support?
- Conduct periodic brief cognitive assessments throughout the day to determine presence of waxing and waning of symptoms; e.g., orientation, attention and concentration, memory, thought processes; do not rely on orientation findings alone to determine extent or presence of acute confusion.
- Collaborate with physician to determine contributing factors to current findings.

— Patient Outcomes and Nursing Interventions[1-22]

Patient Outcome: Differentiate Between Reality and Unreality

- Call patient by preferred name; introduce self each time; use clear and specific verbal communication; stand or sit within easy viewing by the patient; avoid sudden, rapid physical movement.

- Give a brief, simple explanation of the purpose for being with the patient; avoid complex interactions.
- Provide consistency in assigning staff who work with the patient—one nurse per shift, if possible.
- Ensure that any sensory aids used by the patient are available and in working order, e.g., glasses, hearing aids, dentures; encourage the patient to use them.
- Eliminate unnecessary environmental stimuli; keep equipment noise to a minimum; avoid overuse of television and radio.
- Provide appropriate visual cues; e.g., clock and calendar within easy viewing, watch, familiar photos.
- Use appropriate tactile cues; e.g., handshake, place hand on patient's shoulder.
- Provide adequate, nonglare lighting to prevent shadows from distorting visual perceptions.
- Provide privacy.
- Check the patient's orientation at varied intervals; gently correct misinformation without confrontation; incorporate orientation information during course of routine conversation.
- Teach family and friends techniques for reinforcing reality with patient.
- Do not argue or agree with delusional material or hallucinatory experiences; acknowledge recognition of patient's distress with these experiences; assure the patient that he or she will be safe in present environment.
- Encourage the patient and family to report hallucinations, frightening thoughts, and beliefs that the patient experiences.
- Assure the patient and family that distressing mental status changes, delusions, hallucinations, problems with concentration and memory will go away.

Patient Outcome: Experience No Injury to Self or Others in Environment

- Ensure presence of adequate staff to be with the patient.
- Explain safety mechanisms in immediate environment; e.g., call light, side rails, night light.
- Remove unnecessary clutter from immediate environment.
- Ensure provision of adequate lighting in the patient's immediate area.
- Use distraction to decrease aggressive, excited, confused responses.
- Use restraints as needed.
- Teach the patient proper use of equipment, e.g., walker, wheelchair, IV standard.

Patient Outcome: Maintain Adequate Fluid and Nutritional Intake

- Monitor food and fluid intake; document intake and output if necessary.
- Collaborate with dietary department if additional fluid and food supplements are indicated.

- Supervise and assist during mealtimes as needed.
- Observe for signs of dehydration.

Patient Outcome: Maintain Optimal Pattern of Elimination

- Be sure that patient has regular toileting schedule.
- Check for bowel or bladder incontinence to prevent skin breakdown.
- Encourage intake of food and fluids to prevent constipation.
- Give stool softeners as needed.

Patient Outcome: Experience Improved Sleep-Wakefulness Cycle

- Provide scheduled periods of undisturbed rest, particularly at night.
- Discourage daytime naps.
- Facilitate a day and night activity pattern.
- Collaborate with the patient and family to assist in identification of techniques for promoting rest and sleep (back rub, soothing music, routine hygiene activities).
- Minimize or eliminate unnecessary, unfamiliar environmental noise, e.g., loud radio or television, conversations by staff.

Patient Outcome: Meet Self-Care Needs to Extent Possible

- Give one-step, simple commands, allowing for completion of one task at a time.
- Encourage the patient to do as much for self as possible; assist as needed with hygiene, bathing, grooming.
- Allow reasonable time for completing activities; do not rush patient.

Patient Outcome: Maintain Personal and Social Integrity

- Include family and significant others in the patient's care.
- Recognize the likelihood that the patient and family are experiencing increased distress regarding patient's mental status changes and fluctuations; acknowledge their fears and concerns; provide them with explanations about changes in behavior.
- Encourage family and friends to maintain regular contact with patient and to share ongoing information regarding family activities and plans, particularly those that involve the patient.
- Incorporate recognition of the patient's past strengths and accomplishments during the course of brief conversations with patient and family.
- Reinforce appropriate behaviors.

—— Evaluation/Outcome Criteria

- Reports satisfactory sleep pattern
- Increased orientation to time, place, and person
- Increased ability to concentrate and attend to environmental stimuli
- Initiates and follows through with goal-directed activities
- Regains optimal self-care and role functioning

■ REFERENCES

1. Abraham IL, Fox JM, Harrington DP, et al: A psychogeriatric nursing assessment: protocol for use in multidisciplinary practice. Arch Psychiatr Nurs 4(4):242–259, 1990
2. American Psychiatric Association: Diagnostic and Statistical Manual of Mental Disorders, 3rd ed, rev. Washington, DC, American Psychiatric Association, 1987
3. Batt LJ: Managing delirium: implications for geropsychiatric nurses. J Psychosoc Nurs Ment Health Serv 27(5):22–25, 31, 32, 1989
4. Blank K, Perry S: Relationship of psychological processes during delirium to outcome. Am J Psychiatry 141(7):843–847, 1984
5. Brady PF: Labeling of confusion in the elderly. J Gerontol Nurs 13(6):29–32, 1987
6. DeBoer G, Wilson HS: Applying the nursing process for clients with organic mental syndromes and disorders. In Wilson HS, Kneisl CR: Psychiatric Nursing, 3rd ed. Menlo Park, CA, Addison Wesley, 1988
7. Eklund ES: Perception/cognition, altered (confusion). In McFarland GK, Thomas MD: Psychiatric Mental Health Nursing. Philadelphia, JB Lippincott, 1991
8. Foreman MD: Acute confusional states in hospitalized elderly: a research dilemma. Nurs Res 35(1):34–38, 1986
9. Foreman MD: Confusion in the hospitalized elderly: incidence, onset, an associated factors. Res Nurs Health 12:21–29, 1989
10. Francis J, Kapoor WN: Delirium in hospitalized elderly. J Gen Int Med 5:65–79, 1990
11. Francis J, Martin D, Kapoor WN: Prospective study of delirium in hospitalized elderly. JAMA 263(8):1097–1101, 1990
12. Gomez GE, Gomez EA: Delirium. Geriatr Nurs 8(6):330–332, 1987
13. Inouye SK, van Dyck CH, Alessi CA, Balkin S, Siegal AP, Horwitz RI: Clarifying confusion: the confusion assessment method. Ann Int Med 113(12):941–948, 1990
14. Lipowski ZJ: Delirium: Acute Confusional States. New York, Oxford University Press, 1990
15. Luna-Raines M: The confused response. In Riegel B, Ehrenreich D (eds): Psychological Aspects of Critical Care Nursing. Rockville, MD, Aspen Publishers, 1989
16. Nelson MK: Organic mental disorders. In Hogstel MO (ed): Geropsychiatric Nursing. St Louis, CV Mosby, 1990
17. Rockwood K: Acute confusion in elderly medical patients. J Am Geriatr Soc 37:150–154, 1989
18. Stuart GW, Sundeen SJ: Principles and Practice of Psychiatric Nursing, 3rd ed. St Louis, CV Mosby, 1987
19. Williams MA, Ward SE, Campbell EB: Confusion: testing versus observation. J Gerontol Nurs 14(1):25–30, 1988
20. Wise MG: Delirium. In Hales RE, Yudofsky SC (eds): The American Psychiatric Press Textbook of Neuropsychiatry. Wash DC, American Psychiatric Press, 1987
21. Wolanin MO, Phillips LRF: Confusion: Prevention and Care. St Louis, CV Mosby, 1981
22. Yazdanfar DJ: Assessing the mental status of the cognitively impaired elderly. J Gerontol Nurs 16(9):32–36, 1990

■ THOUGHT PROCESS, ALTERED (DELUSIONS)

— Definition

Altered thought processes (delusions) are fixed, false personal beliefs that are inconsistent with reality.[9,13]

— General Principles[1–13]

- Beliefs may encompass many aspects of the patient's life or may be circumscribed to one particular area.
- The patient may be resistive to seeking or accepting treatment.
- Preoccupation with beliefs may interfere with the ability to successfully maintain relationships with family, friends; it may prevent gainful employment and lead to other personal distress.
- Content and consistency of delusions may be influenced by cultural beliefs, as well as biological and psychosocial factors.
- Research suggests that a prefrontal system disorder may be a factor in patients with schizophrenia who are delusional.

— Related Factors[9,13]

Severe threats to physiological integrity
    Nutritional disturbances
    Metabolic disturbances
    Neoplasms
    Infections
    General paresis
Alcohol or drug intoxication
Severe psychosocial stressors
Perception of personal inadequacy
Anxiety
Loneliness
Aggressive feelings

— Defining Characteristics[9,13]

Incorrect inferences about external reality
Belief that there is direct relationship between events or activities of
    others and threat to self
Beliefs of being under control by an external person or force
    through thought insertion (beliefs that others put ideas into
    one's head) or thought withdrawal (beliefs that others remove
    thoughts from one's head)
Beliefs that one's thoughts are being broadcast and can be heard by
    others
Feelings of persecution and victimization
Erroneous somatic beliefs about alterations in body or bodily
    functions
Resistive to treatment
Grandiose beliefs about self and abilities
Preoccupation with belief(s)

Impaired ability to evaluate own perceptions and thoughts
Easily irritated when others do not subscribe to beliefs
Impaired relationship with others
Difficulties with work role

— Nursing Assessment[1–13]

- Is the patient at risk for acting on delusional beliefs, e.g., harming self or others?
- Has the patient acted on delusional beliefs in past?
- Verify that the patient's statements are indeed delusional.
- Obtain accurate drug history, including prescription and over-the-counter drugs, as well as street drugs.
- Obtain information about alcohol use and abuse.
- Use family and significant others for gathering and verifying information about delusional beliefs.
- Review findings from medical work-up to rule out organic causes for delusional thinking.
- Evaluate the extent that delusional beliefs affect meeting self-care needs, e.g., nutritional needs (food is "poisoned"), hygiene and grooming (believes the body is made of cardboard and will disintegrate in water).
- How long has the patient experienced delusions?
- In what ways do delusions interfere with role performance, employment, living arrangements, attentiveness to health needs and problems, financial management?
- Does the patient indicate awareness of problem and desire help?
- What are patient's beliefs about psychotropic medication?
- Determine availability of social support and services, family, friends, community.

— Patient Outcomes and Nursing Interventions[1–13]

Patient Outcome: Experience Decreased or No Distortion of False Beliefs

- Listen for description of delusional thinking during initial assessment period; avoid encouragement of further descriptions in subsequent interactions.
- Give feedback concerning a delusion in terms of feeling tone expressed, such as the fear it may generate for the patient, or the loneliness the patient is experiencing.
- Convey recognition that beliefs are real to the patient, if the patient requests opinion, but express doubt, e.g., "I realize those thoughts are very real to you, but they sound *very* unusual to me."
- Do not expect rational explanations to change the patient's mind and correct delusion.
- Avoid arguing with, challenging, or trying to convince the patient of erroneous thinking and conclusions.
- Refocus conversation to another topic after listening carefully to delusion.

- Provide experiences in the here and now that the patient can talk to others about and have experiences validated by others.
- Observe for possible precipitant of delusional conversation; assist the patient to begin to recognize possible stressors; help the patient learn ways to avoid or eliminate factors that contribute to delusional thinking.
- Teach the patient the following:
  - Ways to control thoughts (i.e., to distract self from thinking same thought over and over, to become involved in concrete activities)
  - To recognize when thoughts are becoming disorganized (i.e., finding self jumping from subject to subject)
  - To anticipate increased anxiety in a new situation and to think of a way to decrease the anxiety
  - To check out ideas and thoughts with others
  - To practice thought-stopping technique
  - To engage in thought-switching technique
  - To dispute irrational thoughts
  - To use problem-solving process
  - To learn when, where, and with whom delusional talk can be shared
- Teach patient's family how to respond to and manage the patient's delusions.

Patient Outcome: Avoid Harming Self or Others

- Ask the patient about thoughts of harming self or others.
- Inform appropriate professional staff, family, or significant others if the patient seems to be a danger to self or others because of delusional beliefs.
- Inform the patient that potential harmfulness to self or others has been shared with appropriate staff and others.
- Encourage compliance with recommendations for prescribed psychotropic medication.

Patient Outcome: Engage in Self-Care Activities

- Elicit verbalization of fears and concerns regarding factors that impede self-care activities such as eating, bathing, grooming.
- Try to negotiate/arrive at some sort of compromise in areas in which the patient expresses reluctance; that is, try to provide foods the patient sees as safe to eat, allow distance at meal time, have the patient choose a time when bathing is least frightening.
- Convey recognition of progress in attending to self-care needs.

Patient Outcome: Engage in Socially Acceptable and Rewarding Activities

- Collaborate with the patient to determine realistic goals for socialization.
- Respect needs for solitude and isolation.
- Suggest that the patient choose small, realistic goals, preferably

one at a time, to ensure success; e.g., identifying and engaging in one pleasurable activity during the coming week.

- Do not attempt to force the patient to engage in an activity that is contrary to delusional beliefs.
- Assist the patient in developing a daily schedule that minimizes environmental factors that trigger delusional thinking and stimulates interest in what is occurring in real world.

— Evaluation/Outcome Criteria

Demonstrates decrease in delusional thinking
Demonstrates improved ability to relate with others
Meets self-care needs
Absence of harm to self or others

■ REFERENCES

1. Benson DF, Stuss DT: Frontal lobe influences on delusions: a clinical perspective. Schizophr Bull 16(3):403–411, 1990
2. Chesla C: Clients with schizophrenia and other psychotic disorders. In Wilson HS, Kniesl CR: Psychiatric Nursing, 3rd ed. Menlo Park, Addison-Wesley, 1988
3. Hemsley DR, Garety PA: The formation and maintenance of delusions: a Bayesian analysis. Br J Psychiatry 149:51–56, 1986
4. Houseman C: The paranoid person: a biopsychosocial perspective. Arch Psychiatr Nurs 4(3):176–181, 1990
5. Lindner R: The jet-propelled couch. In The Fifty-Minute Hour: A Collection of True Psychoanalytic Tales. New York, Holt, Rinehart, Winston, 1961
6. Mitchell J, Vierkant AD: Delusions and hallucinations as a reflection of the subcultural milieu among psychotic patients in the 1930s and 1980s. J Psychol 123(3):269–274, 1989
7. Riley B: Schizophrenia, paranoid disorders, anxiety disorders, and somatoform disorders. In Hogstel MO (ed): Geropsychiatric Nursing. St Louis, CV Mosby, 1990
8. Rosenthal TT, McGinness TM: Dealing with delusional patients: discovering the distorted truth. Issues Ment Health Nurs 8:143–154, 1986
9. Scheideman J: Perception/cognition, altered (delusions). In McFarland GK, Thomas MD: Psychiatric Mental Health Nursing. Philadelphia, JB Lippincott, 1991
10. Sinha VK, Chaturvedi SK: Consistency of delusions in schizophrenia and affective disorder. Schizophr Res 3:347–350, 1990
11. Stein MB, Forbes RD: Delusional disorder in mother and daughter: a case report. Can J Psychiatry 32:387–388, 1987
12. Tousley MM: The paranoid fortress of David J. J Psychosoc Nurs Ment Health Serv 22(2):8–16, 1984
13. Whitley G: Clients with delusional (paranoid disorder). In McFarland GK, Thomas MD: Psychiatric Mental Health Nursing. Philadelphia, JB Lippincott, 1991

■ THOUGHT PROCESSES, ALTERED (HALLUCINATIONS)

— Definition[9]

Altered thought processes (hallucinations) are false sensory experiences not based on reality that may be triggered by external or internal stimuli.

— General Principles[5,7,8,10]

- Although neuroleptics may decrease the anxiety associated with hallucinations, medications do not always eliminate their presence.
- Hallucinations are frequently of sudden onset, which can be very frightening to the patient.
- The age of onset varies, beginning as early as age 6.
- Patients with frightening, especially persecutory auditory hallucinations, may harm themselves or others.
- Auditory hallucinations occur most commonly, but any sensory organ can be involved.
- Attempts to cope with auditory hallucinations may evolve through phases.
  1. The startle phase in which the person is frightened;
  2. The organization phase in which the person selects and communicates with the voice(s);
  3. The stabilization phase in which the person adopts a pattern of dealing with the voices.
- Auditory hallucinations can be perceived as positive or negative, e.g., with positive hallucinations the person can feel strengthened and view self positively. The "good-bad" trajectory of auditory hallucinations is very complex and is not totally understood.
- The duration of hallucinations varies from brief periods to several decades.
- The onset of hallucinations requires a thorough evaluation to rule out organic causes.
- Variables that affect individual responses in coping with auditory hallucinations include
  1. Attributed meaning and level of friendliness in voice and message;
  2. Degree of acceptance of voice as part of self versus alien to self;
  3. Nature of voice (e.g., spiritual) and reaching a peaceful acceptance of voice as part of self.
- An explanatory model for auditory hallucinations includes four factors:
  1. Internal arousal or mood disturbance;
  2. Predisposition or presence of critical threshold for hallucinatory experience;
  3. External stimulation—determines whether the patient experiences the hallucination in consciousness;

    4. Positive reinforcement occurs as the hallucinatory experience results in successful relief of tension.

—— Related Factors[2,4,5,9,10]

Sleep deprivation
Sensory deprivation
Substance abuse
Organic syndromes
Psychiatric disorder
Traumatic emotional event
Severe interpersonal difficulties
Dissociated emotional difficulties
Psychodynamic factors
Social isolation
Loneliness

—— Defining Characteristics[2,4,5,9,10]

Inability to attend to self-care needs, e.g., unkempt hair, disheveled, dirty clothes, malnourished
Suicidal thought, suicide attempt
Inattention to daily role responsibilities, e.g., absence from work, inability to complete housekeeping tasks
Sense of bewilderment
Feeling of helplessness
Loss of control over focal awareness
Diffuse thinking
Nonresponse to external stimuli
Misinterpretation of external reality
Listening posture and attitude
Averted gaze, often at some elevated point
Nonreality-based behaviors, e.g., lips moving, talking or mumbling to self
Autistic reverie
Decreased arousal level
Increasingly more restricted lifestyle
Feelings of dependency on voices
Distancing or alienation from significant others
Anxiety in presence of others
Social withdrawal
Problems with the law
Shame and embarrassment
Negative auditory hallucinations:
    Inner turmoil and chaos
    Loss of energy because of intrusive nature of hallucinations
Helpful auditory hallucinations:
    Feelings of recognition and trust
    Increased self-esteem
    Increased self-strength

—— Nursing Assessment[1-10]

- Assess for suicidal potential or other intentions to harm self, homicidal intent, or plans to inflict injury to others.
- Evaluate for actual presence of hallucinations by direct questioning of the patient.
- Observe for antecedents of hallucinatory experience, e.g., traumatic emotional event, anxiety-producing situation.
- Thoroughly explore evolution and experience of hallucinations for the patient; i.e., to evaluate role of hallucinations in the patient's individual dynamics and to identify areas of conflict and concern. Identify major themes and affect related to themes.
- Are command hallucinations present? What is the nature of them? Does patient follow the commands? What time of day and in what circumstances do hallucinations tend to occur?
- Has the patient previously experienced hallucinations? For how long? When did the patient have the initial experience of hallucinations? How has patient responded to, coped with, and attempted to control them in the past? What has been the patient's affective response to hallucinations?
- To what extent does the patient actually experience the hallucinations as real, and to what extent can he or she differentiate the experience from reality?
- Evaluate the degree of impact of hallucinations on role performance and activities of daily living.
- Assess the patient's level of fear and anxiety.
- If patient is on medication, note the actual effects on patient; obtain information about actual compliance with medication schedule.

—— Patient Outcomes and Nursing Interventions[1-10]

Patient Outcome: Experience Decrease in Frequency and Intensity of Hallucinations

- In collaboration with psychiatrist, administer neuroleptics to reduce anxiety and hallucinations.
- Assist the patient to decrease fear. Assure the patient that he or she is in a safe environment and will be protected.
- Involve the patient in a supportive one-to-one relationship, with goal of strengthening ego functions.
- Find out the patient's past coping strategies for dealing with hallucinations.
- Explore the patient's frame of reference and underlying feelings and dynamics of hallucinations.
- After initial assessment, focus attention on the underlying feelings and dynamics of the hallucinations and avoid undue attention on the description of the actual content.
- According to the patient's response, redirect attention and involve the patient in interesting and meaningful activities, especially those involving a verbal response or those involving information-processing activities.
- Introduce meaningful auditory stimulus for those patients whose

hallucinations decrease in response. Base these activities on what the patient has found helpful in the past.
- For those patients experiencing increased hallucinations with increased stimulation, identify ways to lessen interpersonal stress and environmental exposure to stimuli.
- Refer the patient for psychotherapy.

Patient Outcome: Acquire Increased Understanding of and Ability to Manage Hallucinations

- Promote self-esteem (see *self-esteem disturbance* in this chapter).
- Explore with the patient the meaning of hallucination for the patient; e.g., is the patient attempting to escape from something?
- Help the patient differentiate between "good" and "bad" voices.
- Teach the patient to monitor symptoms that may be warning signs of relapse; e.g., sleep disturbance, decreased concentration.
- Explore with the patient the helpfulness of a variety of strategies for dealing with hallucinations; e.g., ignoring them; listening, understanding, and talking to positive voices; accepting hallucinations as part of self.
- Teach the patient dismissal intervention, which may be helpful to some patients. Care must be used, however, since extinguishing hallucinations in patients with chronic mental illness may be counterproductive. Steps include (1) Validate whether the patient is hearing voices; e.g., "Mrs. Jones, are you hearing voices right now?" (2) Say to patient, "I can tell you how to stop those disturbing voices." (3) Tell the patient to say loudly and clearly several times, "Go away and leave Mrs. Jones alone."
- Help the patient to develop self-monitoring and self-regulatory strategies to deal with the hallucinations. Assist the patient in recognizing anxiety and other signs and symptoms prodromal to hallucinations. Teach the patient strategies for dealing with anxiety (see *anxiety* in this chapter). Use dismissal intervention, if appropriate. Identify with the patient other self-regulatory strategies; e.g., self-instruction, increased involvement in meaningful activities (jogging, seeking company of others, sports), decreased involvement in stressful activities, strategies to deal with emotions (sleep, relaxation techniques, music). (See Chapter 5—*stress management.*)
- Teach the patient information about hallucinatory experiences and help the patient understand and realize that these experiences are part of the illness.
- Teach the patient to limit hallucinatory experiences to a private place so as not to upset others.
- Encourage the patient to discuss hallucinations with other patients experiencing them so as to decrease sense of isolation, carefully timing readiness for this.

—— Evaluation/Outcome Criteria

Verbalizes decrease in hallucinations
Meets self-care needs

Describes effective coping strategies for living with auditory hallucinations

Describes purpose, dosage, side effects, and scheduled time of medication accurately

▬ REFERENCES

1. Benjamin LS: Is chronicity a function of the relationship between the person and the auditory hallucination? Schizophr Bull 15(2):305–310, 1989
2. Carpenito LJ: Altered thoughts or altered perceptions? AJN 11:1283, 1985
3. Eastwood MR, Corbin S: Hallucinations in patients admitted to a geriatric psychiatry service: review of 42 cases. J Am Geriatr Soc 31(10):593–597, 1983
4. Field WE: Hearing voices. J Psychosoc Nurs Ment Health Serv 23(1):9–14, 1985
5. Romme MAJ, Escher DMAC: Hearing voices. Schizophr Bull 15(2):209–216, 1989
6. Schwartz MS, Shockley EL: The Nurse and the Mental Patient. New York, Russell Sage Foundation, 1956
7. Slade PD: The external control of auditory hallucinations. An information theory analysis. Br J Clin Soc Psychol 6:123–132, 1976
8. Slade PD: Towards a theory of auditory hallucinations: outline of an hypothetical four-factor model. Br J Soc Clin Psychol 15:415–423, 1976
9. Thomas MD: Perception/cognition, altered (hallucinations). In McFarland GK, Thomas MD: Psychiatric Mental Health Nursing. Philadelphia, JB Lippincott, 1991
10. Williams CA: Perspectives on the hallucinatory process. Issues Ment Health Nurs 10:99–119, 1989

▬ THOUGHT PROCESSES, ALTERED (SUSPICIOUSNESS)

— Definition

Suspiciousness is a mode of interacting manifested by pervasive mistrust of others.[6,8]

— General Principles[1–10]

- Persons who mistrust others are often viewed as being untrustworthy.
- While a sense of trust is developed in early years, later encounters can shape a person's level of trust or suspiciousness.

— Related Factors[6,8]

Sensory organ impairment
Organic mental disorder

Psychoactive substance disorder
Fears of loss of autonomy or loss of self-control
Aggression
Crisis, maturational and situational
Anxiety
Psychiatric disorder
Low self-esteem

—— Defining Characteristics[6,8]

Poor interpersonal relationships
Guarded affect
Flat affect
Inflexible thinking
Overuse of projection
Difficulty sharing knowledge of self with others
Withdrawal from others
Frequent isolation from others; conveyance of a superior attitude
Belief in conspiracy; feelings of being persecuted and misjudged
Misinterpretation of another's intentions
Misinterpretation of acts of others followed by an aggressive
    response
Alienation
Tense manner
Impaired problem solving
Discomfort with own motivation and goals
Difficulty in accepting other's viewpoint, especially if different from
    own
Difficulty in accepting new experiences
Ineffective use of resources

—— Nursing Assessment[1-10]

- Determine if there is a relationship between expression of
  suspiciousness and potential for aggression.
- Ascertain the impact of suspiciousness on areas of daily activities
  and lifestyle.
- Find out any history of legal problems and occupational
  difficulties relative to the mistrust of others.
- Assess the patient's history of family interactions.
- Determine the extent and quality of contact with significant
  others.
- Identify the patient's assessment of strengths and limitations.
- Examine the patient's fear of loss of control.
- Assess the perception of need for help.
- Identify areas in which the patient accepts help.
- Evaluate use of health resources and compliance with treatment
  regimen.
- Assess reasons, meanings, dynamics, for underlying
  suspiciousness.

—— Patient Outcomes and Nursing Interventions[1-10]

Patient Outcome: Develop an Increasing Sense of Trust of the Environment and Others

- Give clear, concise information when answering questions or offering explanations of what is occurring.
- Avoid whispering.
- Establish trusting interpersonal relationship with the patient (see Chapter 2).
- Establish a milieu in which the patient feels safe and protected (see Chapter 5—*milieu therapy*).
- Inform the patient of schedule changes as soon as possible.
- Be extremely honest about all interactions with the patient. Follow through on what you or the staff have promised.
- Avoid talking to others about the patient in the patient's presence.
- Do not try to prove the patient wrong or challenge the patient.
- Acknowledge the plausible aspects of suspiciousness; e.g., "You may not be able to trust all persons; on the other hand, there is no reason to think that *no* one can be trusted."
- Be aware of situations in which the patient attempts to prove his or her expectations of suspiciousness.
- Question gently the beliefs of the patient.
- Respect the client's experience without agreeing with it; e.g., "I am aware that this is distressful for you, but I have no reason to believe that all of the staff on this unit hate you."
- Convey understanding of the patient's dilemma without arguing about beliefs.
- Respond to the patient's suspiciousness by reflecting on theme or feeling symbolically expressed: "It must be very distressing for you to believe that . . . ;" "I have not experienced him as threatening."
- Question the logic behind suspiciousness; e.g., "You think Sue is against you?"
- Avoid putting the patient on defensive so that he or she has to protect self.
- Refrain from correcting misinterpretations through reasoning.
- Once the dynamics of the suspiciousness are understood, do not encourage repetitive talk about it. Focus instead on the underlying feelings or process.
- Note inconsistency between actual behavior and verbal statements of "everything is fine."
- Acknowledge awareness for process and feelings behind the suspiciousness; e.g., "You must feel really lonely to believe that all your friends are against you."
- Give positive feedback when the patient demonstrates trust of another.

Patient Outcome: Experience Decreased Mistrust and Improved Interpersonal Relationships

- Initially, make frequent, short interpersonal contacts. Minimal number of staff should make these initial contacts.

- Assist the patient in identifying people with whom it is appropriate to share thoughts.
- Discuss consequences to the patient of continued suspiciousness of others.
- Give assurance that the environment is safe.
- Listen, demonstrating an accepting attitude.
- Set limits on aggressive acts toward others.
- Give feedback when patient is noted to be insulting and threatening towards others.
- Respect the patient's privacy.
- Teach the patient the following:
  - To become consciously aware of feelings of suspiciousness and to make an effort to check them out objectively or to act appropriately despite the fear
  - The importance of dealing with feelings and personal space and not with the whole environment
  - Problem solving as one way of dealing with misinterpretations of reality
  - Steps in the formation of a trusting relationship, such as introducing self, spending time with another, being aware of the other's needs, sharing something in common
  - To validate perceptions with others
  - To recognize the consequences of suspiciousness on the patient's life and activities of daily living
- Encourage the patient to participate in group therapy, after level of suspiciousness has lessened

— Evaluation/Outcome Criteria

Participates in activities of daily living
Makes appropriate appraisals of situations and people
Enjoys adequate role responsibility
Demonstrates increased levels of trust

■ REFERENCES

1. Barefoot JC, Siegler IC, Nowlin JB, Peterson BL, Haney TL, Williams RB: Suspiciousness, health, and mortality: a follow-up study of 500 older adults. Psychosom Med 49:450–457, 1987
2. DiBella GAW: Educating staff to manage threatening paranoid patients. Am J Psychiatry 136(3):333–335, 1979
3. Kendler KS, Heath A, Martin NA: A genetic epidemiologic study of self-report suspiciousness. Compr Psychiatry 28(3):187–196, 1987
4. Knowles RD: Control your thoughts. AJN (2):353, 1981
5. Knowles RD: Disputing irrational thoughts. AJN 81(4):735, 1981
6. Scheideman J: Suspiciousness. In McFarland GK, Thomas MD: Psychiatric Mental Health Nursing. Philadelphia, JB Lippincott, 1991
7. Shroder RJ: Nursing intervention with patients with thought disorders. Perspect Psychiatr Care 17(1):32–39, 1979

8. Thomas MD: Trust in the nurse-patient relationship. In Carlson CC (ed): Behavioral Concepts and Nursing Intervention. Philadelphia, JB Lippincott, 1970
9. Thorne SE et al: Reciprocal trust in health care relationships. J Adv Nurs 13(6):782–789, 1988
10. Tousley MM: The paranoid fortress of David J. J Psychosoc Nurs Ment Health Serv 22(2):8–16, 1984

Major Nursing Interventions

5

■ ADVOCACY[9,15,33,65,67,79,84,89,93,94,97,103,114,129,136, 169,189,206,240,245]

—— Definition

Advocacy is a goal-directed nursing action based on knowledge of the responsibility and accountability for the psychiatric patient's rights, dignity, freedom, and safety; it may involve risk taking on behalf of the welfare of the patient or family of the patient, within the mental health care delivery system.

—— Purpose

The purpose of advocacy is to ensure the rights, dignity, safety, and protection of the psychiatric patient and/or family of the patient who are experiencing difficulty in exercising the freedom of self-determination or who are unable to exercise the freedom of self-determination within the mental health care delivery system.

—— Specific Nursing Interventions

1. Identify vulnerable populations who are at risk for obtaining appropriate treatment within the mental health care delivery system; e.g., the chronically mentally ill, homeless patients and families, male and female patients within the correctional system, patients with acquired immune deficiency syndrome patients with dual diagnoses of mental illness and substance abuse.
2. Obtain information about the patient's and family's needs, preferences, and goals for mental health care.
3. Determine the availability of resources and provide the patient or family with this information.

4. Assist the patient and family to learn how to maximize their use of these resources.
5. Ensure that systems are in place to help the patient and family make informed decisions regarding their rights to accept or to refuse mental health treatment; e.g., somatic therapies, hospitalization.
6. Assist the family of an incapacitated psychiatric patient (e.g., a patient with senile dementia) to make informed decisions regarding participation in research and treatment that requires informed consent.
7. Ensure that patient's rights (e.g., to refuse treatment, to privacy, to send and receive mail, to make and receive telephone calls) are protected.
8. Ensure that patients are routinely informed of possible side effects from prescribed psychotropic medications.
9. Collaborate with the mental health team to ensure the use of the least restrictive alternatives for the patient; e.g., use, level, and form of antipsychotic medication, seclusion.
10. Demonstrate a sensitivity to the psychiatric patient's personal values, beliefs, and hopes.
11. Assist in the interpretation of the psychiatric patient's needs that may not always be seen as rational by some of the mental health team.
12. Collaborate with the mental health team to assure that treatment plans for all patients, including controversial patients (such as violent adolescents, the homeless, patients with substance abuse, patients who manipulate to meet their needs for control) are based on the identification of individual patient needs, as opposed to staff needs and biases.
13. Contribute to community efforts to improve resources for psychiatric patients and their families.
14. Participate in activities that have an impact on the legislation of psychiatric mental health care resources and treatment.

■ ASSERTIVENESS TRAINING[11,33,49,91,128,163,166,170, 171,203,247]

— Definition

Assertiveness training involves teaching patients, families, and groups to achieve personal goals by using communication techniques that enable them to directly express their opinions, thoughts, and feelings in a manner that fosters and maintains self-respect in both the sender and the receiver of the communication.

— Purpose

The purpose of assertiveness training is to achieve personal goals in a manner that increases feelings of self-worth and self-respect, decreases feelings of helplessness and powerlessness in interpersonal communication, and preserves the dignity and self-respect of the receiver.

— Specific Nursing Interventions

1. Identify patients who are likely to benefit from assertiveness training; e.g., patients who have difficulty using "I" statements, giving and re-

ceiving compliments, making eye contact, and patients with passive or aggressive patterns of interaction.

2. Determine the patient's motivation to change.
3. Assist the patient to identify behaviors that the patient would like to change.
4. Emphasize the importance of recognizing that the patient cannot change others, but that the patient can change his or her *own* behaviors in order to achieve feelings of self-worth and self-respect.
5. Suggest that the patient focus on changing one behavior at a time.
6. Help the patient formulate realistic goals.
7. Assist the patient to identify examples of what needs to be accomplished in order to achieve desired goal; e.g., the statement, "I really appreciated your help," contributes to achievement of the goal of giving positive comments.
8. Encourage the patient to set up a time frame for achieving goals.
9. Teach the patient to use statements that begin with "I" when expressing own viewpoint.
10. Teach the patient to clearly convey information needs, expectations, or desired behaviors from others.
11. Facilitate the patient's ability to accept praise and to give compliments.
12. Teach the patient to differentiate among passive, assertive, and aggressive behaviors.
13. Use role-playing techniques and group feedback to help the patient to become aware of strengths and difficulties in the use of assertive communication.
14. Help the patient reexamine assumptions that can hinder assertive responses.
15. Teach the patient to become aware of nonverbal behaviors (e.g., facial expression, body posture, tone of voice) that are congruent with the verbal message.
16. Teach specific assertive techniques; e.g., agreeing with truth, selective ignoring, sorting issues.
17. Teach the patient how to deal with anger in self and from others.
18. Provide opportunities for the patient to practice self-praise and recognition.

■ COMMUNICATION TECHNIQUES[6,20,26,46,47,62,73,76,107,112, 113,157,178,184,187,188,211,217]

— Definition

Communication techniques are goal-directed verbal and nonverbal interventions that are based on a working knowledge of communication theories that foster constructive relationships.

— Purpose

The purpose of communication techniques is to create and maintain a therapeutic nurse-patient alliance; to minimize obstacles that can impede, distort, and complicate the achievement of a mutual understanding between the patient and the nurse; and to assist the patient to identify and explore relationship problems with others.

—— Specific Nursing Interventions

1. Keep communication clear and direct by using short, simple sentences that focus on what the patient is dealing with.
2. Keep in mind that all verbal communication with the patient can be evaluated as having either a therapeutic influence on the patient's emotional growth or a nontherapeutic influence that reinforces psychopathology.
3. Recognize the influence of factors such as nonverbal communication, culture, and anxiety on the communication process between nurse and patient.
4. Keep in mind that specific communication techniques are only *tools* for enhancing the communication process in the nurse-patient relationship and that the effectiveness of these tools is based on the judicious use of specific techniques.
5. Use *questioning* to obtain specific information, clarify, and offer assistance.
6. Avoid closed questions in which the nurse implies what the answer is that is expected.
7. *Encourage description* by using verbal and nonverbal means to assist the patient to keep talking; e.g., open-ended statements and questions, such as "Go on," "Tell me more," "When did you . . . ?" "Where were you?" or nodding head.
8. Use *reflection*, repeating the same key words used by the patient, to let the patient know what the nurse has heard the patient overtly or covertly say.
9. Use *restating*, repeating main thought, by using words similar to those used by the patient, in order to encourage expansion.
10. Use *focusing*, to help the patient stick to important subject matter or theme, for example, "What did you say that you did after you became angry?" or "You were saying that . . ."
11. Use *active listening*, attending to the patient's communications (not on the nurse's personal responses to be made), to interpret what is communicated and to respond selectively.
12. Share *observations*, by verbalizing what the nurse observes about a patient's behavior, for example, "You appear to be feeling sad."
13. Use *clarifying* to request feedback to make certain that the patient's communications are accurately understood, for example, "By telling me . . . are you saying that . . . ?" or, "To whom are you referring when you say *they*?"
14. Use *silence* to observe, to reflect, and to interpret possible meanings of the patient's prior verbal and current nonverbal communication. Avoid switching to a superficial topic or introducing a new topic.
15. Use *confrontation*, only after basic trust has been established, to assist the patient in becoming aware of specific aspects of the behavior or problems.
16. Use *humor*, in selected situations, to decrease anxiety and tension by changing the patient's perception of an anxiety-producing situation.
17. Seek *consensual validation* by requesting feedback from the patient to check understanding and interpretation of the patient's communication and perceptions.

18. Use *summarization*, in the form of a condensed version, of the general content and theme of the conversation to give the patient feedback and allow for further clarification and validation.

■ CONTRACTING[62,86,93,130,135,137,155,162,182]

— Definition

Contracting is the establishment between patient and nurse of mutually agreed-upon expectations, actions, or goals about the psychiatric patient's treatment or health care. The expectations, actions, or goals that emphasize the patient's behavior and the accountability of the nurse and/or other members of the mental health team are clearly stated.

— Purpose

The purpose of contracting is to increase the psychiatric patient's adherance to a therapeutic regimen; to increase the patient's sense of control; to increase the patient's motivation; to minimize staff splitting; to set limits; and to maximize consistency among the treatment team.

— Specific Nursing Interventions

1. Prior to contracting, assess the patient's cognitive ability to understand and to remember the contract.
2. Assess the patient's motivation for participating in a treatment plan that includes contracting.
3. Respect the patient's right to make decisions about psychiatric treatment.
4. Promote the patient's participation in the identification of desired behavioral changes and specific goals.
5. Help the patient to identify realistic, attainable, and measurable goals.
6. Use the patient's own words, whenever possible, to describe target behaviors and goals.
7. When appropriate, give the patient the option of writing a contract that specifies the behaviors and goals that the patient intends to accomplish.
8. Determine the need for including a reinforcer or reward in the contact.
9. Describe the responsibilities and expected activities of both the patient and the nurse or other members of the treatment team.
10. Incorporate a time-dated component within the contract, e.g., specify when the patient will begin to work on the behavioral changes, goals, a time line, and when the contract will be terminated.
11. Provide the patient with a copy of the contract, after it has been signed by both the patient and the nurse, and include a copy in the patient's chart.
12. Collaborate with other members of the mental health team to ensure consistency in implementation and adherence to the patient's contract.
13. Evaluate the contract with the patient at agreed-upon time intervals to determine the need for renegotiation and revision of the terms.

■ CRISIS INTERVENTION[2,32,60,90,123,133,149,165,215,223,234,235,241]

— Definition

Crisis intervention is the systematic process, based on a working knowledge of crisis theory, of assessment, planning, intervention, and evaluation for a patient, family, or group experiencing perceptual-cognitive-emotional disequilibrium following a stressful situation, event, or turning point in life.

— Purpose

The purpose of crisis intervention is to restore perceptual-cognitive-emotional equilibrium, to maximize potential for learning and growth, and to prevent or reduce ineffective and dysfunctional responses to biopsychosocial stressors.

— Specific Nursing Interventions

1. *Assessment*
   - Determine the patient's level of anxiety, anger, distress.
   - Help the patient clarify motivation for seeking help.
   - Help the patient identify and describe the precipitating event.
   - Help the patient maintain focus on the here and now.
   - Facilitate the patient's expression of feelings, thoughts, and behaviors aroused by crisis.
   - Assist the patient to describe perceptions of ability to cope with the current problematic situation.
   - Determine the patient's current social support and available resources, e.g., family, community.
   - Determine the patient's ability to participate in planning for therapeutic interventions.
   - Evaluate for suicidal or homicidal intent.
   - Determine the influence of alcohol and drug use on the current crisis.
   - Help the patient identify, describe, and analyze past coping behaviors during problematic situations.
2. *Planning*
   - Decrease the patient's anxiety to a level that allows the patient to participate in mutual planning.
   - Help the patient explore various alternatives for coping with the current situation.
   - Help the patient become aware of hidden strengths, e.g., spiritual beliefs, personal philosophy, and situational supports such as family, friends, community.
   - Help the patient to develop realistic plans for coping with the situation.
   - Collaborate with other health care providers in the development of a plan.
   - Assist the patient in evaluating possible outcomes of the proposed solutions.

3. *Intervention*
   - Initiate actions to minimize physical danger for the patient and/or significant others; e.g., arrange for protection from abusive spouse, notify appropriate persons of the patient's verbalization of intent to harm self or others.
   - Facilitate the patient's regaining emotional control by
     - acknowledging the intense feelings and fears generated by crisis;
     - assisting the patient to redefine the situation by adding additional information or reorganizing existing information.
- Convey recognition of the patient's constructive contributions in the generating of possible solutions.
- Based on the individual situation, enlist the patient's family or other support groups as a resource in the implementation of therapeutic strategies.
- Convey hope for the patient's ability to successfully resolve crisis.
- Initiate referrals, based on individual patient need and desire, to other treatment programs, e.g., alcohol and drug treatment, marital or group therapy.
4. *Evaluation*
   - Facilitate the patient's evaluation of the plan that was implemented; i.e., have the patient compare the current level of psychological coping and comfort compared to the level prior to the precipitating event.
   - Help the patient develop realistic plans for the future, based on the patient's perceptions of progress and support system.
   - Consider the need for referral for brief or long-term psychotherapy or for hospitalization.

■ DECISION-MAKING[14,52,71,111,131,164,170,183,201]

— Definition

Decision-making nursing interventions focus on the psychiatric patient's use of an organized, systematic process for choosing a specific course of action.

— Purpose

Decision-making interventions are used to promote patient choice and autonomy in psychiatric mental health settings; to help the psychiatric patient make informed decisions that are consistent with the patient's personal beliefs, values, and goals; to help the patient avoid high-risk situations during a crisis state by making intelligent and informed decisions; to decrease the psychiatric patient's conflict in making choices about life events (e.g., health treatment, relationships, living arrangements); and to decrease feelings of helplessness and unnecessary dependency.

— Specific Nursing Interventions

1. Determine if the patient wants or needs to make a decision or if the patient is seeking advice.

2. Assess the patient's cognitive abilities (e.g., consistency in orientation, memory, reality testing, judgment) and the patient's level of anxiety to determine ability to comprehend and make independent decisions.
3. Based on individual assessment and the patient's preference, evaluate the benefit of including patient's family, significant others, other professionals, or resource persons in the decision-making process.
4. Convey respect for the patient's concerns.
5. Help the patient to identify and clarify as precisely as possible the problem that requires a course of action; i.e., state the problem in clearly understood language.
6. Facilitate the patient's identification of factors that interfere with the decision-making process.
7. Encourage the patient to focus on one decision at a time, in order to minimize feeling overwhelmed.
8. Teach the patient to recognize limitations of making passive, nonreflective decisions without obtaining adequate, factual information.
9. Have the patient identify and describe desired goals as well as alternate goals.
10. Teach the patient to consider a variety of approaches for arriving at a decision, by using techniques such as the following:
    - Brainstorming to generate a written list of potential solutions without taking time to evaluate how good or bad they are, in order to identify as many solutions as possible and to avoid rejecting any alternatives too hastily
    - Changing the point of view or frame of reference by imagining that the patient is advising another patient or friend about what to do
    - Adapting, modifying a solution that has worked for the patient in previous similar situations.
11. Have the patient prioritize alternatives according to the patient's criteria of importance.
12. Avoid imposing own values and beliefs on the patient's decision, selection, and ranking of alternatives.
13. Facilitate the patient's comprehension of complex aspects of alternatives by breaking down choices into smaller, more understandable components.
14. Assist the patient to compare and contrast the positive and negative consequences that could result from each alternative.
15. Help the patient reexamine positive and negative consequences of identified alternatives, including original unacceptable choices, before making final decision.
16. Assist the patient to identify barriers or impediments to implementing decision or alternatives, e.g., patient's knowledge, motivation, and availability of resources.
17. Help the patient develop contingency plans for dealing with the consequences of the chosen course of action.
18. Assist the patient in communicating decision-making needs, values, and plans to family and members of mental health team.
19. Support the patient's implementation of the decision.
20. Provide the opportunity for the patient to evaluate the effectiveness of the decision by having the patient review original goals and compare

current outcomes in terms of the successful achievement of or failure to achieve original goals.

21. Support the patient's analysis of decision-making outcomes as preparation for selection of new solutions or modification of previous decisions.

■ DISCHARGE PLANNING[10,35,37,66,77,124,181,202,205,226,245]

— Definition

Discharge planning as an intervention involves systematic nursing actions that focus on the process of the psychiatric patient's transition or discharge from the current psychiatric mental health treatment setting to the community.

— Purpose

Discharge planning prepares the psychiatric patient for resocialization and reintegration into the community and minimizes the occurrence of relapse or rehospitalization by ensuring the availability and accessibility of community resources for the psychiatric patient and family.

— Specific Nursing Interventions

1. Identify patients who are at risk for experiencing problems in their resocialization and reintegration in the community, e.g., patients with a history of substance abuse, the homeless and unemployed, the organically mentally disordered, the chronically mentally ill.
2. Develop individualized discharge plans in collaboration with the patient that are based on an assessment that includes demographic information, the patient's financial resources, past medical, psychiatric, and psychosocial history, as well as the patient's current level of functioning.
3. Develop specific discharge plans in collaboration with the patient that are based on an individual assessment of patient's needs, e.g., understanding of diagnosis, medication monitoring, day treatment program, nursing home, diet, emergency call-back numbers.
4. Encourage the patient to identify anticipated problems associated with discharge as soon as possible after entry into psychiatric treatment.
5. Have the patient describe perceptions of current support system, e.g., family, friends, community resources.
6. Help the patient describe plans for discharge and to develop measurable goals to be achieved prior to and following discharge.
7. Convey recognition of the patient's abilities to anticipate and avoid problems after discharge.
8. Collaborate with the treatment team in the use of therapeutic passes to prepare inpatients for transition to community living.
9. Use the family as a resource in identifying problems associated with discharge and suggesting possible solutions for these problems; help the family identify their needs and expectations.

10. Teach the patient and significant others about lifestyle changes, maintaining motivation for change, and symptom monitoring and management.
11. Collaborate with the mental health team in the use of patient/family meetings to formulate discharge plans and identify potential problems.
12. Contribute to discharge plans that are based on a realistic assessment of community resources for special populations, such as children with psychiatric disorders, the chronically mentally ill, and organically mentally impaired patients.
13. Coordinate referrals to appropriate community mental health resources that are available to the patient after discharge, e.g., psychotherapy resources, halfway house, day treatment program, nursing home.
14. Maintain ongoing collaboration with the mental health team to clarify and coordinate discharge plans.
15. Based on evaluation of outcome criteria, revise the nursing care plan prior to discharge.
16. Provide the patient and family with information about available medical, social, and vocational community resources.
17. Provide the patient and family with specific information regarding mental health aftercare appointments.
18. Assist the patient in working through the termination process associated with discharge, e.g., loss.

■ EDUCATION, PATIENT EDUCATION[5,7,8,25,33,36,43,53,62,64, 72,74,77,80,98,100,180,185,186,197,238,242,245,246]

— Definition

Patient education is goal-directed formal and informal teaching that is based on an assessment of the psychiatric patient's learning needs, learning ability, and resources to meet these needs.

— Purpose

Patient education maximizes the psychiatric patient's understanding and management of health care and promotes the achievement of a satisfactory and productive pattern of self care and daily living; it decreases anxiety about health problems and promotes adherence to treatment recommendations and plans.

— Specific Nursing Interventions

1. Determine the psychiatric patient's learning needs and resources
   - Identify the patient's knowledge about psychiatric illness, e.g., cause, treatment, symptoms (including early signs of relapse), prevention, and medication management.
   - Have the patient give examples of problems related to the management of psychiatric illness.
   - Identify the patient's motivation for learning, e.g., patient's personal health beliefs and values, fears about mental illness, pressure from peers or family.

- Find out the patient's preferred style of learning, e.g., reading, individual or group education, television.
- Identify possible impediments to learning, e.g., impaired vision or hearing; limited formal education; if patient is functionally illiterate; developmental or learning disabilities; presence of intrusive hallucinations; moderate, severe, or extreme anxiety; memory loss, confusion.
- Determine the influence of cultural factors or language barriers.
- Obtain information about the patient's emotional support system and current living conditions.
- Assess the patient's learning goals.

2. Collaborate with the patient in development of realistic and measurable leaning goals.

3. Develop an individualized teaching plan that is congruent with information obtained during assessment of learning needs, abilities, and emotional state.

4. During initial, acute phase of inpatient treatment, collaborate with other members of the mental health team to help the patient begin to recognize and learn that symptoms are manifestations of an illness that can be treated; gradually provide patient with additional information about psychiatric illness and treatment.

5. Use simple, understandable words to explain treatment regimens; ask the patient to use own words to describe understanding of verbal and written instructions.

6. Use a variety of teaching tools, based on availability of resources, that take into consideration the patient's individual educational needs, learning abilities, and emotional state

- Consider using programmed and computer-assisted instruction to accommodate patients who are slow learners, or patient's with poor tolerance for lengthy interpersonal contract.
- Provide books and pamphlets that the patient can easily read and understand; printed materials should include questions to direct patient's focus and maintain attention; use printed materials that primarily contain pictures and words with one or two syllables for patients who are having reading difficulty; and use materials that are culturally relevant and written in patient's own language.
- Use techniques such as puppetry, art work, and posters, to enhance the teaching-learning process for children.
- Use videotapes to enhance understanding of communication skills.
- Use television for role playing and social skills modeling.
- Use audiotapes to provide the patient with ready access for reviewing content previously presented, for example, assertive communication techniques.
- Use bibliotherapy (e.g., books for lay people and articles from current news magazines and journals) as a means for explaining psychiatric illness and treatment in understandable terms and for decreasing some of the stigma that may be associated with mental illness.

7. Use specific techniques to maximize patient's self care:

- Use reframing to teach the patient to manage side effects of medication by viewing signs of side effects as an indication that the medication is working.

- Have the patient keep a diary to monitor medication side effects.
- Use an individual or small group approach to teach the patient about the potential effects of psychiatric and medical illness (as well as certain medications) on their sexuality.
- Assign homework (e.g., specific reading assignments, television programs, practicing of new skill) prior to individual or group meetings.
- Use homogeneous groups for teaching self-monitoring and coping strategies and to provide psychological support, e.g., lithium group.
- Use role play of potential problematic situations to prepare patients for reentry into the community.
- Use contracting to reinforce application and follow-up of specific educational content; include the learning behaviors, teaching methodology to achieve goals, patient and nurse's responsibilities, and plans for follow-up and evaluation.

8. Incorporate patient teaching on risk and prevention of AIDS and other sexually transmitted diseases for both inpatients and outpatients in the psychiatric treatment setting. Discuss the use and/or plan for access to condoms.
9. Encourage regular check-ups including breast self-exam and pap smears for women, testicular self-exam for men.
10. Collaborate with other members of the mental health team in both inpatient and community mental health programs to provide classes that focus on activities of daily living in preparation for planned place of residence:
    - Meeting self-care needs for grooming and personal hygiene, clothing selection, and care of clothing
    - Planning for and preparing meals, storing food, making grocery lists, and shopping for food and other basic necessities
    - Money management, budgeting, using a bank, and managing a checking account
    - Leisure planning and use of available community resources for leisure activities
    - Effective communication techniques and stress management
11. In day treatment and continuing treatment programs, collaborate with medical-surgical clinical nurse specialists and nurse practitioners, as well as other members of the mental health team, to develop a health education program that focuses on issues such as
    - AIDS risk and prevention;
    - Assessment and management of safety hazards in the environment, e.g., group homes, private residences;
    - Management of physical problems, e.g., hypertension, diabetes, obesity, emphysema and smoking-related disorders;
    - Healthy lifestyle practices: e.g., good nutrition, adequate sleep.
12. Conduct home-based patient/family education meetings, when appropriate, to strengthen teaching that was initiated during inpatient treatment.
13. Evaluate the effectiveness of patient education on an ongoing basis by

- Having the patient provide self-report of achievement of identified learning goals, e.g., management of side effects of medication, ability to meet self-care needs; improved symptom management;
- Making ongoing, direct observations of the patient's achievement of identified goals, e.g., remission or decrease in psychiatric symptoms, development of effective coping strategies, management of self-care needs and activities of daily living;
- Evaluating the patient's adherence to a recommended treatment regimen;
- Using the patient's family as a resource to provide information about patient's progress in achieving educational goals, where it is appropriate and the client consents;
- Discussing mutual observations of the patient's progress with other members of the patient's treatment team

14. When patient education goals are not met, evaluate the following:
    - The patient's acceptance of learning goals versus nurse's priorities of the patient's learning needs
    - Clarity and appropriateness of goals in terms of the patient's individual needs, learning readiness, motivation, and abilities
    - Effectiveness and appropriateness of teaching tools for the patient (e.g., too complex; too elementary; culturally relevant)
    - Effectiveness and appropriateness of teaching techniques for patient
    - Unrealistic time frame for accomplishment of educational goals

15. Revise patient teaching goals and plans, based on findings from evaluation.

■ EDUCATION, FAMILY EDUCATION[5,10,13,25,48,72,74,80,81,87, 100,110,141,169,197,245]

— Definition

Family education encompasses goal-directed formal and informal teaching of the psychiatric patient's family or individual members within the family, based on an assessment of the patient's and/or family's learning needs, learning ability, and available resources.

— Purpose

Family education enlists the support of the psychiatric patient's family in maximizing the patient's ability to manage health problems, self-care needs, and activities of daily living; decreases family members' anxiety about the patient's health problems and treatment needs; promotes patient/family adherence to treatment recommendations; assists family members of the psychiatric patient to become familiar with the inpatient unit or outpatient clinic and the therapeutic process; clarifies the family's misconceptions about psychiatric illness; promotes realistic expectations about the patient's recovery from mental illness; reduces the risk of relapse for the psychiatric patient; and improves the coping skills of family members.

— Specific Nursing Interventions

1. Conduct a learning assessment of the family's learning needs, abilities, and resources related to the patient's psychiatric illness; include children in this assessment:
   - Find out the family's perception of and personal beliefs about the patient's psychiatric problems and mental illness, e.g., causes, manifestations, course of illness, and appropriate treatment.
   - Look for indications of the family placing blame on themselves or patient, stigmatization, denial, fears about hereditary aspects of mental illness.
   - Have the family identify perceptions of skills necessary to successfully attend to their needs as a family and as individual family members, as well as the patient's needs.
   - Observe for unrealistic expectations a family might have about the patient's recovery and needs following discharge, e.g., living arrangements, financial support, emotional support, medication management.
   - Identify possible learning impediments of individual family members, e.g., impaired vision or hearing, limited formal education, functional illiteracy, developmental or learning disabilities.
   - Assess for influence of cultural factors on family learning needs.
2. Encourage the family to participate in decisions about the educational approach that would be most helpful to them, e.g., individual, group, meeting with patient and family in home setting, meeting with or without patient present.
3. Collaborate with nursing peers and other members of the mental health team to implement a plan for family psychoeducation that begins immediately following the identified patient's entry into the psychiatric mental health care system:
   - Orient the family to the culture of the inpatient unit and its resources, e.g., physical environment, functions of different members of the patient's mental health team and how they can be contacted.
   - Acknowledge the presence of feelings, including varying levels of anxiety in family members, and use techniques to promote stress management.
   - Clarify the roles of the patient's mental health team.
   - Inform the family of inpatient unit rules and practices.
   - Provide the family with concrete basic information about the nature of the patient's illness and its treatment, to decrease feelings of anxiety, helplessness, and isolation, e.g., discuss the patient's diagnosis, a description of patient's experience with the illness, up-to-date information about the course of the illness and expected outcome, and institutional and community resources for the patient and family.
   - Provide the family with written material that explains the patient's psychiatric illness, treatment, early signs of relapse, and availability of local, regional, and national resources. Provide an

opportunity for the family to participate in the patient's treatment.

4. Collaborate with nursing peers and other members of the mental health team to offer psychoeducational groups to families, with a focus on interactive instructional activities, e.g., symptoms of illness, communication skills, medication management, and strategies for home management of stress and disruptive behavior.

5. Provide opportunities for family members to discuss the psychopharmacologic management of the patient's illness, e.g., target symptoms, dosage, side effects, and resources for obtaining medication.

6. Ensure that the family receives written information regarding specific therapies the patient is receiving.

7. Prior to discharge, provide the family with information about treatment options and community resources for patient and family outside the hospital, e.g., day hospitals, day treatment programs, sheltered workshops, medication clinics.

8. Provide the family with factual information about patient's needs after discharge, including the patient's responsibilities and aftercare plans; when possible, include the patient in discussions of the patient's strengths, current and future needs, and plans for managing health and psychiatric problems.

9. Teach the family to differentiate between residual symptoms in the patient and symptoms that are indicative of recurrence of psychiatric illness.

10. When appropriate, use home-based family education meetings that include the patient in order to
    - Discuss the family's ongoing information needs about the nature, course, and treatment of patient's psychiatric illness and health-related problems;
    - Correct misconceptions about the patient's illness and symptoms;
    - Elicit ongoing patient/family concerns and hopes regarding the patient's recovery from and living with mental illness.

11. Teach the family to recognize and pay attention to their own needs, in addition to the patient's needs, to prevent burnout in themselves.

12. Evaluate the effectiveness of family education on an ongoing basis by
    - Asking family members to report on the fulfillment of their learning needs and goals;
    - Asking the family to identify any additional learning needs;
    - Making direct observations of the family's ability to process educational information and to apply it to themselves and the identified patient.

13. When family education goals are not met, evaluate the following:
    - The family's identification, acceptance, and priorities of learning goals versus the nurse's identification and priorities
    - Clarity and appropriateness of goals in terms of family's and patient's needs, learning readiness, motivation, and abilities
    - Effectiveness and appropriateness of educational approaches, e.g., too complex, too elementary, culturally relevant
    - Unrealistic time frame for accomplishment of educational goals

14. Evaluate need for referral to other resources.

15. Revise family education goals and plans, based on findings from evaluation.

■ MILIEU THERAPY[1,13,33,50,69,74,107,126,138,194,204,232]

—— Definition

Milieu therapy, as a nursing intervention, uses nursing strategies that capitalize on aspects of the psychiatric patient's environment to promote growth or effect changes in patient behaviors.

—— Purpose

Milieu therapy provides a safe and growth-promoting environment; helps psychiatric patients learn new and socially appropriate behaviors; increases or maintains the patient's use of skills in managing own self care; and increases or maintains the patient's use of social and emotional skills in relating to others, in order to facilitate the transition to community living.

—— Specific Nursing Interventions

1. Ensure that the patient's bill of rights is posted within easy viewing and discuss the meaning of its content with the individual patient or with a group of patients.
2. Promote orientation to the inpatient unit by ensuring that directional signs, clocks, and calendars are provided and that written communication regarding rules of conduct, patient guidelines and expectations, and activity schedules is clear and easily seen. Use color to differentiate areas, individualizing bedrooms. Use name tags that can be easily read to identify staff.
3. Assess the patient's orientation to the actual environment as well as environmental boundaries, e.g., rules of conduct, patient guidelines, and activity schedules.
4. Based on individual assessment, encourage patient participation in decisions related to the environment, such as on room assignment.
5. Collaborate with nursing peers and other members of the mental health team to ensure that the environment is adapted to meet the developmental and therapeutic needs of patient populations; furniture and play equipment of appropriate size for children, communal area for peer interaction for adolescents, structure and support for regressed adults and children, adequate lighting, nonskid surfaces, brighter colors for the aged.
6. Collaborate with nursing peers and other mental health team members to provide individualization of milieu approaches for special populations; for example, patients on psychiatric intensive care benefit from minimal stimulation and a focus on reality orientation during the initial admission; patients in addictions' treatment benefit from a structured treatment program that includes negative consequences when the patient does not fulfill expected responsibilities. Address and work

through staff attitudes that have a potential adverse effect on the patients.

7. Ensure that the physical environment for suicidal or psychotic patients is free from harmful objects or conditions.
8. Assess for environmental stressors, such as loud and intrusive conversations, loud radio, television, or musical instruments, and decrease the noise level as needed. Assess also for temperature, ventilation, etc.
9. Provide privacy in sleeping areas and bathrooms.
10. Ensure that privacy is provided for patient interactions with staff and families.
11. Use open report with entire treatment team present, as a tool to facilitate staff-patient communication (when deemed appropriate) by
    - Preventing distorted communications;
    - Clarifying treatment goals;
    - Assisting patients to have a better understanding of their treatment and procedures as well as treatment approaches for other patients.[194]
12. Be judicious in the use of open report in potentially problematic situations, such as legal issues.[194]
13. Ensure that the nursing staff, as well as other members of the mental health team, are accessible and available for interactions with patients and families.
14. Use supportive interventions such as recognition and listening to provide the opportunity for developing a sense of well-being and self-esteem.
15. Use community meetings to promote problem solving by discussing issues that pertain to both patients and staff, e.g., the use of therapeutic passes, patient threats, suicide precautions, meal and bedtime schedules, patient privileges, access to visitors.
16. Promote the patient's understanding of what it means to live with another, mutual goals, the responsibility for another, giving recognition.
17. Assist the patient to meet spiritual needs by providing time in the patient's schedule as well as a place for meditation, solitude and reflection; facilitate the patient's access to clergy or spiritual advisors and religious services.
18. Ensure that psychoeducation for the patient and family is provided.
19. Collaborate with the mental health team to create an environment in which patients and families have opportunities for engaging in formal and informal activities with other patients and/or staff, e.g., meals, movies, discussion groups, recreational activities, community activities.

■ PROTECTIVE INTERVENTIONS: ACTIVITY AREA RESTRICTION[92,118]

— Definition

Activity area restriction is a therapeutic method of limiting the movement of a psychiatric patient to a specific room or area, such as a patient's room, dayroom, or ward.

—— Purpose

Activity area restriction protects the patient from self-injury or injury to others, assists the patient to control impulsive behaviors, provides time for the patient to reevaluate the current situation and develop alternate responses for coping.

—— Specific Nursing Interventions

1. Explain the procedure to the patient, including the purpose and anticipated length of time for the restriction.
2. Ensure that the patient's treatment team is informed of the rationale for room or ward restriction.
3. Provide the patient with support to remain within the area, e.g., staff to help the patient focus on behaviors and actions that necessitated restriction.
4. Continue with selected activities, e.g., personal hygiene needs, exercise, individual therapy, based on individual assessment.
5. Give the patient immediate feedback about inappropriate behavior; help the patient explore ways to modify behavior.

▬ PROTECTIVE INTERVENTIONS: OBSERVATION FOR SUICIDE PREVENTION[40,63,147,153,172,174,209,222,233]

—— Definition

Observation for suicide prevention employs continuous use of the nurse-patient relationship to prevent suicide in a patient who has been evaluated to be at risk for self-injury or suicide.

—— Purpose

The goal of observation for suicide is to prevent the patient from self-injury or death; to increase patient's control of self-destructive impulses; and to provide opportunity for the patient to talk about feelings associated with self-destructive behavior, e.g., anger towards self and others, hopelessness, helplessness.

—— Specific Nursing Interventions

1. Provide a safe environment for the patient:
   - Place the patient in an area that permits constant observation, even in the bathroom, by nursing staff on a 24-hour basis.
   - Inspect the patient's belongings in the patient's presence and remove items that the patient could use for self-harm, e.g., belts, scarves, pills, razors, glass, knives, matches.
   - Remain within arm's length of the patient.
   - Have the patient sleep in a room or area that facilitates constant observation.
   - Ensure that the patient swallows oral medications.
   - Provide meals on a tray that contains no metal utensils and no glass items, based on individual assessment of lethality potential

with these items; if the patient is allowed to have a regular tray, be sure to check for missing silverware or glass items when tray is collected.

2. Establish a dependable relationship with patient:
   - Introduce self, explain purpose for being with the patient and ongoing availability.
   - Encourage description of thoughts and feelings about suicidal ideation or attempt.
   - Convey empathy for the patient's feelings and views of life.
   - Convey expectation that the patient will not harm self.
   - Develop a nursing plan of care with the patient that includes the patient making a verbal or written "no self-harm" contract.
3. Monitor current suicidal risk:
   - Presence of suicidal ideation, verbalized intent
   - Suicidal behavior or change in suicidal plans
   - Patient's perception of effects of suicidal ideation/attempt on others
   - Presence of command hallucinations to harm self or others
   - Prevailing feelings of hopelessness, helplessness, worthlessness, guilt
   - Patient's perception of a support system, e.g., spouse, other family, friends, church
   - Patient's ability to consider alternatives other than suicide as solutions for problems
5. Help the patient contact friend, spouse, parent, or other significant person; maintain one-to-one supervision during their visits; be sure that visitors do not inadvertently leave harmful objects with the patient.
6. Collaborate with the mental health team on a daily basis to evaluate continuance of suicide precautions and observation.

■ PROTECTIVE INTERVENTIONS: SECLUSION[3,12,68,85,105,115, 145,154,161,199,202,224,227,228,231,248]

— Definition

Seclusion is a therapeutic process of limit setting that involves the removal of a patient from an open environment (in contact with patients, staff, or others) to a private and secured room from which the patient can be observed through a window or video monitor.

— Purpose

Seclusion provides a physical means of control and containment to prevent the psychiatric patient from harming self or others; it is an appropriate method for decreasing the stimulation the patient is receiving in the immediate environment or for helping the patient regain control of unacceptable verbal and nonverbal behaviors; it prevents destruction of the physical environment and prevents disruption of the ongoing treatment program.

—— Specific Nursing Interventions

1. Assess behaviors indicative of the need for use of seclusion, e.g., increasing levels of agitation, hyperactivity, confusion, impulsivity, and intrusiveness; a patient who has not responded to de-escalation techniques or medications; a patient who is at risk for harming self or others; a patient who is unwilling or unable to agree to a verbal contract to control the intent to harm self or others.
2. Provide a protected room, e.g., empty cubicle with soundly constructed walls and floor, a door that cannot be opened from the inside, protected window and ventilation equipment, recessed light fixtures, and no furnishings other than a durable mattress that is not flammable. Try to have a clock and calendar within sight of the patient.
3. Clear the immediate area of other patients and physical obstructions to the seclusion room.
4. Select a designated leader to give the patient clear, brief explanations for seclusion, e.g., "You must spend some time in a room by yourself until you can control your dangerous behavior."
5. Give the patient the option of walking quietly to the room, accompanied by staff. If the patient refuses, initiate the seclusion procedure.
6. Form a team of at least four staff and a designated leader, and clarify the responsibility of each staff member (e.g., who will grasp and control each extremity, who will control the patient's head, the method of transporting the patient to the seclusion room.
7. Use a team approach to hold and control the patient's extremities at the joint, and to control the patient's head to prevent neck injury or biting.
8. Bring the patient to the floor, using backward motion. Call for additional staff if needed, before taking the patient to the seclusion room.
9. Keep the patient's arms pressed tightly to sides and hold legs tightly at knees when lifting. Control and lift the patient's head at the same time as the patient's back, hips, and legs are lifted.
10. Place the patient on back on seclusion room mattress, with head toward the door and feet in opposite direction.
11. Search the patient for potentially dangerous objects; e.g., belts, ties, scarves, knives, matches.
12. Restate the reason for seclusion and list necessary behaviors for release; inform the patient of the availability of staff and tell how to ask for help with toileting or other additional needs.
13. Have the team exit one at a time, releasing the patient's legs first and arms last. Have the last team member quickly leave the seclusion room in a backward fashion, being sure that door to the seclusion room is locked.
14. Notify the patient's physician immediately, if this has not previously been done, keeping in mind that a physician's order is necessary for the patient to remain in seclusion.
15. Follow institutional guidelines for frequency of monitoring the patient (usually a minimum of every 15 minutes) and determine if constant observation is necessary.
16. Observe for patient behaviors indicative of exhaustion or self harm as a result of agitation and for other medical problems.
17. As soon as feasible, schedule a time for the staff to evaluate the cir-

cumstances leading to seclusion, discuss their reactions, and identify possible strategies for prevention of seclusion in the future.

18. Verbally acknowledge the nurse's presence at each check by calling the patient by name. Provide the patient with information such as time of day, when to expect the next meal, and disposition of clothing and valuables.

19. Collaborate with the team to be sure that a direct visit in the seclusion room is scheduled at least every 2 hours.

20. Provide for an adequate number of staff to accompany anyone who enters the seclusion room, e.g., to talk with the patient, take vital signs, and help with meals and toileting.

21. Take vital signs a minimum of every 2 hours.

22. Instruct the patient to sit in the corner of the seclusion room when serving food or providing fluids. Serve food in paper containers. Use blunt eating utensils. Promptly remove unused portions, containers, and utensils.

23. Offer fluids frequently, to prevent dehydration.

24. Offer bathroom facilities every 2–3 hours.

25. Provide ongoing brief interactions to decrease the patient's feeling abandoned and to minimize worsening of psychosis secondary to decreased sensory stimulation.

26. Avoid exploration of conflicts, feelings, and ideas during the initial period of seclusion.

27. Collaborate with the physician and other team members regarding appropriate use of p.r.n. medication for agitation, to avoid overmedicating.

28. Check the room on a regular basis for temperature, cleanliness, and safety of environment.

29. Provide for the patient's personal hygiene needs, e.g., daily bath, teeth brushing and individual grooming needs.

30. Determine the patient's need for continued treatment and ability to be weaned from seclusion by evaluating the patient's
    - Responsiveness to verbal directions;
    - Behavior during feeding, bathing, toileting activities;
    - Level of agitation and aggression;
    - Ability to wait for things requested;
    - Ability to remain oriented;
    - Behaviors indicative of hallucinatory experiences or delusional thinking.

31. Following removal from seclusion room, help the patient describe issues that lead to the need for seclusion intervention, discuss benefits of the intervention, and identify alternate ways to avoid use of this intervention in the future.

■ PROTECTIVE INTERVENTIONS: RESTRAINTS[3,68,85,105,106,154,199,202,224,227,228,248]

— Definition

Use of restraints is the process of applying or maintaining specialized equipment that restricts and limits a patient's physical activity and mobility. Restraints include

- *Wristcuffs*—wide, padded, leather cuffs secured with a leather strap and locking device, that can be attached to the wrists or ankles of the patient and then secured to the patient's waist or to the patient's bed;
- *Waist restraints*—three belts, one of which is fastened around the patient's waist with the other two being looped through each side of the waist belt and then secured to the bed frame.

—— Purpose

Use of restraints provides a physical means of control for preventing an out-of-control patient from harming self or others, prevents destruction of the physical environment, and prevents disruption of the ongoing treatment program.

—— Specific Nursing Interventions

1. Assess behaviors indicative of the need for restraints, e.g., inability or unwillingness of the patient to respond to staff attempts to control the patient's behavior with verbal interventions to prevent the patient from injuring self, patients, and others; a patient in seclusion who is determined to be at high risk for harming self or others.
2. Use a team approach of at least four staff and one leader to initiate the application of physical restraints after unsuccessful attempts to control the patient's behavior with verbal interventions.
3. Clear the immediate area of other patients and physical obstructions.
4. Gather around the designated leader, to convey confidence and control of the situation, to clarify type of restraint, to clarify the responsibility of each staff member (e.g., who will hold and control each extremity and who will control the patient's head; and to determine if restraints will be applied before or after the patient is placed in seclusion room, if the latter is necessary).
5. If the patient is restrained on the bed, place in prone position to decrease the chance of aspiration.
6. If patient is placed in wrist restraints, place hands behind back and straps through waist loops of pants. Have the leader explain to the patient the type of restraint that will be used to help the patient achieve control of behavior.
7. Allow the patient a few seconds to comply; do not allow further negotiation or discussion.
8. Following a prearranged signal, have staff grasp and control patient's extremities at the joint and control the patient's head to prevent neck injury or biting.
9. Bring the patient to the floor, using backward motion. Call for additional staff if needed, before taking the patient to the seclusion room. (Restraints may be applied at this time).
10. Use uniform lifting of patient's body and support the extremities and head while carrying the patient to seclusion room. (Apply restraints, if not previously done, being sure that they are securely fastened and locked).
11. Search the patient for dangerous objects, such as matches, jewelry, belts, ties, and scarfs.

12. Notify the patient's physician immediately, if this has not previously been done.
13. Follow institutional guidelines for frequency of monitoring the patient's response to restraints, usually a minimum of every 15 minutes.
14. Convey recognition of patient's need for dignity and self-esteem.
15. Check skin areas for signs of irritation, or impaired circulation; assure some movement of extremities every fifteen minutes; check vital signs.
16. Release restraints one at a time as needed and at least every 2 hours, (frequency is determined by institutional parameters, usually every 2 hours) or to allow the patient to eat and go to the bathroom. Be sure that adequate staff are available during these times.
17. If the patient's level of agitation does not permit an active exercise for the limbs, then do passive range of motion as the patient's condition permits.
18. Provide 1:1 constant observation when the patient is in four-point restraints.
19. Collaborate with the physician and other team members regarding appropriate use of medication, to avoid over medicating.
20. Schedule time with the treatment team to evaluate the circumstances leading to use of restraints, staff reactions to the situation, and possible strategies for prevention in future.
21. Provide the opportunity for other patients to verbalize their fears and concerns about the incident.
22. Collaborate with the team to determine when restraints can be removed or if some type of restraint device is needed when the patient returns to the open ward.
23. After removal of restraints, help the patient describe the issues that led to the need for this intervention, discuss the benefits from the use of restraints, and identify alternate ways to avoid the use of this intervention in the future.

■ PROTECTIVE INTERVENTIONS: SEIZURE MANAGEMENT[23,34, 42,82,101,104,142,167]

— Definition

Seizure management is a nursing intervention for the psychiatric patient who experiences, has had, or is at risk for having a seizure.

— Purpose

Seizure management interventions are initiated to prevent and minimize injury to the patient during an actual seizure and to reduce or prevent the occurrence of a seizure by collaborating with the psychiatric patient's physician in pharmacologic management.

— Specific Nursing Interventions

1. Ascertain patients who are at risk for having seizures, e.g., patients taking psychotropic medications that can lower the seizure threshold, patients who are at risk for alcohol or drug withdrawal, patients with

previous seizure history, patients taking antiepileptic medication irregularly.
2. Assess the patient's thoughts and feelings associated with risk factors for seizure, e.g., known prodromal signs, fears about injury during seizure, knowledge about seizure control, as well as thoughts and feelings associated with psychosocial issues of seizure management, such as the social network, social isolation, discrimination.
3. Interventions for the patient having an actual seizure:
   - Assist the patient to a lying position.
   - Protect and support the head with a pad or small, flat pillow if the patient is on floor; remove pillows if the patient is in bed.
   - If possible, have the patient lie on his or her side with head flexed forward to allow the tongue to fall forward and to promote drainage of secretions.
   - Do not attempt to force anything into the patient's mouth.
   - Remove the patient's glasses.
   - Loosen clothing.
   - Remove furniture or objects that the patient might strike during a seizure.
   - Do not attempt to restrain the patient (restraint during strong muscular contractions can cause fracture).
   - Provide privacy from onlookers.
   - Observe and report the type of movements and body part affected, size of pupils, state of consciousness, duration, incontinence, and behavior following seizure.
4. Interventions after seizure:
   - Keep the patient on his or her side to prevent aspiration.
   - Maintain a patient airway.
   - Determine the need for oxygen.
   - Do not offer liquids or solid food until the patient is fully awake.
   - Have a staff member remain with the patient until the patient regains consciousness and is fully awake and oriented; reorient the patient to the environment as necessary.
   - Provide an opportunity for the patient to discuss thoughts and feelings associated with the seizure.
   - Ascertain if the patient experienced aura prior to the seizure.
5. Based on individual assessment, ensure that safety measures are taken to prevent injury from subsequent seizures, e.g., quiet environment for the patient who is at risk for seizures; a bed that is close to floor.
6. Monitor vital signs.
7. Collaborate with the patient's physician regarding pharmacologic management for prevention of seizures.
8. Assess for possible contributing factors of seizure, e.g., history of alcohol and/or drug abuse, lack of understanding of the importance of compliance with medication regimen.
9. Develop an individualized patient education plan that incorporates information for prevention and control of future seizures, such as the following:
   - Importance of abstinence from alcohol and drug abuse
   - Importance of taking anticonvulsant medication at prescribed times

- Name of anticonvulsant medication, purpose, and common side effects
- Keeping seizure record—using seizure calendar, for example
- Name of health care provider and aftercare plans for seizure management

10. Ensure that patients with seizure disorder wear medic alert bracelets.

▬ REALITY ORIENTATION[38,39,78,107,108,117,156,225]

— Definition

Reality orientation is an individual or group approach that directs the cognitively impaired or disoriented psychiatric patient to be cognizant of time, place, and persons by systematically focusing on these dimensions.

— Purpose

Reality orientation strives to reduce or halt disorientation, to decrease social withdrawal and increase social interaction, develop and increase feelings of self-esteem, and to promote the cognitively impaired psychiatric patient's adherence to a recommended therapeutic regimen.

— Specific Nursing Interventions

1. Identify patients who are disoriented or are at risk for becoming disoriented, e.g., patients who are delusional, hallucinating; patient's who are experiencing acute or chronic confusion; older patients who are moderately confused; and patients who experience loss of memory.
2. Greet the patient by giving own name and calling the patient by preferred name.
3. Use touch, such as handshake, when appropriate.
4. Determine the patient's contact with reality by asking the patient to give information such as, "Tell me what today's date is?" "Tell me what day of the week this is?" "What time is your next meal?" "How long have you been in the hospital?" "What is the name of this place?"
5. Provide the patient with ongoing brief and simple explanations; e.g., "I want to help you to improve your memory"; "I want to be sure that you know who I am and where you are."
6. Provide the patient with brief and simple explanations and reminders about where the patient is, the reason for being in that environment, and what is expected from the patient. Work only on a selected number of things at a time. Identify with the patient's treatment team the essential aspects of the environment or expected behaviors that the patient is not aware of or is having difficulty in remembering.
7. Ensure that physical props, e.g., clocks, calendars, directional signs, and orientation boards (containing current information on date, season, weather, next meal) are within easy access and printed in large easy-to-read print for the patient's viewing; periodically reorient the patient to these props. Use environmental cues, e.g., floor and wall different colors, individual pictures and indicators outside of rooms, large symbols on bathroom, one end of hall different from the other.

8. Provide the patient with information about current events, building upon recognition of the patient's past interests, skills, and knowledge.
9. Give recognition for positive responses, e.g., "Good, your memory is getting better"; "You are remembering more information today than you were able to recall last week."
10. Acknowledge the patient's environmental observations, e.g., "That's correct, your next meal will be dinner"; "Yes, that lawn mower is making a great deal of noise."
11. Engage the patient in simple memory games, such as discussion of holidays (favorite, last one celebrated, next holiday).
12. Gently correct misinformation without arguing or confrontation.
13. Ensure consistency of reality orientation techniques throughout the day by collaborating with peers and other members of the mental health team.
14. Use a short weekly mental status assessment test to assist in the evaluation of the effectiveness of reality orientation interventions.

■ SOCIAL SKILLS TRAINING[18,30,31,143,151,170,192]

— Definition

Social skills training is a therapeutic group or individual approach that uses social learning principles to teach psychiatric patients, usually those with chronic mental illness, how to overcome interactional deficits by developing interpersonal skills for successful social and community adaptation.

— Purpose

Social skills training teaches the psychiatric patient skills for effectively interacting with others (e.g., family, friends, peers, employers), teaches ways to decrease or avoid stressful situations that may lead to exacerbation of mental illness, increases the psychiatric patient's self-confidence and self-esteem, and teaches daily living skills.

— Specific Nursing Interventions

1. Identify patients who might benefit from social skills training:
   - Chronically mentally ill patients who have difficulty initiating or maintaining relationships with others
   - Patients who have difficulty initiating and participating in routine day-to-day conversations
   - Patients who speak only when spoken to
   - Patients who are unable to express disapproval without resorting to overt aggression (e.g., yelling, swearing, hitting)
   - Patient's with inappropriate sexual behaviors (e.g., sexual verbalizations or advances to peers or staff)
   - Patients who report having difficulties in specific interpersonal situations (e.g., job interview skills, job maintenance; friendship and dating; conversing with others)
2. Collaborate with patient and treatment team in matching particular social skills training group to patient outcome desired, keeping in mind the following attributes:

- The ability to follow instructions
- An attention span of 15–90 minutes in a structured situation
- The ability to form and understand simple sentences
- The ability to give their name, date of birth, and current date when asked

3. Obtain specific information about the patient's problematic social interactions
   - Have the patient give real-life examples to illustrate interpersonal problems.
   - Have the patient keep a daily diary to monitor difficult situations.
   - Use role-playing techniques to assess the patient's social skills in specific situations (e.g., discussing side effects from medication, obtaining information about social security benefits).
   - Talk with the patient's caregivers or family.
   - Compile observations from other team members.
   - Review the patient's previous medical and social service records.
   - Observe and evaluate the patient's social skills during unstructured interactions with others.

4. Have the patient actively participate in the selection of specific and attainable goals that focus on positive, constructive, and functional behaviors in the patient's current life situation.

5. In a group setting, use techniques for group social skills in training[151]
   - Allow for individual differences in learning new skills.
   - Begin and end group on time.
   - Welcome members and describe the purpose of group; introduce new members.
   - Have returning patients introduce themselves and explain social skills training to new patients.
   - Inquire about absent members, to convey the value of *all* members.
   - Have the patients describe the results of previous homework assignments.
   - Inquire about interpersonal difficulties during the past week or anticipated problems during the coming week.
   - Help each individual patient identify a specific problem and goal that will be focused on during the meeting.
   - Engage the group in a discussion of the benefits associated with learning the identified desired skill.
   - Assist each individual patient to select and plan the situation for role play e.g., daily living skill such as using public transportation, job interviews, discussing medication side effects with health care provider; enlist other patients in setting up role-playing scenes and participating as role players; help the patient and other role player to focus on the patient's specific short- and long-term goals.
   - Give positive feedback through immediate praise and encourage group participation in giving positive feedback and praise; facilitate corrective feedback from members; use flip chart or blackboard to record ratings and general group feedback.
   - In order to assess cognitive and perceptual deficits, ask the patient to describe understanding of feedback, short- and long-

term goals, and other alternative approaches that could have been used.

- Select a patient to model a "real" person in the patient's life. Ask the patient to role play response behavior to the "real person," concentrating on the targeted behaviors; coach the patient on the desired behaviors.
- Give appropriate positive feedback on desired behaviors, encouraging group participation.
- At the conclusion of the training session, give the patient specific homework that focuses on practicing the new responses in the patient's actual environment.

6. In a one-to-one situation, use techniques adapted from the above, for social skills training.

7. In a family situation, use techniques adapted from above, for social skills training.

▬ Stress Management[22,24,27,33,37,51,54,94,97,109,119, 125,127,146,159,170,191,197,207,211,212,218,221,225,229, 236,237,239]

—— Definition

Stress management nursing strategies incorporate nonpharmacologic techniques and therapies in the management of the psychiatric patient's counterproductive physiological and psychological responses to stressful situations and life events.

—— Purpose

The purpose of stress management strategies is to decrease the patient's nonadaptive responses to stressors and to reduce tension in specific situations (e.g., job interview or performance); to decrease the patient's overall level of daily tension; to decrease tension associated with sleep pattern disturbance; to increase the patient's ability to solve problems in stressful situations; to decrease or eliminate the need for addictive behaviors (e.g., overeating, smoking, substance abuse); to alter the patient's response to chronic pain; to increase the patient's cognitive abilities (e.g., concentration, learning, and study habits); to increase the patient's sense of control in anxiety-producing situations; to decrease emotions to a level in which the patient can function effectively.

—— Specific Nursing Interventions

1. Identify patients whose level of stress interferes with their ability to function and to be productive and who would particularly benefit from learning stress management techniques or therapies (e.g., patients who are experiencing anxiety, fear, anger, powerlessness, post-trauma response, impaired social interaction, self-esteem disturbance, or chronic pain).

2. Conduct an organized assessment that includes the patient's description of the most troublesome symptoms, family history of similar difficulties, what has and has not helped in the past, the reason for seeking

help at this time, prescribed and over-the-counter medications, physical illness and limitations, previous use of stress management techniques, substance use or abuse, dietary habits (including caffeine use), sleep and activity patterns, daily routines, perceptions of current stressors, psychiatric history, motivation for learning stress management, and willingness to practice the techniques in the absence of the direct supervision of the nurse.[208]

3. Conduct a careful review of the patient's medical and psychiatric problems and treatment, in order to identify patients who are at risk for experiencing untoward effects from progressive relaxation or imagery techniques (e.g., the depressed patient who might become more withdrawn, patients who hallucinate or are delusional and who might experience loss-of-reality-contact reactions, patients whose pharmacologic regimen leaves them at risk for experiencing a temporary hypotensive or hypoglycemic state; and patients with medical problems such as arthritis or lower back pain).

4. Collaborate with the patient's physician before initiating progressive relaxation or imagery techniques with these populations and exercise caution in using progressive relaxation techniques with them.

5. Collaborate with the patient to develop an individualized plan for stress management.

6. Use a small group or individual approach to teach specific relaxation techniques, e.g., diaphragmatic breathing techniques, active and passive progressive relaxation, autogenic training, yoga, meditation, imagery, and affirmations (positive self-statements, such as, "I am relaxed").

7. Use a small group or individual approach to discuss common maladaptive ways for dealing with stress, e.g., substance abuse, overwork, overeating.

8. Teach the patient that the relaxation response is a learned response that requires practice and work and that it can be elicited in almost any person.

9. Use concrete techniques with psychotic patients who have loose associations.

10. Emphasize the importance of incorporating four essential elements to elicit relaxation response: a quiet environment with minimal distractions; the use of a mental device, word, or phrase that is repeated over and over in a consistent manner as a stimulus for shifting the mind from externally oriented thought; adopting a passive attitude that excludes worrying about how well the patient is doing; and achieving a comfortable position (not lying down—which may lead to sleep).

11. Inform the patient that relaxation techniques are tools for developing alternative responses to stress, that the techniques are easy to use once they are learned, that it may take weeks or months before the patient experiences the full desired results, and that the overall goal is improvement and not the achievement of perfection.

12. Explain that the patient needs to practice techniques for 15–20 minutes one to two times a day in a quiet environment, with emphasis on the fact that the actual environment where the patient strives to elicit a relaxation response may not always be a quiet place.

13. Help the patient to recognize situations, interpretations, and self-talk that trigger a stress response and subsequent response patterns. Teach

the patient to begin to learn measures for control of these responses and patterns:

- Control events by defining limits and refusing to become involved in a situation that causes stress (such as by physically or emotionally removing self from stressful situation).
- Control the interpretation of a stressful event by relabeling the meaning of the experience.
- Control self-talk by replacing irrational, negative ideas and beliefs with more realistic and accurate observations and statements.

14. Use visualization and imagery to decrease the emotional intensity associated with an actual or potential stress event or situation:
    - Confer with the patient's psychiatrist prior to use of visualization and imagery.
    - Teach the patient to create a positive mental picture of the desired experiences and/or situations.
    - Have the patient select a pleasurable image (e.g., lying on a warm beach, fishing at a secluded lake, walking through the woods on a sunny day) to create a relaxed state for visualization.
    - Use caution, e.g., more concrete techniques, in implementation of these techniques with psychotic patients.

15. Engage the patient in musical activities to decrease stress response; identify the patient's past associations with music that can influence the use of this modality for stress management:
    - Identify the role that music has played in the patient's life.
    - Obtain information about music with which the patient is familiar and the patient's form of participation with music (e.g., singing, listening, playing an instrument).
    - Assess factors that can influence the psychiatric patient's response to music (e.g., cultural, spiritual, and religious beliefs; educational preparation; presence of delusional thinking and hallucinations).
    - Encourage the use of soothing, unobtrusive music as a pre-bedtime ritual for patients with sleep pattern disturbance that is associated with anxiety.
    - Use unobtrusive and preferably unrecognized background music in the inpatient setting to create a calming effect during mealtime.
    - Have the patient use music as an adjunct for visualization and imagery in conjunction with chronic pain management and control; have the patient monitor breathing while listening to music, emphasizing the importance of slow and deep breathing to enhance the relaxing effects from music.
    - When appropriate, arrange for the patient to have access to an individual headset to use for listening to audiotapes of music for stress reduction; be judicious in use of headsets for patients who are actively experiencing auditory hallucinations.

16. Promote the use of humor as an emotion-focused coping strategy for relieving tension and anxiety.
    - Determine the patient's past use of humor to deal with stressful situations.

- Identify topics the patient finds amusing.
- When appropriate, encourage the patient to talk about events or topics that evoke humorous responses in the patient, nurse, or others.
- Facilitate patient's use of humorous audiovisuals (e.g., audiotapes of old radio comedies, movies, videotapes, or books).

17. Have the patient keep a stress-awareness diary for a minimum of 2 weeks to tract responses to stressful events and situations:
    - Have patient record information such as time of occurrence and physical and emotional responses.
    - Schedule time for the patient to review the findings with the nurse.

18. Evaluate the patient's response to stress management techniques and therapies by determining the extent to which patient outcomes for stress reduction have been achieved (e.g., improved sleep pattern, reduced anxiety, increased sense of control, increased ability to cope with chronic pain).

19. Based on the evaluation findings, collaborate with the patient, peers, and other members of the mental health team to revise and modify the original plan for stress management or to continue with the current plan.

■■■ SUPPORTIVE THERAPY: GRIEF COUNSELING[16,45,67,90,94-96, 120,122,132,134,165,190,193,195,200,214,234,243,244]

— Definition

Grief counseling involves individual or group psychotherapeutic interventions for patients who have experienced the loss of a significant object of value, e.g., a person, body part, or prized possession.

— Purpose

The goal of grief counseling is to facilitate the experience of normal grieving and to prevent dysfunctional grieving.

— Specific Nursing Interventions

1. Assist the patient to recognize that responses to the current loss are influenced by the patient's past experiences with loss.
2. Assist the patient to recognize the influence of socioeconomic background, education, and cultural and spiritual beliefs on the ability to cope with the current loss.
3. Determine the length of time since the patient learned of the loss.
4. Encourage the patient to verbalize thoughts and feelings about the loss.
5. Assist the patient to talk about past or present memories of the person, body part, or prized possession.
6. Monitor for possible suicidal ideation or intent; initiate protective action if the patient is at risk for suicide.
7. Encourage a description of the patient's perceptions of the current and anticipated problems associated with the loss.
8. Help the patient clarify factual information about the loss.

9. Help the patient to recognize the universality of the need for normal grieving.
10. Encourage the patient to identify and describe past as well as current strengths in coping with loss.
11. Help the patient recognize normal behaviors that accompany the experience of loss.
12. Facilitate the constructive expression of feelings (e.g., anger, sadness, guilt).
13. Assist the patient and significant others to talk about their thoughts and feelings of stigma that may be associated with potentially "unspeakable losses," (e.g., suicide, abortion, divorce, AIDS).
14. Emphasize the importance of maintaining good health habits.
15. Encourage the patient to develop or to resume constructive social relationships.
16. Evaluate the need for referral to community resources, such as support groups or self-help groups.
17. Evaluate the need for referral for brief psychodynamic individual, group, or family therapy.

▬ Supportive Therapy: Offering Hope[17,27,55,75,107,116, 144,165,196,210,211,216,239]

— Definition

Offering hope is a goal-directed nursing action that conveys the expectation that the psychiatric patient will be able to alter perceptions of futility or hopelessness associated with an actual or potential event or situation.

— Purpose

The purpose of offering hope is to help the psychiatric patient mobilize previous coping strengths and skills; to increase the patient's sense of hopefulness during a crisis; to prevent suicide; to facilitate normal grieving during an actual or potential loss; to prevent dysfunctional grieving; and to facilitate adaptation to the disabling effects of chronic mental illness.

— Specific Nursing Interventions

1. Assess for stressful life events that involve loss and change.
2. Have the patient describe perceptions of these stressful life events.
3. Assess the patient's cognitive and affective levels of functioning and developmental level and needs.
4. Evaluate the influence of physical problems and medical interventions on the patient's perceptions of hopelessness.
5. Determine the adequacy of the patient's social support system.
6. Assess the patient's personal and formal spiritual beliefs (e.g., philosophy of life, religious activities, association with people with similar spiritual or religious beliefs).
7. Collaborate with appropriate clergy or spiritual counselors.
8. Convey hope that is grounded in the belief that patient is able to prevent potential difficulties or overcome difficulties in current situation.

9. Use statements that convey realistic hope for patient, for example:
   "One of the things that I have to offer as your nurse is that. . . ."
   "I can offer you hope that you will be able to return to your family."
   "I can offer you hope that you will begin to feel better about yourself."
   "I can offer you hope that you will be able to identify other solutions for your problems besides ending your life."
   "I can offer you hope that you will recover from your loss and be able to find meaning in your life."
   "I am spending time with you because I believe that you are able to identify solutions that will help you to feel more optimistic about the future."
10. Use therapeutic humor to help the patient reframe the actual or potential situation or event in more positive terms.
11. Encourage the patient to emphasize strengths rather than weaknesses.
12. Convey recognition of the patient's past and present strengths and accomplishments.
13. Help the patient identify irrational beliefs in self and others and to recognize self-defeating behaviors.
14. Encourage the patient to use affirmations that are congruent with current goals to overcome feelings of hopelessness (e.g., "I am hopeful for the future"; "I am feeling optimistic.")
15. Encourage the patient to set realistic daily goals.
16. Promote positive expectations of the future by having the patient identify problems that can be resolved; help the patient develop realistic future goals for resolving these problems.
17. Facilitate the patient's recognition of realistic future achievements.
18. Use the patient's family as a resource in conveying hope for the present and the future (e.g., encourage the patient to share goals with the family; encourage the family to express positive feelings to the patient and to convey recognition of the patient's ability to change).

■ SUPPORTIVE THERAPY: PRESENCE[88,152]

— Definition

Presence is the verbal and nonverbal therapeutic use of self by being physically and psychologically available to meet the psychiatric patient's needs for help, comfort, and support.

— Purpose

This technique is intended to establish a therapeutic relationship, decrease anxiety, convey empathy, decrease loneliness, decrease social isolation, increase social interaction, provide emotional support, and encourage verbalization of perceptions.

— Specific Nursing Interventions

1. Observe for behavioral manifestations of avoidance of social interactions, withdrawal from interpersonal contacts, solitary activities, withdrawal from and avoidance of anxiety-producing situations.

2. Convey a calm, accepting, and nondemanding approach.
3. Communicate empathy and unconditional positive regard to the patient (e.g., "I have come to spend some time with you, because I am aware that this is a difficult experience for you.")
4. Specify availability of the nurse, including length of time during each contact with the patient.
5. Respect the patient's need for silence to examine thoughts and feelings.
6. Sit quietly with the patient and explain that the nurse will remain with the patient whether or not the patient converses with the nurse.
7. Use periods of silence to unobtrusively observe the patient's behaviors and to reflect on the possible meanings of these behaviors.
8. Inform the patient of the nurse's ongoing availability, how the patient can contact the nurse, and the resources the nurse can provide.

■ REFERENCES

1. Adler WN: Milieu therapy. In Lion JR, Adler WN, Webb WL (eds): Modern Hospital Psychiatry. New York, WW Norton & Co, 1988
2. Aguilera DC, Messick JM: Crisis Intervention: Theory and Methodology, 6th ed. St Louis, CV Mosby, 1989
3. Alexander DI: Aggression (mild, moderate, extreme/violence). In McFarland GK, Thomas MD: Psychiatric Mental Health Nursing. Philadelphia, JB Lippincott, 1991
4. Allen JG, Deering CD, Buskirk KJR, Coyne L: Assessment of therapeutic alliances in the psychiatric hospital milieu. Psychiatry 51(3):291–299, 1988
5. American Nurses' Association, Division on Psychiatric and Mental Health Nursing Practice: Standards of Psychiatric and Mental Health Nursing Practice. Kansas City, American Nurses' Association, 1982
6. Anderson ML: Nursing Interventions: What did you do that helped? Perspect Psychiatr Care 21(1):4–8, 1983
7. Antai-Ontong D: Concerns of the hospitalized and community psychiatric client. Nurs Clin North Am 24(3:665–672, 1989
8. Armstrong ML: Orchestrating the process of patient education: methods and approaches. Nurs Clin North Am 24(3):597–604, 1989
9. Baier M: Case management with the chronically mentally ill. J Psychosoc Nurs Ment Health Serv 25(6):17–20, 1987
10. Baker AF: How families cope. J Psychosoc Nurs Ment Health Serv 27(1):31–36, 1989
11. Bara M, Rugg M: Assertive communication for effective leadership. Can Nurse 85(9):19–20, 1989
12. Baradell JG: Humanistic care of the patient in seclusion. J Psychosoc Nurs Ment Health Serv 23(2):8–14, 1985
13. Baskerville BH: Milieu therapy. In McFarland GK, Thomas MD: Psychiatric Mental Health Nursing. Philadelphia, JB Lippincott, 1991
14. Baumann A: Decision making during a crisis state. In Baumann A, Johnston NE, Antai-Otong D: Decision Making in Psychiatric and Psychosocial Nursing. Toronto/Philadelphia, BC Decker, 1990
15. Bawden EL: Reaching out to the chronically mentally ill homeless. J Psychosoc Nurs Ment Health Serv 28(3):6–13, 1990

16. Beal G: Helping men cope with divorce. J Psychosoc Nurs Ment Health Serv 27(8):30–32, 1989
17. Beck AT, Steer RA, Kovacs M, Garrison B: Hopelessness and eventual suicide: a 10-year prospective study of patients hospitalized with suicidal ideation. Am J Psychiatry 142(5):559–563, 1985
18. Bellack AS, Turner SM, Hersen M, Luber RF: An examination of the efficacy of social skills training for chronic schizophrenic patients. Hosp Community Psychiatry 35(10):1023–1028, 1984
19. Benfer BA, Schroder PJ: Nursing in the therapeutic milieu. Bull Menninger Clin 49(5):451–465, 1985
20. Benjamin A: The Helping Interview: With Case Illustrations. Boston, Houghton, Mifflin, 1987
21. Benson DF, Stuss DT: Frontal lobe influences on delusions: a clinical perspective. Schizopr Bull 16(3):403–411, 1990
22. Benson H: The Relaxation Response. New York, Avon Press, 1976
23. Bernat JL: Getting a handle on an adult's first seizure. Emerg Med 21(1):20–24, 27,28, 1989
24. Bishai M: Visualization and guided imagery. In Baumann A, Johnston NE, Antai-Otong: Decision Making in Psychiatric and Psychosocial Nursing. Toronto/Philadelphia, BC Decker, 1990
25. Blackford KA: The children of chronically ill parents. J Psychosoc Nurs Ment Health Serv 26(3):33–36, 1988
26. Bleathman C, Morton I: Validation therapy with the demented elderly. J Adv Nurs 13:511–514, 1988
27. Bloch D: Words That Heal: Affirmations and Meditations for Daily Living. New York, Bantam, 1990
28. Blumenthal SJ: Suicide: a guide to risk factors, assessment, and treatment of suicidal patients. Med Clin North Am 72(4):937–971, 1988
29. Blumenthal SJ: Youth suicide; risk factors, assessment, and treatment of adolescent and young adult suicidal patients. Psychiatr Clin North Am 13(3):511–556, 1990
30. Brady JP: Social skills training for psychiatric patients, I: concepts, methods and clinical results. Am J Psychiatry 141(3):333–340, 1984
31. Brady JP: Social skills training for psychiatric patients, II: clinical outcome studies. Am J Psychiatry 141(4):491–498, 1984
32. Brownell MJ: The concept of crisis: its utility for nursing. Adv Nurs Sci 6(4):10–21, 1984
33. Browning MA: Depression. In Hogstel MO (ed): Geropsychiatric Nursing. St Louis, CV Mosby, 1990
34. Brunner LS, Suddarth DS, Bare BG, Boyer MJ, Smeltzer SCO: Textbook of Medical-Surgical Nursing, 6th ed. Philadelphia, JB Lippincott, 1988
35. Buckwalter KC, Abraham IL: Alleviating the discharge crisis: the effects of a congitive-behavioral nursing intervention for depressed patients and their families. Arch Psychiatr Nurs 1(5):350–358, 1987
36. Buckwalter KC, Kerfoot KM: Teaching patients self care: a critical aspect of psychiatric discharge planning. J Psychosoc Nurs Ment Health Serv 20(5):15–20, 1982
37. Buckwalter KC, Hartsock J, Gaffney J: Music therapy. In Bulechek GM, McCloskey JC: Nursing Interventions, Treatments for Nursing Diagnoses. Philadelphia, WB Saunders, 1985

38. Burnside I: Nursing and the Aged: A Self Care Approach. New York, McGraw-Hill, 1988

39. Burnside I: Working with the Elderly: Group process and Techniques, 2nd ed. Monterey, CA, Wadsworth Health Science Division, 1984

40. Bydlon-Brown B, Billman RR: At risk for suicide . . . nobody cares if I live or die! Will someone please help me? AJN 88(10):1358–1361, 1988

41. Campbell L: Hopelessness: a concept analysis. J Psychosoc Nurs Ment Health Serv 25(2):18–22, 1987

42. Campbell VG: Neurologic system. In Thompson JM, McFarland GK, Hirsch JE, Tucker SM, Bowers AC: Mosby's Manual of Clinical Nursing, 2nd ed. St Louis, CV Mosby, 1989

43. Carmen E, Brady SM: AIDS risk and prevention for the chronic mentally ill. Hosp Community Psychiatry 41(6):652–657, 1990

44. Carser DL: Primary nursing in the milieu. J Psychiatr Nurs Ment Health Serv 19(2):35–41, 1981

45. Carter SL: Themes of grief. Nurs Res 38(6):354–358, 1989

46. Chapman AH: The Treatment Techniques of Harry Stack Sullivan. New York, Brunner/Mazel, 1978

47. Chapman GE: Reporting therapeutic discourse in a therapeutic community. J Adv Nurs 13(2):255–264, 1988

48. Chesla C: Parents' illness models of schizophrenia. Arch Psychiatr Nurs 3(4):218–225, 1989

49. Clark CC: Assertive Skills for Nurses. Rockville, MD, Aspen Publishers, 1978

50. Cohen S, Khan A: Antipsychotic effect of milieu in the acute treatment of schizophrenia. Gen Hosp Psychiatry 12:248–251, 1990

51. Cook JD: The therapeutic use of music: a literature review. Nurs Forum 20(3):253–266, 1981

52. Corcoran S: Decision-making strategies for choosing nursing interventions. In Snyder M (ed): Independent Nursing Interventions. New York, Wiley, 1985

53. Corrigan PW, Liberman RP, Engel JD: From noncompliance to collaboration in the treatment of schizophrenia. Hosp Community Psychiatry 41(11):1203–1211, 1990

54. Courtright P, Johnson S, Baumgartner MA, Jordan M, Webster JC: Dinner music: does it affect the behavior of psychiatric inpatients? J Psychosoc Nurs Ment Health Serv 28(3):37–40, 1990

55. Cousins N: Head First: The Biology of Hope. New York, EP Dutton, 1989

56. Craig C, Ray F, Hix C: Seclusion and restraint: decreasing the discomfort. J Psychosoc Nurs Ment Health Serv 27(7):16–19, 1989

57. Critchley DL: Clinical supervision as a learning tool for the therapist in milieu settings. J Psychosoc Nurs Ment Health Serv 25(8):18–22, 1987

58. Critchley DL: Providing a therapeutic milieu experience for a patient diagnosed with AIDS. Arch Psychiatr Nurs 1(6):441–443, 1987

59. Critchley DL, Berlin IN: Parent participation in milieu treatment of young psychotic children. Am J Orthopsychiatry 51(1):149–155, 1981

60. Cunningham JM: Crisis intervention. In McFarland GK, Thomas MD: Psychiatric Mental Health Nursing. Philadelphia, JB Lippincott, 1991

61. Curtis RC (ed): Self-defeating Behaviors: Experimental Research, Clinical Impressions, and Practical Implications. New York, Plenum Press, 1989

62. Deering CG: Developing a therapeutic alliance with the anorexia nervosa client. J Psychosoc Nurs Ment Health Serv 25(3):10–17, 1987

63. Dingman CW, McGlashan TH: Characteristics of patients with serious suicidal intentions who ultimately commit suicide. Hosp Community Psychiatry 39(3):295–299, 1988

64. Dixon E, Park R: Do patients understand written health information? Nurs Outlook 38(6):278–281, 1990

65. Donahue MP: Advocacy. In Bulechek GM, McCloskey JC: Nursing Interventions: Treatments for Nursing Diagnoses. Philadelphia, WB Saunders, 1985

66. Donner LL, Kopytko EE, McFolling SD, et al: Increasing psychiatric inpatients' community adjustment through therapeutic passes. Arch Psychiatr Nurs 4(2):93–98, 1990

67. Dugan DO: Death and Dying; emotional, spiritual, and ethical support for patients and families. J Psychosoc Nurs Ment Health Serv 25(7):21–29, 1987

68. Eichelman B: Toward a rational pharmacotherapy for aggressive and violent behavior. Hosp Community Psychiatry 39(1):31–39, 1988

69. Ekland ES: Hopelessness. In McFarland GK, Thomas MD: Psychiatric Mental Health Nursing. Philadelphia, JB Lippincott, 1991

70. Ellis NK, Krch-Cole E: Providing a therapeutic milieu experience for a patient diagnosed with AIDS. Arch Psychiatr Nurs 1(6):436–440, 1987

71. Eraker SA, Politser P: How decisions are reached: physician and patient. In Dowie J, Elstein A (eds): Professional Judgment: A Reader in Clinical Decision-making. New York, Cambridge University Press, 1988

72. Falloon IRH, Boyd JL, McGill CW: Family Care of Schizophrenia: A Problem-solving Approach to the Treatment of Mental Illness. New York, Guilford Press, 1984

73. Farran CJ, Keane-Hagerty E: Communicating effectively with dementia patients. J Psychosoc Nurs Ment Health Serv 27(5):13–16, 1989

74. Farran CJ, Carr V, Maxson E: Goal-related behaviors in short-term psychiatric hospitalization. Arch Psychiatr Nurs 2(3):159–164, 1988

75. Farran CJ, Popovich JM: Hope: a relevant concept of geriatric psychiatry. Arch Psychiatr Nurs 4(2):124–130, 1990

76. Field WF: The Psychotherapy of Hildegard E. Peplau. New Braunfels, TX, PSF Productions, 1979

77. Fishel AH: A community-based program for emotionally disturbed children and youth. J Child Adolesc Psychiatr Ment Health Nurs 3(4):128–133, 1990

78. Fitzpatrick JJ: Gerontological counseling. In Lego S (ed): The American Handbook of Psychiatric Nursing. Philadelphia, JB Lippincott, 1984

79. Floyd J: Research and informed consent: the dilemma of the cognitively impaired client. J Psychosoc Nurs Ment Health Serv 26(3):13–21, 1988

80. Foster SW: The pragmatics of culture: the rhetoric of difference in psychiatric nursing. Arch Psychiatr Nurs 4(5):292–297, 1990
81. Fran CJ, Carr V, Maxson E: Goal-related behaviors in short-term hospitalization. Arch Psychiatr Nurs 2(3):159–164, 1988
82. Friedman D: Taking the scare out of caring for seizure patients. Nursing 18(2):52–60, 1988
83. Friis S: Measurements of the perceived ward milieu: a reevaluation of the Ward Atmosphere Scale. Acta Psychiatr Scand 73(5):589–599, 1986
84. Gadow S: Clinical subjectivity: advocacy with silent patients. Nurs Clin North Am 24(2):535–541, 1989
85. Gair DS: Guidelines for children and adolescents. In Tardiff K (ed): The Psychiatric Uses of Seclusion and Restraint. Wash DC, American Psychiatric Press, 1984
86. Gallop R: The patient is splitting: everyone knows and nothing changes. J Psychosoc Nurs Ment Health Serv 23(4):6–10, 1985
87. Gant AB, Goldstein G, Pinsky S: Family understanding of psychiatric illness. Community Ment Health J 25(2):101–108, 1989
88. Gardner DL: Presence. In Bulechek GM, McCloskey JC: Nursing Interventions: Treatments for Nursing Diagnoses. Philadelphia, WB Saunders, 1985
89. Garritson SH: Characteristics of restrictiveness. J Psychosoc Nurs Ment Health Serv 25(1):10–19, 1987
90. Gavoni LA: Psychosocial issues of AIDS in the nursing care of homosexual men and their significant others. Nurs Clin North Am 23(4):749–765, 1988
91. Geeting B, Geeting C: How to Listen Assertively. New York, Simon & Shuster, 1976
92. Gentilin J: Room restriction: a therapeutic prescription. J Psychosoc Nurs Ment Health Serv 25(7):13–16, 1987
93. Gerace LM: The patient needing long-term supportive therapy. In Durham JD, Harden SB (eds): The Nurse Psychotherapist in Private Practice. New York, Springer Publishing, 1986
94. Gerety EK: Grieving, anticipatory grieving, dysfunctional grieving. In McFarland GK, Thomas MD: Psychiatric Mental Health Nursing. Philadelphia, JB Lippincott, 1991
95. Gerety EK, McFarland GK: Dysfunctional grieving. In McFarland GK, McFarlane EA: Nursing Diagnosis and Intervention: Planning for Patient Care. St Louis, CV Mosby, 1989
96. Gerety EK, McFarland GK: Dysfunctional grieving. In Thompson JM, McFarland GK, Hirsch JE, Tucker SM, Bowers AC: Mosby's Manual of Clinical Nursing, 2nd ed. St Louis, CV Mosby, 1989
97. Gerety EK, McKim JD, Sosnovec PA, Cowan ME: Instructor's Manual to Accompany McFarland and Thomas's Psychiatric Mental Health Nursing. Philadelphia, JB Lippincott, 1991
98. Gessner BA: Adult education: the cornerstone of patient teaching. Nurs Clin North Am 24(3):589–595, 1989
99. Goldberg K: The quilt work theory: a milieu approach. New Dir Ment Health Serv Summer(38):5–21, 1988
100. Goldwyn RM: Educating the patient and family about depression. Med Clin North Am 72(4):887–896, 1988
101. Graham O, Naveau I, Cummings C: A model for ambulatory care of

patients with epilepsy and other neurological disorders. J Neurosci Nurs 21(2):108–112, 1989

102. Grunebaum H, Friedman H: Building collaborative relationships with families of the mentally ill. Hosp Commun Psychiatry 39(11):1183–1187, 1988

103. Gullberg PL: The homeless chronically mentally ill: a psychiatric nurse's role. J Psychosoc Nurs Ment Health Serv 27(6):9–13, 1989

104. Gummit RJ: The Epilepsy Handbook: The Practical Management of Seizures. New York, Raven Press, 1983

105. Gutheil TG: The therapeutic milieu: changing themes and theories. Hosp Commun Psychiatry 36(12):1279–1285, 1985

106. Gutheil TG, Tardiff K: Indications and contraindications for seclusion and restraint. In Tardiff K (ed): The Psychiatric Uses of Seclusion and Restraint. Wash, DC, American Psychiatric Press, 1984

107. Hamilton GP: Promotion of mental health in older adults. In Hogstel MO (ed): Geropsychiatric Nursing. St Louis, CV Mosby, 1990

108. Hanley I: Reality orientation in the care of the elderly patient with dementia—three case studies. In Hanley I, Gilhooly M (eds): Psychological Therapies for the Elderly. New York, New York University Press, 1986

109. Hansen PA, Rhode JM, Wolf-Wilets V: Stress management. In McFarland GK, Thomas MD: Psychiatric Mental Health Nursing. Philadelphia, JB Lippincott, 1991

110. Harter L: Multi-family meetings on the psychiatric unit. J Psychosoc Nurs Ment Health Serv 26(8):18–22, 1988

111. Hawks JH: Should nurses give moral advice? Image: J Nurs Scholar 16(1):14–16, 1984

112. Hays JS, Larson K: Interacting with Patients: Communications for General and Psychiatric Nurses. New York, Macmillan, 1963

113. Helms J: Active listening. In Bulechek GM, McCloskey JC: Nursing Interventions: Treatments for Nursing Diagnoses. Philadelphia, WB Saunders, 1985

114. Herrick CA, Smith JE: Ethical dilemmas and AIDS: nursing issues regarding rights and obligations. Nurs Forum 24(3,4):35–46, 1989

115. Heyman E: Seclusion. J Psychosoc Nurs Ment Health Serv 25(11):8–12, 1987

116. Herth K: Relationship of hope, coping styles, concurrent losses, and setting to grief resolution in the elderly widow(er). Res Nurs Health 13:109–117, 1990

117. Hogstel MO: Mental illness in the nursing home. In Hogstel MO (ed): Geropsychiatric Nursing. St Louis, CV Mosby, 1990

118. Holnsteiner MG: Elopement, potential for. In McFarland GK, Thomas MD: Psychiatric Mental Health Nursing. Philadelphia, JB Lippincott, 1991

119. Hoover RM, Parnell PK: An inpatient educational group on stress and coping. J Psychosoc Nurs Ment Health Serv 22(6):16–22, 1984

120. Horsley GC: Baggage from the past. Am J Nurs 88(1):58–63, 1988

121. Houseman C: The paranoid person: a biopsychosocial perspective. Arch Psychiatr Nurs 4(3):176–181, 1990

122. Houseman C, Pheifer WG: Potential for unresolved grief in survivors of persons with AIDS. Arch Psychiatr Nurs 2(5):296–301, 1988

123. Hradek EA: Crisis intervention and suicide. J Psychosoc Nurs Ment Health Serv 26(5):24–27, 1988

124. Hughes L, Joyce B, Staley D: Does the family make a difference? J Psychosoc Nurs Ment Health Serv 25(8):8–13, 1987

125. Hyman RB, Feldman HR, Harris RB, Levin RF, Malloy GB: The effects of relaxation training on clinical symptoms: a meta-analysis. Nurs Res 38(4):216–220, 1989

126. Jack LW: Use of milieu as a problem-solving strategy in addiction treatment. Nurs Clin North Am 24(1):69–80, 1989

127. Jacobson E: Progressive Relaxation. Chicago, University of Chicago Press, 1974

128. Jakubowski P, Lange AJ: The Assertive Option: Your Rights and Responsibilities. Champagne, IL, Research Press, 1978

129. Janosik EH, Davies JL: Psychiatric Mental Health Nursing. Boston, Jones and Bartlett, 1989

130. Jensen DP: Patient contracting. In Bulechek GM, McCloskey JC. Nursing Interventions: Treatments for Nursing Diagnoses. Philadelphia, WB Saunders, 1985

131. Jiwani GN: Problem solving. In Baumann A, Johnston NE, Antai-Otong: Decision Making in Psychiatric and Psychosocial Nursing. Toronto/Philadelphia, BC Decker, 1990

132. Johnson J: Psychiatric nursing in a crisis center: standards and practice. Nurs Management 17(8):81, 82, 1986

133. Johnson S: The grieving patient. In Durham JD, Hardin SB (eds): The Nurse Psychotherapist in Private Practice. New York, Springer, 1986

134. Johnson SE: After a Child Dies: Counseling Bereaved Families. New York, Springer, 1987

135. Johnson SW, McSweeney M, Webster RE: Leisure: how to promote inpatient motivation after discharge. J Psychosoc Nurs Ment Health Serv 27(9):29–31, 1989

136. Johnstone MJ: Professional ethics and patients' rights: past realities, future imperatives. Nurs Forum 24(3,4):29–34, 1989

137. Jones RN, O'Brien P: Unique interventions for child inpatient psychiatry. J Psychosoc Nurs Ment Health Serv 28(7):29–31, 1990

138. Kahn EM, White EM: Adapting milieu approaches to acute inpatient care for schizophrenic patients. Hosp Community Psychiatry 40(6):609–614, 1989

139. Kahn EM, Fredrick N: Milieu-oriented management strategies on acute care units for the chronically mentally ill. Arch Psychiatr Nurs 2(3):134–140, 1988

140. Kalogjera IJ, Bedi A, Watson W, Meyer A: Impact of therapeutic management on use of seclusion and restraint with disruptive adolescent inpatients. Hosp Commun Psychiatry 40(3):280–285, 1989

141. Kane CF, DiMartino E, Jimenez M: A comparison of short-term psychoeducational and support groups for relatives coping with chronic schizophrenia. Arch Psychiatr Nurs 4(6):343–353, 1990

142. Kaufman DM: Clinical Neurology for Psychiatrists, 3rd ed. Philadelphia, WB Saunders, 1990

143. Kelly JA: Social-skills Training: A Practical Guide for Interventions. New York, Springer, 1982

144. Kennison MM: Faith: an untapped health resource. J Psychosoc Nurs Ment Health Serv 25(10):28–30, 1987

145. Kirkpatrick H: A descriptive study of seclusion: the unit environment, patient behavior, and nursing inteventions. Arch Psychiatr Nurs 3(1):3–9, 1989

146. Kneisl CR: Stress management. In Wilson HS, Kneisl CR: Psychiatric Nursing, 3rd ed. Menlo Park, CA, Addison-Wesley, 1988

147. Kneisl CR, Zangari ME: Crisis intervention. In Wilson HS, Kneisl CR: Psychiatric Nursing, 3rd ed. Menlo Park, CA, Addison-Wesley, 1988

148. Knight MM, Wigder KS, Fortsch MM, Polcari A: Medication education for children: is it worthwhile? J Child Adolesc Psychiatr Ment Health Nurs 3(1):25–28, 1990

149. Kus RJ: Crisis intervention. In Bulechek GM, McCloskey JC: Nursing Interventions: Treatments for Nursing Diagnoses. Philadelphia, WB Saunders, 1985

150. Liberman RP, Wong SE: Behavior analysis and therapy procedures related to seclusion and restraint. In Tardiff K (ed): The Psychiatric Uses of Seclusion and Restraint. Washington, DC, American Psychiatric Press, 1984

151. Liberman RP, DeRisi WJ, Mueser KT: Social Skills Training for Psychiatric Patients. New York, Pergamon Press, 1989

152. Liehr PR: The core of true presence: a loving center. Nurs Sci Q 2(1):7–8, 1989

153. Lion JR: Violence and suicide within the hospital. In Lion JR, Adler WN, Webb WL (eds): Modern Hospital Psychiatry. New York, Norton, 1988

154. Lion JR, Soloff PH: Implementation of seclusion and restraint. In Tardiff K (ed): The Psychiatric Uses of Seclusion and Restraint. Washington, DC, American Psychiatric Press, 1984

155. Loomis ME: Levels of contracting. J Psychosoc Nurs Ment Health Serv 23(3):8–14, 1985

156. Love C: Applying the nursing process with the elderly. In Wilson HS, Kneisl CR: Psychiatric Nursing, 3rd ed. Menlo Park, CA, Addison-Wesley, 1988

157. Magnan MA: Listening with care. Am J Nurs 89(2):219–221, 1989

158. Manderino MA, Bzdek VM: Social skill building with chronic patients. J Psychosoc Nurs Ment Health Serv 25(9):18–23, 1987

159. Mast DE: Effects of imagery. Image: J Nurs Scholar 18(3):118–120, 1986

160. Masterman SH, Reams R: Support groups for bereaved preschool and school-age children. Am J Orthopsychiatry 58:562–570, 1988

161. McCoy SM, Garritson SH: Seclusion: the process of intervening. J Psychosoc Nurs Ment Health Serv 21(8):8–15, 1983

162. McEnany GW, Tescher BE: Contracting for care: one nursing approach to the hospitalized borderline patient. J Psychosoc Nurs Ment Health Serv 23(4):11–18, 1985

163. McFarland GK, Gerety EK: Self-concept, disturbance in: self esteem. In Kim MJ, McFarland GK, McLane AM: Pocket Guide to Nursing Diagnoses, 4th ed. St Louis, CV Mosby, 1991

164. McFarland GK, Leonard HS, Morris MM: Nursing Management and Leadership and Management: Contemporary Strategies. New York, John Wiley & Sons, 1984

165. McGee RF: Hope: a factor influencing crisis resolution. Adv Nurs Sci 6(4):34–44, 1984
166. McQuade K: Assertiveness training. In Lego S (ed): The American Handbook of Psychiatric Nursing. Philadelphia, JB Lippincott, 1984
167. Madden JF: Calming the storms of alcohol withdrawal. Emerg Med 22(7):22–24, 27, 28, 1990
168. Mitchel J, Vierkant AD: Delusions and hallucinations as a reflection of the subcultural milieu among psychiatric patients of the 1930s and 1980s. J Psychol 123(3):269–274, 1989
169. Moffet MJ: Evolution of psychiatric community care. J Psychosoc Nurs Ment Health Serv 26(7):17–21, 1988
170. Monti PM, Abrams DB, Kadden RM, Cooney NL: Treating Alcohol Dependence: A Coping Skills Training Guide. New York, Guilford Press, 1989
171. Moore JB: Effects of assertion training and first aid instruction on children's autonomy and self-care agency. Res Nurs Health 10:101–109, 1987
172. Morofka V: Mental health. In Thompson JM, McFarland GK, Hirsch JE, Tucker SM, Bowers AC: Mosby's Manual of Clinical Nursing, 2nd ed. St Louis, CV Mosby, 1989
173. Mosher LR, Kresky-Wolff M, Matthews S, Menn A: Milieu therapy in the 1980s. A comparison of two residential alternatives to hospitalization. Bull Menninger Clin 50(3):257–268, 1986
174. Motto J, Heibron DC, Juster RP: Development of a clinical instrument to estimate suicide risk. Am J Psychiatry 142(6):680–686, 1985
175. Muesner KT, Levine S, Bellack AS, Douglas MS, Brady EU: Social skills training for acute psychiatric inpatients. Hosp Community Psychiatry 41(11):1249–1251, 1990
176. Mulvihill D: Milieu therapy in a children's unit. Can J Psychiatr Nurs 24(4):17–18, 1983
177. Mulvihill D: Therapeutic relationships in milieu therapy. Can J Psychiatr Nurs 30(1):21–22, 1989
178. Naschinski C: The communication process. In McFarland GK, Thomas MD: Psychiatric Mental Health Nursing. Philadelphia, JB Lippincott, 1991
179. Niemeier DF: A behavioral analysis of staff patient interactions in a psychiatric setting. West J Nurs Res 5(4):269–281, 1983
180. Nigro A, Maggio J: A neglected need: health education for the mentally ill. J Psychosoc Nurs Ment Health Serv 28(7):15–19, 1990
181. Norris J: Chronically mentally ill patients. In McFarland GK, Thomas MD: Psychiatric Mental Health Nursing. Philadelphia, JB Lippincott, 1991
182. O'Brien P, Caldwell C, Transeau G: Destroyers: written treatment contracts can help curb self-destructive behavior. J Psychosoc Nurs Ment Health Serv 23(4):11–18, 1985
183. O'Connor AM, D'Amico MJ: Decisional conflict. In McFarland GK, Thomas MD: Psychiatric Mental Health Nursing. Philadelphia, JB Lippincott, 1991
184. O'Toole AW, Welt SR (eds): Interpersonal Theory in Nursing Practice: Selected Works of Hildegard E. Peplau. New York, Springer, 1989
185. Parios R: Activities of daily living groups. In Lego S (ed): The Amer-

ican Handbook of Psychiatric Nursing. Philadelphia, JB Lippincott, 1984

186. Pelletier LR: Psychiatric home care. J Psychosoc Nurs Ment Health Serv 26(3):22–27, 1987
187. Peplau HE: Interpersonal Relations in Nursing. New York, GP Putnam's Sons, 1952
188. Peplau HE: Talking with patients. AJN 60(7):964–966, 1960
189. Petr C, Poertner J: Protection and advocacy for the mentally ill: new hope for emotionally disturbed children? Community Ment Health J 25(2):156–163, 1989
190. Pheifer WG, Houseman C: Bereavement and AIDS: a framework for intervention. J Psychosoc Nurs Ment Health Serv 26(10):21–26, 1988
191. Philips C: The psychological management of chronic pain: a treatment manual. New York, Springer, 1988
192. Plante TG: Social skills training: a program to help schizophrenic clients cope. J Psychosoc Nurs Ment Health Serv 27(3):6–10, 1989
193. Poncar PJ: The elderly widow: easing her role transition. J Psychosoc Nurs Ment Health Serv 27(2):6–11, 1989
194. Puskar KR, McAdam D: Use of open report as a staff-patient model of communication on a schizophrenia research unit: a case report. Arch Psychiatr Nurs 2(5):274–280, 1988
195. Rando TA (ed): Loss and Anticipatory Grief. Lexington, MA, Lexington Books, 1986
196. Rawlins RP: Hope-despair. In Beck CK, Rawlins RP, Williams SR (eds): Mental Health-Psychiatric Nursing: A Holistic Life-Cycle Approach, 2nd ed. St Louis, CV Mosby, 1988
197. Redman BK: The Process of Patient Education, 6th ed. St Louis, CV Mosby, 1988
198. Romoff V, Kane I: Primary nursing in psychiatry: an effective and functional model. Perspect Psychiatr Care 20(2):73–78, 1982
199. Roper JM, Coutts A, Sather J, Taylor R: Restraint and seclusion: a standard and standard care plan. J Psychosoc Nurs Ment Health Serv 23(6):18–32, 1985
200. Rossiter AB: A model for group intervention with preschool children experiencing separation and divorce. J Orthopsychiatry 58:387–396, 1988
201. Rothert ML, Talarczyk GJ: Patient compliance and the decision-making process of clinicians and patients. J Compliance Health Care 2(1):55–71, 1987
202. Roy B, Helt A: Clinical forum. J Child Adolesc Psychiatr Ment Health Nurs 2(3):110–112, 1989
203. Sadler AG: Assertiveness training. In Bulechek GM, McCloskey JC: Nursing Interventions: Treatments for Nursing Diagnoses. Philadelphia, WB Saunders, 1985
204. Saifnia JA: Milieu therapy. In Beck CK, Rawlins RP, Williams SR (eds): Mental Health-Psychiatric Nursing: A Holistic Life-Cycle Approach, 2nd ed. St Louis, CV Mosby, 1988
205. St. Germain L: Discharge planning. In Lego S (ed): The American Handbook of Psychiatric Nursing. Philadelphia, JB Lippincott, 1984
206. Salladay SA, McDonnell MM: Spiritual care, ethical choices, and patient advocacy. Nurs Clin N Am 24(2):543–549, 1989

207. Samuels M, Samuels N: Healing with the Mind's Eye: A Guide for Using Imagery and Visions for Personal Growth and Healing. New York, Summit Books, 1990
208. Scandrett S, Uecker S: Relaxation training. In Bulechek GM, McCloskey JC: Nursing Interventions: Treatments for Nursing Diagnoses. Philadelphia, WB Saunders, 1985
209. Schachter SO: Threats of suicide. J Contemp Psychother 18(2):145–163, 1988
210. Sideleau BF: Irrational beliefs and intervention. J Psychosoc Nurs Ment Health Serv 25(3):18–24, 1987
211. Simon JM: Therapeutic humor: who's fooling who? J Psychosoc Nurs Ment Health Serv 26(4):8–12, 1988
212. Simonton C, Matthews-Simonton S, Creighton J: Getting Well Again. New York, Bantam Books, 1978
213. Sinha VK, Chaturvedi SK: Consistency of delusions in schizophrenia and affective disorders. Schizophr Res 3:347–350, 1990
214. Skeen P, Walters L, Robinson B: How parents of gays react to their children's homosexuality and to the threat of AIDS. J Psychosoc Nurs Ment Health Serv 26(12):6–10, 1988
215. Slaby AE, McNamara ME: The psychiatric emergency room. In Lion JR, Adler WN, Webb WL (eds): Modern Hospital Psychiatry. New York, Norton 1988
216. Slusher MP, Anderson CA: Belief perseverance and self-defeating behavior. In Curtiss R (ed): Self-Defeating Behaviors: Experimental Research, Clinical Impressions, and Practical Implications. New York, Plenum Press, 1989
217. Smith BJ, Cantrell PJ: Distance in nurse-patient encounters. J Psychosoc Nurs Ment Health Serv 26(2):22–26, 1988
218. Snyder M: Biofeedback. In Snyder M (ed): Independent Nursing Interventions. New York, John Wiley & Sons, 1985
219. Snyder M: Progressive relaxation. In Snyder M (ed): Independent Nursing Interventions. New York, John Wiley & Sons, 1985
220. Snyder M: Progressive relaxation as a nursing intervention: an analysis. Adv Nurs Sci 6(3):47–58, 1984
221. Sodergren KM: Guided imagery. In Snyder M (ed): Independent Nursing Interventions. New York, John Wiley & Sons, 1985
222. Spillers GM: Suicide potential. In McFarland GK, Thomas MD: Psychiatric Mental Health Nursing. Philadelphia, JB Lippincott, 1991
223. Stelzer J, Elliott CA: A continuous-care model of crisis intervention for children and adolescents. Hosp Community Psychiatry 41(5):562–564, 1990
224. Straker M: Guidelines for the elderly. In Tardiff K (ed): The Psychiatric Uses of Seclusion and Restraint. Wash, DC, American Psychiatric Press, 1984
225. Stuart GW, Sundeen SJ: Principles and Practice of Psychiatric Nursing, 3rd ed. St Louis, CV Mosby, 1987
226. Swearingen L: Transitional day treatment: an individualized goal-oriented approach. Arch Psychiatr Nurs 1(2):104–110, 1987
227. Tardiff K: Concise Guide to Assessment and Management of Violent Patients. Wash, DC, American Psychiatric Press, 1989
228. Tardiff K: Management of the violent patient an emergency situation. Psychiatr Clin North Am 11(4):539–549, 1988

229. Titlebaum HM: Relaxation. Holistic Nurs Practice 2(3):17–25, 1988
230. Tousley MM: The paranoid fortress of David J. J Psychosoc Nurs Ment Health Serv 22(2):8–16, 1984
231. Tsemberis S, Sullivan C: Seclusion in context: introducing a seclusion room into a children's unit of a municipal hospital. Am J Orthopsychiatry 58(3):462–465, 1988
232. Vaglum P, Friis S, Karterud S: Why are the results of milieu therapy for schizophrenic patients contradictory? An analysis based on four empirical studies. Yale J Biol Med 58(4):349–361, 1985
233. Valente SM: Adolescent suicide: assessment and intervention. J Child Adolesc Psychiatr Ment Health Nurs 2(11):34–39, 1989
234. Van Dongen CJ: The legacy of suicide. J Psychosoc Nurs Ment Health Serv 26(1):8–13, 1988
235. van Servellen G, Nyamathi AM, Mannion W: Coping with a crisis: evaluating psychological risks of patients with AIDS. J Psychosoc Nurs Ment Health Serv 27(12):16–21, 1989
236. Varcarolis EM: Relaxation. In Lego S (ed): The American Handbook of Psychiatric Nursing. Philadelphia, JB Lippincott, 1984
237. Vissing V, Burke M: Visualization techniques for health care workers. J Psychosoc Nurs Ment Health Serv 22(1):29–32, 1984
238. Walsh J: Psychoeducational program evaluation: one practical method. J Psychosoc Nurs Ment Health Serv 25(3):25–31, 1987
239. Watzlawick P: The Situation Is Hopeless, But Not Serious (the Pursuit of Unhappiness). New York, WW Norton, 1983
240. Werner JS, Gibbs LE: Clinicians' fallacies in psychiatric practice. J Psychosoc Nurs Ment Health Serv 25(8):14–17, 1987
241. Williams SR, Aguilera DC: Crisis intervention. In Beck CK, Rawlins RP, Williams SR (eds): Mental Health-Psychiatric Nursing: A Holistic Life-Cycle Approach, 2nd ed. St Louis, CV Mosby, 1988
242. Wistrom FE: Role playing. J Psychosoc Nurs Ment Health Serv 25(6):21–24, 1987
243. Woolsey SF: Support after sudden infant death. AJN 88(10):1347–1351, 1988
244. Worden JW: Grief Counseling and Grief Therapy, 2nd ed. New York, Springer, 1991
245. Worley NK, Albanese N: Independent living for the chronically mentally ill. J Psychosoc Nurs Ment Health Serv 27(9):18–23, 1989
246. Young EW: Sexual needs of psychiatric clients. J Psychosoc Nurs Ment Health Serv 25(7):30–32, 1987
247. Zappe C, Epstein D: Assertive training. J Psychosoc Nurs Ment Health Serv 25(8):23–26, 1987
248. Zillman MA: Use of seclusion and restraints. In Lego S (ed): The American Handbook of Psychiatric Nursing. Philadelphia, JB Lippincott, 1984

■ GROUP TREATMENT[1–37]

—— Therapeutic Groups

Overall goal is re-education, prevention of health problems, development of potentials, and enhancement of quality of life. Such groups

1. Emphasize the repressive inspirational approach, in which negative/maladaptive feelings and behaviors are replaced by more constructive ones;
2. Rely heavily on techniques of support, counseling, and re-education;
3. Are frequently self-help groups (e.g., Al-Anon, Alateen, Alcoholics Anonymous, Recovery, Gamblers Anonymous, Parents Without Partners).

—— Adjunctive Groups

The goal is to encourage perceptual or sensory stimulation, reality orientation, or resocialization. Examples include the following:

1. *Remotivation groups*—utilize a five-step technique to aid in resocializing withdrawn or regressed patients.
2. *Reorientation groups*—foster orientation to self, others, and environment and aim to increase the awareness of very disoriented or regressed patients.
3. *Bibliotherapy*—The patient achieves the goals of perceptual stimulation and interpersonal interaction by reading and discussing books, poems, and newspapers.
4. *Music therapy*—fosters sensory stimulation and getting in touch with feelings as the patient listens to music or plays an instrument.
5. *Social skills groups*—teach basic social skills. Videotaping may be utilized to increase the patient's information about self.

—— Group Psychotherapy Groups

The overall goal is problem solving, insight without personality reconstruction, or personality reconstruction.

A. Personality reconstruction
Major goals are to modify personality, to modify behavior patterns, and to reduce the use of previously used defense mechanisms where indicated.
1. Groups are characterized by an intensive analytic focus on each patient in the group (i.e., each member is analyzed within the group context).
2. Interpersonal problems occurring among group members are worked through with an emphasis on analyzing the historical roots of these problems. Group fosters multiple opportunities for catharsis.
3. Group is long-term and membership to new members is closed.
4. An example is analytical group psychotherapy.

B. Insight without reconstruction
The goal is to help members gain emotional integration and intellectual insight that increases understanding of the problem and decreases maladaptive behaviors without attempting to achieve major personality reconstruction.
1. Groups are characterized by emphasis on the interpersonal problems of members in the "here and now."
2. Goals are achieved through analysis of communications and interpersonal relationships with others.

3. Problems are explored in greater depth than in problem-solving groups.
4. The group helps group members gain greater insight about their effect on others, how others affect them in turn, and about alternative behavioral options.

C. Problem solving
The goal is to help group members resolve circumscribed problems and gain problem-solving skills.
1. Groups are characterized by emphasis on circumscribed problems experienced by a group member (e.g., problems associated with discharge, relating to other patients, and coping with the institutional regimen).
2. Goals are achieved by means of isolating individual patient problems for discussion in the group.
3. Group members contribute ideas for resolving a given problem based on their own education or experience or both. The patient may report the results of the implemented plan of action back to the group.

── Influencing Factors

Factors in group therapy, therapeutic groups, and/or adjunctive groups that facilitate the patient's development of more adaptive behavioral patterns include the following:[4]

1. *Universality*—Patients discover that they are not alone and that others in the group may experience problems similar to their own.
2. *Instillation of hope*—Patients develop hope for their own improvement as they sees others in the group coping more adaptively.
3. *Corrective reexperiencing of the primary family group*—Group experiences provide patients with the opportunity to work through conflicts stemming from their primary family groups.
4. *Information gained*—The group provides patients with the opportunity to learn about mental health and mental illness.
5. *Altruism*—Patients benefit from being helpful to other group members (e.g., their self-esteem may be improved).
6. *Group cohesiveness*—Group members are attracted to the group with a sense of "we-ness." Patients in the group develop a sense of belonging, acceptance, individual validation, and ability to express—but tolerate—intermember hostility.
7. *Catharsis*—Patients are able to ventilate their emotions.
8. *Imitative behavior*—Patients observe the behavior of others in the group and experiment with the behavior's usefulness for themselves.
9. *Gaining socializing techniques*—The group experience provides patients with the opportunity to acquire social skills.
10. *Interpersonal learning*—Patients display their behavior and through feedback and self-observation gain understanding of their impact on others and about the opinions others have of them. Patients gain awareness of their own responsibility in developing their interpersonal world.
11. *Existential factors*—Patients experience being able to "be" with others and to belong to the group.

—— Characteristics of Effective Groups

1. Problem solving is frequently evidenced.
2. Creativity and innovation are supported.
3. Conflict is tolerated, examined, and resolved.
4. High levels of trust, open and two-way communication, support, and inclusion facilitate cohesion.
5. The group atmosphere is relaxed and comfortable.
6. Group members participate in the evaluation of the group's functioning.
7. Decisions are made by consensus.
8. Objectives and tasks are clarified and modified to foster group member commitment.
9. The three group functions emphasized are—internal maintenance, developmental change, and goal achievement.
10. The leadership role changes among group members over time.

—— Initiating Group Therapy, Therapeutic Groups, and Adjunctive Groups

1. Decide on the type of group to be conducted: delineate the major emphasis and group goals. The specificity of the group goals depends on the type of group.
2. In selecting group members for the type of group, consider the following:
   a. The diagnosis and the degree of mental illness of the patient before placing the patient in group therapy as opposed to group psychotherapy
   b. Potential therapeutic value to patient (i.e., whether the group helps the patient develop more adaptive behavioral patterns)
   c. Motivation and willingness
   d. Factors such as age, sex, intelligence
   e. The size of the group—depends to some extent on the type of group and the type of patients. A good range is from 6 to 10 members.
3. Select an adequate meeting area. It should be an adequate size for the group and free from interruptions, have good ventilation, and be attractively furnished.
4. Select the time and frequency of meeting:
   a. The actual frequency depends on type of group. A common frequency is once per week.
   b. In selecting the time, work around other patient therapies with less flexibility in scheduling, such as industrial therapy.
   c. Changes in meeting place, time, and frequency can adversely affect the group process.

—— Therapist's Role in Preparing the Patient for Group Therapy

1. The therapist's role and interventions will be influenced by the type of group, the type of patients, and the therapist's own theoretical orientation.

2. Preparation of the patient for group can vary as follows:
   a. Information about time, place, and frequency
   b. Individual therapy followed by group therapy/psychotherapy
   c. Brief individual orientation
      (1) Time, place, frequency
      (2) Purpose of group
      (3) Brief description of group members
      (4) What is expected of the patient group (e.g., attendance)
      (5) Behavior that will not be tolerated
   d. In an open group (one in which new members can be added at any time), assist the new members in feeling comfortable.
      (1) Introduce the new member to the group and have group members introduce themselves.
      (2) Summarize what the group has been currently discussing.
      (3) Facilitate group support of the new member. For example, "Mrs. Jones may need our support in becoming a member of this group. We remember how we felt on our first day."

── Phases of Group Development

A. Beginning phase
1. Tasks confronting the group members include the following:
   a. Developing a method for achieving the purpose for which they joined the group
   b. Managing the social relationships so that all members gain comfortable roles for themselves
2. Patient behavioral characteristics include
   a. Seeking to clarify the meaning of group therapy and what group membership entails
   b. Evaluating and testing other group members and seeking a viable personal role
   c. Seeking acceptance, approval, domination, or respect
   d. Demonstrating dependency on the leader and seeking guidance, approval, and direction
   e. Using restricted and stereotyped communication
   f. Searching for member similarities
   g. Providing description of symptoms, medications, and former treatment
   h. Showing anxiety among members

B. Second (middle) phase
   Patient behavioral characteristics include the following:
1. Searching for power, control, and dominance
2. Engaging in conflicts between members and between members and leader
3. Searching for appropriate amount of personal power; struggling for control
4. Expressing criticism and negative comments
5. Giving advice, judgments, and criticism as means of jockeying for position
6. Expressing hostility and rebellion towards therapist
7. Engaging in fantasies of getting rid of leader.

C. Third (termination) phase
Patient behavioral characteristics include the following:
1. Development of group cohesiveness
2. Increase in self-disclosure and mutual trust
3. Increased concern about each other and missing members
4. Appearance of issues of intimacy and closeness among group members
5. Increased awareness of interpersonal interactions as they evolve in the group
6. Final movement of the third phase: teamwork and focus on the purpose and work of the group
7. Feelings about termination (emerge as group comes to the end)

—— Interventions

A. Beginning phase
1. Serve as a role model to demonstrate the behavior expected in group.
2. Discuss with group members what is expected of them in group. Offer structure and direction.
3. Have members introduce themselves.
4. Foster and facilitate interaction.
   a. Do not permit monopolizing.
   b. Intervene to reduce *social* roles and interaction.
   c. Demonstrate congruence, empathy, and unconditional positive regard.
5. Answer questions in relation to time, place, frequency, and purpose of the group.
6. Do not reinforce a group need for dependency on leader.
7. Reduce high anxiety.

B. Second (middle) phase
1. Permit expression of criticism and hostility toward the therapist.
2. Support the fragile group member, when needed, during intermember conflict.
3. Foster and facilitate interaction.
4. Demonstrate congruence, empathy, and unconditional positive regard.
5. Focus on the here-and-now group experiences.
6. Begin to explore themes.

C. Third (termination) phase
1. Foster and facilitate communication.
2. Encourage exploration of behavior, interactions among members, and topic areas discussed.
3. Provide feedback on group process.
4. Support development of group cohesiveness. Support self-disclosure.
5. Support and encourage problem solving and working towards group goals.
6. Offer the opportunity to work through feelings for loss or addition of group member (especially true for open groups).
7. Encourage members to respond to here-and-now experiences in the group.
8. Work through feelings related to termination of the group.

▬ REFERENCES

1. Affonso DD: Therapeutic support during inpatient group therapy. J Psychosoc Nurs Ment Health Serv 23(11):21–25, 1985
2. Akerlund BM, Norberg A: Group psychotherapy with demented patients. Geriatr Nurs 7(2):83–84, 1986
3. Ambrose JA: Joining in: therapeutic groups for chronic patients. J Psychosoc Nurs Ment Health Serv 27(11):28–32, 1989
4. Aronson M, Wolberg L: Group and Family Therapy. New York, Brunner/Mazel, 1980
5. Bion W: Experiences in Groups, and Other Papers. New York, Basic Books, 1961
6. Burnside IM: Working with the Elderly: Group Process and Techniques, 2nd ed. Monterey, Wadsworth Health Sciences, 1984
7. Cartwright D, Zander A: Group Dynamics: Research and Theory. New York, Harper & Row, 1968
8. Corey G, Corey M: Groups, Process and Practice. Monterey, Brooks/Cole Publishing Co, 1982
9. Eggert LL: Individual and group therapy with adolescents. In Critchley D, Maurin J. The Clinical Specialist in Psychiatric Mental Health Nursing: Theory, Research, and Practice. New York: John Wiley & Sons, 1985
10. Grotjahn M, Kline F, Friedmann C: Handbook of Group Therapy. New York, Van Nostrand Reinhold, 1983
11. Janosik E, Phipps L: Life Cycle Group Work in Nursing. Monterey, Wadsworth Health Sciences Division, 1982
12. Kaplan H, Sadock B (eds): Comprehensive Group Psychotherapy. Baltimore, Williams & Wilkins, 1983
13. Lego S: Group therapy. In Lego S (ed): The American Handbook of Psychiatric Nursing. Philadelphia, JB Lippincott, 1984
14. Lego S: Psychoanalytically oriented individual and group therapy with adults. In Critchley D, Maurin J (eds): The Clinical Specialist in Psychiatric Mental Health Nursing: Theory, Research, and Practice. New York, John Wiley & Sons, 1985
15. Lennox D: Residential Group Therapy for Children. London, Tavistock, 1982
16. Lonergan E: Group Intervention, How to Begin and Maintain Groups in Medical and Psychiatric Settings. New York, Aronson, 1982
17. Loomis ME: Group therapy. In McFarland GK, Thomas MD: Psychiatric Mental Health Nursing. Philadelphia, JB Lippincott, 1991
18. Marram GD: The Group Approach in Nursing Practice, 2nd ed. St Louis, CV Mosby, 1978
19. Mullan H, Rosenbaum M: Group Psychotherapy: Theory and Practice. New York, Free Press, 1978
20. Naar R: A Primer of Group Psychotherapy. New York, Human Sciences Press, 1982
21. Nickols M: Change in the Context of Group Therapy. New York, Brunner/Mazel, 1984
22. Oatley K: Selves in Relation: An Introduction to Psychotherapy and Groups. London, Methven, 1984
23. Rosenbaum M (ed): Handbook of Short-Term Therapy Groups. New York, McGraw-Hill, 1983

24. Rosenfeld E: Group therapy. In Beck CK, Rawlins RR, Williams SR (eds): Mental Health-Psychiatric Nursing, 2nd ed. St Louis, CV Mosby, 1988
25. Rutan J, Stone W: Psychodynamic Group Psychotherapy. Lexington, MA, Collamore Press, 1984
26. Schaefer C, Johnson L, Wherry J (eds): Group Therapies for Children and Youth. San Francisco, Jossey-Bass, 1982
27. Schiffer M: Children's Group Therapy: Methods and Case Histories. New York, Free Press, 1984
28. Seligman M (ed): Group Psychotherapy and Counseling with Special Populations. Baltimore, University Park Press, 1982
29. Slater P: Microcosm, Structural, Psychological, and Religious Evolution in Groups. New York, John Wiley & Sons, 1966
30. Sullivan HS: The Interpersonal Theory of Psychiatry. New York, WW Norton, 1953
31. Van Servellen G: Group and Family Therapy. St Louis, CV Mosby, 1984
32. Whitaker DS: Using Groups to Help People. Boston, Routledge Kegan Paul, 1985
33. Weiner M: Techniques of Group Psychotherapy. Washington, DC, American Psychiatric Press, 1984
34. Wilson H, Kneisl C: Psychiatric Nursing, 3rd ed. Menlo Park, CA, Addison-Wesley Publishing, 1988
35. Yablonsky L: Psychodrama. Resolving Emotional Problems Through Role-Playing. New York, Basic Books, 1976
36. Yalom I: Inpatient Group Psychotherapy. New York, Basic Books, 1983
37. Zander A: The Purpose of Groups and Organization. San Francisco, Jossey-Bass, 1985

Major Psychiatric Disorders

6

ORGANIC MENTAL SYNDROMES AND DISORDERS

Organic mental syndromes and organic mental disorders are a group of mental disorders with a variety of behavioral and psychological symptoms that primarily involve cognitive loss and that are etiologically related to alterations in the structure or function of the brain.[1]

Organic mental syndromes.[1]

Delirium
Dementia
Amnestic syndrome
Organic delusional syndrome
Organic hallucinosis
Organic mood syndrome
Organic anxiety syndrome
Organic personality syndrome
Intoxication
Withdrawal
Organic mental syndrome not otherwise specified

Organic mental disorders:[1]

Dementias arising in senium and presenium
Psychoactive substance-induced organic mental disorders
Organic mental disorders associated with Axis III physical disorders or
*   conditions or whose etiology is unknown*

Incidence[1,13]

Delirium: Ten percent of hospitalized patients have delirium.
Dementia: Five percent of the population over 65 have dementia to the degree that they are unable to care for themselves; ten percent of the pop-

ulation over 65 have mild dementia. Alzheimer's disease is the most common dementia.

—— Contributing Factors, Clinical Manifestations and Treatments[1-22]

A. Delirium
1. Contributing factors: brain lesions; trauma; prescription, over-the-counter and street drugs; endocrine dysfunction; poisons; infections; nutritional deficiencies; cardiovascular disorders; urinary disorders; liver disorders; electrolyte imbalances; pulmonary disorders; postoperative states
2. Clinical manifestations
   a. *Onset*: sudden impairment of cognitive functions
   b. *Duration*: brief
   c. *Memory*: impaired recent memory; patient may deny memory problems
   d. *Orientation*: fluctuations throughout a 24-hour period
      Mild: disorientation to time
      Severe: disorientation to time and place; disorientation to self may occur in very severe delirium states.
   e. *Level of consciousness*: fluctuations in level of alertness, ranging from hyper-alertness to stupor
   f. *Attention*: distractable; fluctuations in maintaining concentration
   g. *Perception*: ranges from misinterpretation to blurring of reality, to illusions, to hallucinations (particularly visual)
   h. *Speech*: unintelligible speech at times
   e. *Sleep-wake cycle*: alteration of sleep-wake cycle; day time drowsiness, insomnia at night; increase in cognitive impairment at nighttime
   j. *Psychomotor activity*: fluctuation of activity from hypoactivity and sleepiness to agitation and restlessness
   k. *Emotion*: anxiety and fear; depression
3. Treatment
   a. Biological—focuses on identifying and eliminating the cause(s) of delirium (frequently multifactorial)
   b. Symptomatic measures—focuses on relieving symptoms such as anxiety and fear by providing information about time, place, person, providing a quiet, safe environment, and reassuring patient that problems are of temporary nature.
      - Severe agitation and restlessness may require low dose neuroleptic, e.g., Haloperidol (Haldol).
      - Fluid and electrolyte balance and nutrition maintained
      - Avoid use of benzodiazepines because of their propensity to potentiate delirium; exceptions, however, are benzodiazepines for management of alcohol and drug withdrawal.
      - Minimize environmental stimuli and provide proper lighting and temperature
   c. Prevention of further complications—focuses on protection from falls, self injury, and careful monitoring of condition 24 hours a day.

4. Risk: death; 33% of elderly (over 65 years) who are hospitalized with delirium die within a month.

B. Dementia
1. Contributing factors:
   - 65% of cases by Alzheimer's disease, in which Alzheimer's-type neuropathological brain changes *or*, more specifically, degeneration of cholinergic neurons in the brain are noted at autopsy.
   - 10% of cases are caused by multi-infarct dementia in which blood vessels of the brain have many infarctions.
   - HIV virus
   - 15% of cases are reversible, e.g., hydrocephalus, thiamine deficiency, pneumonia.
2. Clinical features
   a. Slow deterioration occurs in cognitive functioning, causing multiple changes; loss of memory is an early sign.
   b. Anxiety and fatigue increase the severity of symptoms; therefore, the patient experiences more problems at night.
   c. Signs and symptoms:
      - *Memory*: Loss of recent and remote memory
      - *Orientation*: Time problems appear first, then place and person identification are impaired.
      - *Intellectual functioning*: Problems are noted in completing calculations (e.g., keeping check book balanced, completing simple tasks, solving problems, analyzing similarities and differences).
      - *Judgment*: The patient lacks good judgment (e.g., makes inappropriate job or family decisions, "bad" jokes, poor personal appearance and hygiene, ignoring of social conduct rules).
      - *Mood and personality*: Premorbid personality traits may be exaggerated or altered.
      - *Speech*: Patient has problems in communicating (e.g., lack of clarity; perseveration; muteness; blocking).
   d. Avoid misdiagnosis of depression as dementia: The onset of depression is more rapid, and patients with depressive disorder cite their lack of ability or will and their inability to answer questions; whereas patients with dementia will confabulate. Suicide occurs frequently in the elderly.
   e. Course: Many dementias are not treatable and the person becomes increasingly disabled.
      - *Mild*: The patient is able to live independently and take care of personal hygiene but is not able to work or carry on normal social activities; e.g., the patient loses objects, mixes up appointments, is not aware of current events, makes mistakes with money, is inefficient at work, fails to grasp important things at work, tires easily, has poverty of ideas (cliches and set phrases are said repeatedly), shows forgetfulness, irritability, anxiety, displays poor social manners, makes social blunders (stealing, exposing self, bizarre behaviors).

- *Moderate*: Some supervision of daily living activities is needed, e.g., the patient neglects personal hygiene, is untidy in personal appearance, exhibits indifference about eating manners, has incontinence, displays paranoid ideation, is apathetic and disoriented, has broken speech, focuses on food and other physical needs, experiences euphoria at times but is increasingly flat in affect.
- *Severe*: Continuous supervision is needed in all daily living activities. The patient is mute or incoherent, is unable to feed self, to walk, or to perform other motor skills, communicates in a few words or grunts, and may lapse into stupor, then coma.

3. Treatment for reversible forms of dementia
   a. Biological/psychopharmacologic treatment. Focuses on a carefully taken past history; physical examination (especially neurological exam) to rule out and then treat medical causes of dementia; laboratory tests and psychological testing to further identify possible causes.
   b. Identified causes are treated with appropriate medical or surgical measures; i.e., hypothyroidism with thyroid hormone.
   c. Risk factors such as smoking, high fat diet, alcoholism, diabetes, and noncompliance with hypertensive medication are managed.

4. Treatment for nonreversible forms of dementia
   - No specific treatment, but always directed at elimination of any physical cause
   - Symptomatic treatment for anxiety, depression, and insomnia
   - Supportive measures to maintain physical health, self-esteem, social support system, social skills, personal hygiene, and safety in order to maximize level of functioning

5. Treatment of specific forms of dementia: Alzheimer's, primary degenerative dementia of the Alzheimer type, Huntington's chorea, Parkinson's disease
   - No specific treatment, but always directed toward elimination of any physical cause
   - Management of factors known to affect the elderly and the progression of dementia, such as loss of loved ones, malnutrition, lack of sufficient funds, over-medication, and polypharmacy.
   - Management of anxiety, loss, impending death, disturbances in orientation, and changes in lifestyle, through individual, group, and family therapy
   - Antipsychotics in low dose range may be necessary to decrease agitation. They are used with extreme caution, because of side effects that leave patient at risk for falls, problems with urinary retention, and vision disturbances.
   - Environmental management to promote safety and security. Most patients will need institutional care as deterioration progresses.
   - Provide assistance to caregivers as follows:
     1. Instruct and demonstrate ways to avoid stress and to maintain good health habits
     2. Show the family ways to offer emotional support to each

other and ways to cope with the stress of seeing an older family member change, with the hurt of not being recognized, and with feelings of grief, fatigue, guilt,and fear.
3. Assist the family in developing ways to combat patient's disorientation (e.g., appointment calendars, clocks, stable routines, set places for important items, identification bands).
4. Assist the family in coping with their loved one's increasing anxiety and suspiciousness, which, may be evidenced by purposeless movements, a desire to leave a situation, silence, decreasing ability to participate in interactions,and fidgeting. Teach the family ways to reduce patient's anxiety (e.g., remaining calm, conversing in a quiet manner, using distraction).
5. Help the family avoid the patient's exposure to anxiety-producing situations or limit the amount of time the person is in anxiety-producing situations.
6. Help the family deal with the depression of a loved one by reminiscing with patient and by encouraging activities that the person is familiar with and has liked to do in the past.
7. Assist the family in the management of the patient's hostility and belligerence by use of distraction and reassuring techniques.
8. Teach family how to ensure a safe environment, such as reduction of clutter and loose rugs to reduce falls, and locks on doors to prevent wandering.
9. Encourage a family member to obtain power of attorney, and to anticipate and plan for an increasing need for supervision and direct care, progressing to total care, as patient's condition deteriorates.
10. Assist the family in planning for respite for the caregiver.
6. Treatment of AIDS Dementia Complex (ADC)
   a. Incidence
      - 10% of AIDS patients initially have cognitive problems.
      - 66% of AIDS patients will have AIDS dementia complex in course of illness.
   b. Treatment
      - Specific drug treatment: AZT, zidovudine
      - Symptomatic treatment:
        Pain management, e.g., carbamazepine for peripheral neuropathy, acyclovir for herpes zoster
        Antidepressants for depression
        Antipsychotics for psychosis and delirium: Low dose is recommended, because of increased sensitivity.
      - Psychotherapy focuses on issues of loss of health, mourning, role change, impending death, denial, attitudes of society towards homosexuality and AIDS and consequences to patient's self-esteem and support system, coping responses.
      - Residential:
        Hospitalization may be indicated for severe depression, suicide attempts, dementia, delirium.
        Issues of protection of patient and others from infection,

confidentiality, patient's rights, and behavior control are complex and sensitive and require discussion and decision by the treatment team.

C.   Amnestic syndrome
This disorder is marked by an impairment of memory related most frequently to the thiamine deficiency found in chronic alcoholism and in head trauma or injuries which cause damage to the diencephalic and medial temporal structure of brain. The cause is identified and treated.

D.   Organic delusional syndrome
This is a disorder with delusions (persecutory ones are the most frequent) related to an organic factor such as amphetamines, alcohol, and cocaine abuse. The cause is identified and treated.

E.   Organic hallucinosis
This is a disorder with persistent hallucinations related to drug abuse, particularly hallucinogens and alcohol, and sensory deprivation as in blindness and deafness. The cause is identified and treated.

F.   Organic mood syndrome
Organic mood syndrome is a disorder with a depressive or a manic mood related most frequently to medication use (e.g., reserpine, methyldopa), endocrine disorders, and structural diseases of the brain. The cause is identified and treated to the extent possible.

G.   Organic anxiety syndrome
This syndrome, with recurring panic attacks and generalized anxiety, is related to the abuse of psychoactive substances (e.g., amphetamine, cocaine), endocrine disorders (e.g., hyperthyroidism), cardiac arrhythmia, mitral valve prolapse, diabetes, adrenal tumor, brain disorder, and many other medical conditions. The cause is identified and treated, to the extent possible.

H.   Organic personality syndrome
This syndrome is marked by a change from the patient's previous personality, especially in the area of emotional expression and impulse control; it is related to damage of the structure of the brain from head injuries or lesions of temporal and/or frontal lobes of the brain. The cause is identified and treated, to the extent possible.

—— Associated Nursing Diagnoses

Aggression
Communication, impaired
Coping, ineffective individual
Depression
Grieving, dysfunctional
Powerlessness
Social interaction, impaired
Suicide, potential

Thought processes, altered (acute confusion)
Thought processes, altered (suspiciousness)

▬ References

1. American Psychiatric Association: Diagnostic and Statistical Manual, 3rd ed. Washington, DC, American Psychiatric Association, 1987
2. AIDS Policy: Guidelines for inpatient psychiatric units. Am J Psychiatry 145(4):542, 1988
3. Batt LJ: Managing delirium: implications for geropsychiatric nurses. J Psychosoc Nurs Ment Health Serv 27(5):22–25, 1989
4. Cournos F et al: The management of HIV infection in state psychiatric hospitals. Hosp Community Psychiatry 40(2):153–157, 1989
5. Curl A: Agitation and the older adult. J Psychosoc Nurs Ment Health Serv 27(12):12–14, 1989
6. Davies P, Wolozin BL: Recent advances in the neurochemistry of Alzheimer's disease. J Clin Psychiatry 48(suppl 5):23–30, 1987
7. Dickinson LR, Ranseen JD: An update on selected organic mental syndromes. Hosp Commun Psychiatry 41(3):290–300, 1990
8. Duffey BD: Demented, old, and alone. AJN 89(2):212–216, 1989
9. Fenton TW: AIDS-related psychiatric disorder. Br J Psychiatry 151(11):579–588, 1987
10. Flaskerud JH: AIDS: neuropsychiatric complications. J Psychosoc Nurs Ment Health Serv 25(12):4, 6, 1987
11. Harvis KA, Rabins PV: Dementia: helping family caregivers cope. J Psychosoc Nurs Ment Health Serv 27(5):7–12, 1989
12. Jordan KS: Assessment of the person with AIDS in the emergency department. Int Nurs Rev 39(2):57–59, 1989
13. Kaplan HI, Sadock BJ: Synopsis of Psychiatry: Behavioral Sciences, Clinical Psychiatry, 5th ed. Baltimore, Williams & Wilkins, 1988
14. Lipowski ZJ: Delirium: Acute Confusional States. New York, Oxford University Press, 1990
15. Matzo M: Confusion in older adults: assessment and differential diagnosis. Nurs Pract 15(9):32–46, 1990
16. Perry SW: Organic mental disorders caused by HIV: update on early diagnosis and treatment. Am J Psychiatry 147(6):696–704, 1990
17. Sarason IG, Sarason BR: Abnormal Psychology: The Problem of Maladaptive Behavior, 6th ed. New Jersey, Prentice Hall, 1989
18. Servellen G, Nyamathi AM, Mannion W: Coping with a crisis: evaluating psychological risks of patients with AIDS. J Psychosoc Nurs Ment Health Serv 27(12):16–21, 1989
19. Sharipa J, Schlesinger R, Cummings JL: Distinguishing the dementias. AJN 86(6):698–702, 1986
20. Sullivan N, Fogel BS: Could this be delirium? AJN 86(12):1359–1363, 1986
21. Tomb DA: Psychiatry for the House Officer, 3rd ed. Baltimore, Williams & Wilkins, 1988
22. Tune EE, Lucas-Blaustein MJ, Rovner BW: Psychosocial interventions. In Jarvik LF, Winograd CH (eds): Treatments for the Alzheimer Patient: The Long Haul. New York, Springer Publishing, 1988

▬ PSYCHOACTIVE SUBSTANCE USE DISORDERS AND PSYCHOACTIVE SUBSTANCE-INDUCED ORGANIC MENTAL DISORDERS[1-25]

Psychoactive substance use disorders
Psychoactive substance use disorders are a group of mental disorders manifested by "symptoms and maladaptive behavioral changes associated with more or less regular use of psychoactive substances that affect the central nervous system."[2, p. 165]

Terms
- *Abuse* is the pattern of use which includes use of the drug for at least a month; several efforts to stop the use of the drug; engaging in a variety of activities throughout the day to obtain the drug; using more of drug or using drug more frequently; having episodes of intoxication; and impairment of everyday functioning which may include not showing up at work, frequent breaks while at work, inability to complete assignments, unemployment, family fights, and loss of social supports.
- *Dependence* is the pattern of use which includes the factors associated with abuse *plus* symptoms of tolerance or withdrawal.
- *Tolerance* is a term used to indicate that more of the substance is needed to obtain the same effect or that the same amount of the substance is not producing the same effect.

Psychoactive substance-induced organic mental disorders
Psychoactive substance-induced organic mental disorders are a group of organic mental disorders caused by a substance which may produce an organic syndrome, e.g., delirium, hallucinosis (see *organic mental disorders*, this chapter), intoxication, and withdrawal.

▬ Contributing Factors (Psychoactive Substance: Alcohol)[2,7,9-11,13,15,17,23-25]
- Specific etiological factor is unknown.
- Genetic factors (e.g., children of alcoholics)
- Biological factors:
  1. Varying levels of neurotransmitters, serotonin, dopamine and GABA
  2. Serotonin hypothesis: Low brain serotonin is modified by alcohol intake. Continued drinking further depletes the brain serotonin deficit which contributes to the drinking cycle. Low brain serotonin levels may also be associated with circadian rhythms and glucose metabolism problems and with abuse of alcohol and aggressive, violent behavior.
  3. Changes in metabolic and central nervous systems occur with continued use of alcohol.
- *Personality types*: Two types have been associated with genetic factors and serotonin levels.

1. *Type I* is characteristically associated with the adult, with increased stress, with personality traits of anxiety, with tolerance building rapidly, and with dependence. Benzodiazepine/GABA receptors are involved.
2. *Type II* is characteristically associated with sons of alcoholic fathers, with young adults, with antisocial personality traits, with the use of alcohol to increase pleasure, with binge drinking, and with being involved in violent or impulsive activities (e.g., brawls). The tendency towards low blood sugar and an uneven sleep-wake cycle is also present; the area of the brain involved is believed to have many serotonin neurons. Antisocial behavior and depression are frequently associated with this group of disorders.

- *Psychoanalytic theory* hypothesizes trauma from neglect or overprotection affecting the meeting of dependency needs occurring in the oral stage of development. Frustration and conflict may be triggered during stress and the symptoms of anxiety, intense anger, and depression develop. Use of alcohol relieves the feelings and conflicts and releases the inhibitions. The person feels more powerful and able to achieve.
- *Behavior theory* hypothesizes the learned use of alcohol to reduce fear of anxiety, which in turn reinforces the drinking behavior.
- Social and cultural factors include male sex, young adult, middle socioeconomic class, Catholic religious affiliation, culture's toleration of alcohol abuse (e.g., USA and Soviet Union), and parental influence.

Contributing Factors (Other Psychoactive Substances)[2,7,9,10,17,19,25-27]

- Specific etiological factor unknown
- Peer pressure
- Sensation-seeking behavior
- Environmental influences (i.e., low socioeconomic class, family disruption, lack of standards of behavior, hopelessness)
- Low self-esteem
- Problems in dealing with physical pain and/or anxiety
- Overprescribed medication
- Ego deficit in self-care function (dysphoria is managed through use of drugs, because the ego does not assess, identify danger, nor seek protective actions)
- Overwhelming stress, anxiety, or tension
- Beliefs and value system which is compatible with drug use

SELECTED ALCOHOL USE DISORDERS[2,5,6,11,12,14-17,19,20,22,24-26]

Incidence

- Alcohol is the number one world-wide substance of abuse.
- 31% of young adults describe taking five or more drinks within 2-week period.

- 13% of the U.S. population has had alcohol abuse or dependence problems.
- Alcohol is the number three health problem in the USA.
- 85% of persons with alcoholism receive no treatment.

—— Effects

1. Alcohol is ingested orally in different amounts in various types of drinks.
2. Alcohol is absorbed directly from the gastrointestinal tract into the blood stream and goes directly to the brain and other areas of body. Tissues containing more water have a greater concentration of alcohol. The rate of absorption is increased by lack of food in the stomach and by drinking water or carbonated beverages.
3. Elimination of alcohol occurs by excretion through kidneys and lungs and by oxidation, which gives energy and heat to the body.
4. Action: central nervous system depressant
5. Nonmedical use: To relax; to be happy; to alleviate anxiety and stress.
6. Drug interaction: alcohol interacts with many other drugs to potentiate their effects—this can be life-threatening.

—— Alcohol Intoxication

1. How soon the effects of ingesting alcohol can be noted, and the duration of intoxication, is related to the amount of beverage, alcohol content of beverage, absorption rate, excretion rate, tolerance, and individual differences.
2. Early signs include a relaxation of inhibitions, hyperactivity, grandiosity, an increase in mental alertness.
3. Later signs include maladaptive behaviors such as increased aggressiveness, uncooperativeness, irritability, emotional lability, impairment of attention and judgment. Other signs are the smell of alcohol on breath, slurred speech, unsteadiness, nystagmus, flushed face. A blackout (amnesia occurring during intoxication) may be experienced.
4. Behaviors associated with blood alcohol levels:

100–150 mg/dl:	Impairment of muscular coordination, irritability
150–250 mg/dl:	Gait disturbance, slurring speech, apathy
250–400 mg/dl:	Alcohol coma
400–700 mg/dl:	Death due to respiratory depression or aspiration of vomitus

5. Legal intoxication range is 0.10–0.15% blood alcohol level.
6. Presenting symptoms are also present in hypoglycemia, infections of central nervous system, schizophrenia, depression, etc., therefore careful monitoring is required.
7. *Treatment* is symptomatic, including environmental management (e.g., quiet area, prevention of falls, prevention of doing harm to self or others); sedation (with caution, because of the danger of increasing a comatose state); maintenance of fluid and electrolyte balance.
8. *Complications* include automobile accidents (50% of traffic deaths are related to alcohol use); criminal acts (50% of homicides are related to

intoxication); suicides (25% are related to alcohol use); occupational accidents; falls causing fractures or trauma to the brain; conditions related to exposure to extremes of weather; and predisposition to infections.

Uncomplicated Alcohol Withdrawal and Alcohol Withdrawal Delirium

1. *Symptoms of uncomplicated alcohol withdrawal* include tremor (coarse tremor of outstretched hands, of tongue [which may interfere with speech], and of eyelids); anxiety or nervousness; sleep disturbances; nausea and vomiting; symptoms of autonomic hyperactivity (increased blood pressure, tachycardia, sweating); delusions or hallucinations.
   a. Occurs 12–18 hours after cessation or reduction of drinking
   b. Seizures may occur within first 48 hours; they generally precede the development of delirium.
2. *Symptoms of alcohol withdrawal delirium or delirium tremens (DTs)* include delirium (e.g., confusion, agitation, disorientation to time, place, person); memory impairment; hallucinations (most frequently visual); autonomic hyperactivity; fever.
   a. Occurs from 2–8 days after cessation of drinking; alcohol may not be detected in blood.
   b. Death occurs in 10–15% of cases.
3. *Treatment*: The withdrawal syndrome may require little or no treatment other than food, fluids, and a quiet environment. More severe symptoms require evaluation, monitoring, and specific treatment or detoxification.
   a. Benzodiazepines are used for seizures and tremors, and to control agitation.
   b. Thiamine, multivitamins, and a high-carbohydrate diet are given to correct vitamin deficiencies.
   c. Physical restraint may be necessary to prevent injury to self or others
   d. Reality orientation and reassurance to assist in management of delirium

Alcohol Abuse/Alcohol Dependence

1. Patterns are
   a. regular, large daily intake of alcohol;
   b. regular weekend, heavy intake of alcohol;
   c. binges of daily, heavy drinking for weeks to months and long periods of sobriety.
2. Complications associated with continued alcohol dependence include
   a. Medical (e.g., gastritis, anemia, high blood pressure, pancreatitis)
   b. Neurological (e.g., peripheral neuropathy, cerebral atrophy)
   c. Psychiatric (e.g., alcohol amnestic disorder)
   d. Fetal alcohol syndrome (The risk for mothers with alcoholism to have a child with this syndrome is 35%. Mental retardation is frequently caused by this syndrome.)

3. Treatment
   a. Biological/pharmacologic
      (1) Disulfiram (Antabuse), an alcohol-sensitizing drug, produces unpleasant symptoms when alcohol is used; these include flushing, hypotension, nausea, coughing, anxiety, and dizziness. Alcohol consumption while on Antabuse can be highly toxic and potentially life-threatening, e.g., severe hypotension, heart failure, and sudden death. The cooperation of the patient is needed in taking the drug daily.
      (2) Antidepressants may be used to treat depression following the withdrawal phase or because of the coexisting problem of major depression.
      (3) Antianxiety drugs, benzodiazepines, are used to treat symptoms of anxiety following withdrawal or coexisting anxiety disorder; caution is advised because of their dependency-producing effects. Buspirone and propranalol do not appear to cause dependence.
   b. *Self help* focuses on the mutual problems of group members and assists them in resolving daily life issues associated with alcohol. Alcoholic Anonymous (AA) is an example of the self-help model and is one of the major forms of treatment of alcoholism. The process is outlined in 12 steps and is frequently referred to as the 12-step program. The person participates in meetings (frequency may be daily, weekly, monthly, or as needed) at which members share, in depth, their experiences with alcoholism; e.g., problems it has caused, periods of sobriety and drinking, how they found AA, and their process of recovery. Members support each other to continue working toward abstinence. AA also emphasizes developing a relationship with a sponsor who gives additional guidance, hints, and direction. The successful outcomes of the approach may be related to a commitment to AA, the intense affiliation for the group, and the role of helper to one another, but reasons for the effectiveness of the program are not specifically known. The philosophy of the self-help group and the medical model have not been compatible in the past; i.e., no medication, no drugs of any kind, versus the use of medications. However, there is a trend in clinical areas towards the integration of the two treatment models. Greater appreciation and understanding of varying views and contributions towards treatment is basic to the beginning of effective working together of the clinicians and the self-help groups.
   c. *Social learning/behavioral*
      (1) Focuses on abusive drinking through chemical aversion therapy in which an alcoholic beverage is paired with a noxious stimulus (e.g., the nausea from an emetic)
      (2) Focuses on the setting (when and where drinking occurs) and the consequences of drinking, through covert sensitization, in which the person is trained to imagine the sequence of drinking, the noxious stimulus when drinking occurs, and the relief when drinking is stopped
      (3) Focuses on a variety of techniques to produce behavior change: stress management, biofeedback, social skills training, contingency management through identifying rewards and punish-

ments for changing targeted behavior, relapse prevention strategies, and self-control training

d. *Psychoanalytic/psychotherapeutic* treatment focuses traditionally on resolving the conflict associated with dependency needs that increase the anger, depression, guilt, and anxiety that the patient tries to avoid with the use of alcohol; the usefulness of this approach is questioned.

(1) Currently, therapy focuses on offering support to deal with daily problems, stresses, and feelings, without alcohol use.

(2) Group psychotherapy focuses on supporting abstinence through sharing of experience; identifying with a positive view of self as a recovering alcoholic; dealing with denial, grandiosity, and manipulation; and in working with reality and learning to be helpful to others.

e. *Biopsychosocial model or the stages of change model*: Theories from other models are integrated into the stages of change model; i.e., the predispositional influences of genetics and early life experiences, the physiological effects of alcohol, the cognitive factors of expectations, assumptions, appraisals, and defenses, and the behavioral skills and resources of the individual. The four stages of the change process are

(1) Precontemplation stage: No change is being considered in the drinking or other addiction pattern.

(2) Contemplation or commitment and motivation stage: The consequences of the drinking or other addiction pattern are considered; no change in drinking behavior or other addiction pattern is thought of. Interventions would include strengthening of the commitment and motivation to change by increasing the positive view of a new lifestyle and behaviors, by decreasing the fear associated with change itself, by supporting the person's evaluation of the problem and selected action, and by noting the discrepancy between the values and beliefs of the person and the addictive behaviors.

(3) Action stage: Change in own behavior or help to change the behavior is sought. Most programs focus on this stage only.

(4) Maintenance stage: Avoidance of relapse is sought. Interventions would include assistance with relapse prevention by identifying major life stresses, the coping processes and skills used to deal with the stresses, and the reaction to relapses.

f. *Interpersonal/familial* treatment focuses on patterns of family interaction and the individual with the alcohol problem, using one of the many family therapy approaches. From a systems approach, the focus is on changing patterns in the family. From a family functioning approach, the focus is on assisting in the restructuring of family roles and responsibilities and in changing maladaptive patterns that drinking behavior has caused (i.e., conflict, disorganization, enmeshment, shifting of roles). Data seem to indicate better treatment outcomes when the family is involved in the treatment process.

g. *Alcohol treatment programs*: Alcohol treatment programs involve three stages: detoxification, rehabilitation, and aftercare—or stated another way, acute intervention, rehabilitation, and maintenance.

Typically a program provides emergency and detoxification services, followed by a 21–28 day inpatient program involving diagnostic evaluation and a treatment program which includes the 12-step process of recovery of Alcoholic's Anonymous, stress management, activity therapies, individual and family counseling, and occupational counseling. Aftercare supports the behavior changes achieved and provides continued involvement in the 12-step process of recovery, individual therapy, or other form of relapse prevention. It may involve sheltered living arrangements.

▬ AMPHETAMINE USE DISORDERS (E.G., BENZEDRINE, PRELUDIN, "SPEED")[1,2,8,17,20,25–27]

— Incidence

- Two percent of the adult population has had an amphetamine abuse problem.

— Effects

1. Taken orally, intravenously, or by inhalation
2. Nonmedical use: to provide relief from fatigue, to assist with studying, to produce euphoria, to recover from hangover
3. Action: central nervous system stimulant

— Amphetamine Intoxication

1. Effects are experienced within a few minutes to an hour, depending on the route of administration.
2. Signs are increased alertness, agitation, speech pressure, elation, increased aggression, and assaultiveness. Associated signs are increased pulse rate and high blood pressure, dilation of pupils, nausea, vomiting, sweating, and chills.
3. A rush is associated with intravenous use, along with feelings of euphoria and extreme satisfaction with self.
4. Amphetamine delirium and amphetamine delusional disorders may develop.
5. Treatment: supportive measures such as benzodiazepines for anxiety and withdrawal; haloperidol for delirium and delusional disorders, and antidepressants for withdrawal and depression
6. Complications:
   a. Death may occur from cardiovascular shock, convulsions, or hyperpyrexia.
   b. Medical conditions include stroke and myocardial infarctions.

— Amphetamine Withdrawal

1. Crash begins when signs of high dose use have stopped.
2. Withdrawal period begins 24 hours after the crash and lasts up to 4 days.

3. Signs include depression with risk for suicide, lethargy, anxiety, irritability, and sleep pattern disturbance. Other signs are headaches, sweating, GI symptoms, muscle spasms, and increased appetite.

── Amphetamine Abuse/Dependence

Treatment is discussed at end of this section.

■ CANNABIS USE DISORDERS (MARIJUANA)[1,2,8,16,17,20,22,25–27]

── Incidence

- 4% of adult population has had a cannabis abuse problem.
- Decline has been noted in daily use as reported by students (10.7% in 1978; 3.3% in 1987).

── Effects

1. Taken by ingestion or smoking
2. Nonmedical use: to obtain "high" and enhance creativity

── Cannabis Intoxication

1. Effect is noted almost immediately and lasts up to 4 hours.
2. Signs include euphoria and relaxation, increased responsiveness to stimuli in environment such as light or music, sensation of slowing down of time, increased appetite, increased pulse, conjunctival injection (bloodshot eyes due to dilation of arterioles).
3. A person may experience a "bad" trip, increased feelings of anxiety, panic, or depression. Cannabis delusional syndrome may develop.
4. Treatment involves supportive measures.

── Cannabis Abuse/Dependence

1. There is little evidence for dependence.
2. Complications from years of use include
   a. Amotivation syndrome: Person is not able to concentrate, attend to, or complete tasks at work or school.
   b. Increased risk for chronic respiratory conditions and cancer
   c. Interference with short-term memory and learning
   d. Interference with production of male hormones
3. Treatment is discussed at end of this section

■ COCAINE USE DISORDERS[1,2–5,8,17–23,25–27]

── Incidence

- 4 million of the adult population has had a cocaine abuse problem.
- Considered an epidemic; in 1974, persons who had used cocaine one time numbered 5.4 million; in 1985, 25 million had used it.

—— Effects

1. Taken by sniffing through the nose (snorting), through injection (subcutaneous or intravenous), and through free-basing (use of pure cocaine in pipe or cigarette)
2. Nonmedical use: to achieve a sense of well-being and confidence, to increase energy level, to increase performance in music and sports.
3. Action: blockade of dopamine re-uptake.

—— Cocaine Intoxication

1. Effects are experienced almost immediately, last 30 minutes to an hour, and are related to route of administration.
2. Signs include a rush of euphoria, improved work performance of work, agitation, increased alertness, poor judgment, and inappropriate behavior involving sex and aggression. Other signs include increased pulse rate and blood pressure, dilation of pupils, sweating and chills, nausea, vomiting, and hallucinations.
3. Treatment: supportive measures such as diazepam for convulsion and/or anxiety, propranolol as antagonist or sympathomimetic effects.
4. Complications
   a. Death from cardiac or respiratory arrest
   b. Cardiovascular conditions (e.g., myocardial infarction, angina, rupture of aorta, hypertension)
   c. Sexual dysfunction
   d. Hepatitis and AIDS following I.V. administration

—— Cocaine Withdrawal

1. Crash begins when signs of high dose use have stopped.
2. The withdrawal period begins 24 hours after crash and lasts up to 4 days.
3. Signs include craving and a searching for drug; depression; and irritability.

—— Cocaine Abuse

Treatment is discussed at the end of this section..

■ HALLUCINOGENS USE DISORDERS (LYSERGIC ACID [LSD], MESCALINE)[1-2,8,16-17,20,25-27]

—— Incidence

- 0.3% of the adult population has had a hallucinogen abuse problem.

—— Effects

1. Taken orally or by smoking
2. Nonmedical use: to achieve some self-learning or social experience: to produce a "high"

3. Action: affects production of dopamine, acetylcholine, serotonin, GABA; also has a sympathomimetic effect

— Hallucinogen Hallucinosis

1. Effect is experienced in an hour and lasts up to 12 hours.
2. Signs include alteration of perceptions, with vivid colors and changing designs, enhancement and alteration of all senses, visual hallucinations, alteration in sense of time and space, distortion of body image, emotional lability, increased suggestibility, depersonalization, recalling of past events, and belief that insight into self is increasing. Signs also involve increased pulse rate, dilated pupils, sweating, tremor, and blurring of vision.
3. A "bad trip" resembles a panic attack that lasts 8–12 hours and may develop into psychosis. Treatment involves protection from harm to self or others, reassurance or "talking down," and use of diazepam or haloperidol to decrease the agitation.
4. *Flashback* is the reliving of the drug-induced experience when no drug has been taken. It may be triggered by cannabis, coming out of a dark area, increased stress, or fatigue.
(NOTE: There is no withdrawal; dependence is rare.)

■ OPIOID USE DISORDERS (E.G., MORPHINE, HEROIN, DEMEROL)[1,2,8,16,17,20,25–27]

— Incidence

- 0.7% of the adult population has had an opioid abuse or dependence problem.
- Heroin is most frequently used; there are 400,000 to 600,00 addicted persons in the U.S.

— Effects

1. Ingested orally, intravenously (note needle tracks), and subcutaneously (note skin pops and nodules)
2. Nonmedical use: to achieve pain relief and euphoria
3. Action: analgesic effect caused by binding at opioid receptors in the brain

— Opioid Intoxication and Overdose

1. Effects are noted in 1–5 minutes after I.V. administration as a rush or euphoria lasting 10–30 minutes, followed by a period of up to 6 hours of dysphoria, apathy, "nodding," pinpoint pupils, slurred speech, impairment of memory and attention.
2. Overdose is characterized by coma, shock, respiratory depression.
3. Treatment: Administration of opioid antagonist, naloxone, is followed by monitoring for signs of withdrawal reaction, and supportive measures to maintain airway and fluid and electrolyte balance.

—— Opioid Withdrawal

1. Effects begin in 6–9 hours after the last dose and peak in 2–3 days.
2. Early signs include craving for the drug, restlessness, and demanding behavior. Other signs include dilation of pupils, sweating, tearing, runny nose, yawning, fever, insomnia, and poor appetite.
3. Later signs include muscle aches and spasms, GI symptoms, agitation and increased blood pressure, pulse rate, and respirations.
4. Treatment: Methadone, a synthetic opioid, is given in progressively decreasing doses to withdraw patient. Aftercare in a residential program or outpatient clinic is encouraged.

—— Opioid Abuse/Dependence

1. Methadone maintenance programs
   a. *Metabolic or adaptive model* views the craving for opioid drugs as a biochemical deficit which can be corrected by administration of methadone. The person is expected to continue on methadone indefinitely. The person is also expected to learn work skills and to obtain a job. Various services and therapies are adjuncts.
   b. *Psychotherapeutic model* places emphasis on the development of a drug-free lifestyle and resocialization as the goals of the program. Methadone is an adjunct to psychotherapy. Assistance is given the person in the process of withdrawal. Aftercare services are part of the program.
2. Complications of long-term use
   a. Involvement in criminal activities to support habit   ·
   b. Death occurs in 1% of heroin addicts from accidental overdose.
   c. Medical conditions (e.g., AIDS, hepatitis B, venereal disease, cellulitis)

■ PHENCYCLIDINE (PCP)[1,2,8,17,20,25–27]

—— Effects

1. Taken orally, intravenously, or by sniffing or smoking
2. Nonmedical use: to relax, to produce euphoria
3. Action: dissociative anesthetic

—— Phencyclidine Intoxication

1. Initial effects are experienced in 5 minutes and last up to six hours. Other effects may last several days.
2. Signs include euphoria, peacefulness, emotional lability, and lack of awareness of environment. With increased amounts of the drug, the signs include hallucinations, depersonalization, delusions, changes in body image and time and space perception, assaultiveness, homicidal and suicidal behaviors. Other signs include increased pulse rate and blood pressure, nystagmus, ataxia, dysarthria, alteration of pain perception, rigidity, and seizures.
3. Other disorders may develop (i.e., PCP delirium or PCP delusional disorder or PCP mood disorder).

4. *PCP psychosis*: Person is frequently first seen in emergency room and may be disoriented and experiencing hallucinations and problems communicating. Other signs include staring, repeating words heard, paranoia, posturing, and inappropriate behavior (e.g., removing clothes, assaultiveness, masturbation).
5. Treatment symptomatic; includes diazepam for seizure and muscle spasms, quiet environment, haloperidol for behavior control, full restraint only when necessary, and maintenance of fluid and electrolyte balance.

—— Phencyclidine Abuse/Dependence

Treatment is discussed at end of this section.

■ SEDATIVE-HYPNOTIC-ANXIOLYTIC (E.G., BARBITURATES, METHAQUALONE, BENZODIAZEPINES)[1,2,8,17,20,25–27]

—— Incidence

- 1.1% of the adult population has had a sedative-hypnotic-anxiolytic abuse or dependence problem.

—— Effects

1. Sedative-hypnotic-anxiolytics are generally ingested orally; IV barbiturate is used as an alternative to heroin.
2. Action: sedative
3. Nonmedical use: to produce a sense of well-being, relaxation
4. Drug interaction: Alcohol interacts with sedative-hypnotic-anxiolytic drugs to produce an additive effect that can be life-threatening.

—— Sedative-Hypnotic-Anxiolytic Intoxication

1. Signs include disinhibition, incoordination, unsteadiness, problems in thinking clearly, memory problems, slowed speech, irritability, nystagmus, and constriction of pupils.
2. Evaluation of intoxication state is essential since suicide attempts are a possibility.
3. Treatment includes lavage or induction of vomiting, maintenance of airway, fluid and electrolyte balance.

—— Sedative-Hypnotic-Anxiolytic Withdrawal

1. Effects are noted in 1–3 days after cessation of drug.
2. Signs range from mild to delirium to death. The withdrawal process is dangerous.
   a. Mild signs include anxiety, hypotension, tremor.
   b. Next level of symptoms include increasing discomfort, insomnia, poor appetite, coarse tremors of the upper extremities, sweating, tachycardia, visual hallucinations, and seizures.
   c. Delirium is similar to alcoholic delirium tremens.

3. Treatment is symptomatic when the patient is in coma. As soon as possible, a determination of the degree of dependence or habitual dose is made. The dose is decreased slowly while a mild withdrawal state is experienced. An aftercare program is recommended.

── Sedative-Hypnotic-Anxiolytic Abuse/Dependence

1. Complications include
   a. Death from accidental overdose or from suicide
   b. Intravenous use increases risk for AIDS, hepatitis B and other conditions.
2. Treatment is discussed at end of section.

▄▄ TREATMENT FOR ABUSE/DEPENDENCE ASSOCIATED WITH AMPHETAMINE, CANNABIS, COCAINE, OPIOIDS, PHENCYCLIDINE, AND SEDATIVE-HYPNOTIC-ANXIOLYTIC[2,6,14-16,19,20,25-27]

1. Abuse patterns and dependence have been identified for specific drugs in the previous sections; however, because many people today abuse more than one drug, treatment programs that focus on polysubstance abuse are indicated for this population.
2. Drug treatment programs, like alcohol treatment programs, have three phases: acute intervention, rehabilitation, and maintenance.
   a. *Inpatient programs* focus on detoxification from the substance(s).
   b. *Residential programs,* as part of the rehabilitation and maintenance phases, have as goals for the person a change of lifestyle, abstinence, development of work skills, a greater sense of responsibility for self, learning to be honest with self and others, and changing antisocial behaviors. Addiction is viewed as a life-long problem. Sensitivity training, encounter groups, problem-solving or task-oriented groups, and the 12-step program of Alcoholics Anonymous are used.
   c. *Outpatient programs* may be used in the rehabilitation and maintenance phases. In change-focused programs, the emphasis is on resocialization through individual and group therapies. Other programs may have an adaptive focus, which assists an individual with crises as they occur, using a variety of services.
3. Research demonstrates that staying in a treatment program for a 6-month period is linked to behavior changes.
4. Outreach efforts to attract the untreated addict into effective programs are important, because only about 10% of intravenous drug abusers enter a program.
5. In addition to problems of abuse and dependence, the person frequently has medical problems, mental disorders, employment problems, and family problems. Referrals for treatment or special services are indicated.

▄▄ ASSOCIATED NURSING DIAGNOSES

Aggression
Anxiety

Coping, defensive (denial)
Coping, ineffective individual
Crisis, situational
Depression
Family processes, altered
Manipulation
Powerlessness
Self-esteem disturbance
Suicide potential
Thought processes, altered (acute confusion)
Thought processes, altered (hallucinations)

■ REFERENCES

1. Adams RD: Drug dependency in hospital patients. AJN 88(4):477–481, 1988
2. American Psychiatric Association: Diagnostic and Statistical Manual, 3rd ed revised. Washington, DC, American Psychiatric Association, 1987
3. Chychula NM, Okore C: The cocaine epidemic: a comprehensive review of use, abuse and dependence. Nurs Pract 15(7):31–39, 1990
4. Chychula NM, Okore C: The cocaine epidemic: treatment options for cocaine dependence. Nurs Pract 15(10):33–40, 1990
5. Cohen S, Callahan JF (eds): The Diagnosis and Treatment of Drug and Alcohol Abuse. New York, Haworth Press, 1986
6. Collen RL, Leonard KE, Searles JS (eds): Alcohol and the Family: Research and Clinical Perspectives. New York, Guilford Press, 1990
7. Compton P: Drug abuse: a self-care deficit. J Psychosoc Nurs Ment Health Serv 27(3):22–26, 1989
8. Donovan DM, Marlatta GA (eds): Assessment of Addictive Behaviors. New York, Guilford Press, 1988
9. Donovan JM: An etiologic model of alcoholism. Am J Psychiatry 143(1):1–11, 1986
10. Franklin D: Hooked, not hooked: why isn't everyone an addict? Health 4(6):39–52, 1990
11. Galanter M, Castaneda R, Salamon I: Institutional self-help therapy for alcoholism: Clinical outcome. Alcoholism 11:424–425, 1987
12. Galanter M, Talbott D, Gallegos K, Rubenstone E: Combined Alcoholic's Anonymous and professional care for addicted physicians. Am J Psychiatry 147(1):64–68, 1990
13. Goodwin FK: Alcoholism research: delivering on the promise. Pub Health Rep 103(6):569–574, 1988
14. Hubbard RL, Marsden ME, Rachal JV, et al: Drug Abuse Treatment: A National Survey of Effectiveness. Chapel Hill, University of North Carolina, 1989
15. Institute of Medicine: Broadening the Base of Treatment for Alcohol Problems. Washington, DC, National Academy Press, 1990
16. Johnston LD, O'Malley PM, Backman JG: National Trends in Drug Use and Related Factors Among American High School Students and Young Adults. 1975–1986. Washington, DC, US Government Printing Office, 1987

17. Kaplan HI, Sadock BJ: Synopsis of Psychiatry: Behavioral Sciences, Clinical Psychiatry, 5th ed. Baltimore, Williams & Wilkins, 1988
18. Kosten TR: Pharmacotherapeutic interventions for cocaine abuse: matching patients to treatments. J Nerv Ment Dis 177(7):379–389, 1989
19. Marlatt GA, Gordon JR (eds): Relapse Prevention: Maintenance Strategies in the Treatment of Addictive Behaviors. New York, Guilford Press, 1985
20. McKelvy MJ, Kane JS, Kellison K: Double trouble: substance abuse and mental illness. J Psychosoc Nurs Ment Health Serv 25(1):20–25, 1987
21. Millman RB: Evaluation and clinical management of cocaine abusers. J Clin Psychiatry 49(2):27–33, 1988
22. National Institute on Drug Abuse: NIDA Capsules: 1985 National Household Survey on Drug Abuse. Rockville, MD, Press Office of the National Institute on Drug Abuse, 1986
23. Pollack MH, Brotman AW, Rosenbaum JF: Cocaine abuse and treatment. Compr Psychiatry 30(1):31–44, 1989
24. Powell AH, Minick MP: Alcohol withdrawal syndrome. AJN 88(3):312–315, 1988
25. Sarason IG, Sarason BR: Abnormal Psychology: The Problem of Maladaptive Behavior, 6th ed. Englewood Cliffs, NJ, Prentice-Hall, 1989
26. Task Force Report of the American Psychiatric Association: Treatment of Psychiatric Disorders, vol 2. Washington, DC, American Psychiatric Association, 1989
27. Tomb DA: Psychiatry for the House Officer. 3rd ed. Baltimore, Williams & Wilkins, 1988

▬ SCHIZOPHRENIA

Schizophrenia[1–48] is a severely disabling, chronic illness generally lasting a lifetime.[2] It represents a group of five subtypes that present varied and severe symptoms of disordered thinking, e.g., hallucinations, delusions, confusion, disorientation, and bizarre behaviors. Periods of remission occur, but there is usually an overall steadily deteriorating course. The five subtypes are as follows:

Catatonic type
Disorganized type
Paranoid type
Undifferentiated type
Residual type

▬ Incidence[2,24,39,47]

- 1% of population
- Age of onset is usually before 25 years of age.
- The majority of patients are 15–54 years of age.
- 50% of mental hospital beds are occupied by schizophrenic patients.
- Lower socioeconomic class has higher prevalence of schizophrenia.

—— Contributing Factors[5,11,15,24,28,30,35,45,47]

Research and theories emphasize several factors:

- The *genetic factor* is significant. First-degree relatives of persons with schizophrenia have ten times the risk for developing schizophrenia. Adoption studies of twins developing schizophrenia provide evidence of the great importance of genetics. The discovery of a genetic marker is predicted for the future.

- *Prenatal disturbances* during the second trimester of pregnancy, causing abnormality in brain structure and functioning related to stress or viral infections, and complications at delivery such as hemorrhage are implicated. The effects may not be noted until adolescence when the effect of information processing is first detected.

- *Brain structure abnormalities*: Factors such as increased size of cerebral ventricles, variations in cerebral blood flow, abnormal EEG, thickening of corpus callosum, etc., have been demonstrated, but there has been no consistent abnormality of structure or function found.

- *Neurotransmitter abnormalities*: Dopamine hypothesis refers to hyperactivity of the dopaminergic system and is validated by research. Other neurotransmitters such as norepinephrine, serotonin, GABA are also involved.

- *Stress-diathesis model* proposes that the person has a genetic predisposition or an intrauterine metabolic condition affecting the developing nervous system. The structures affected are ones associated with being aware of the environment, being aware of the sensations generated, and integrating this into a perception of reality. In other words, there is a deficiency in the information-processing system. The person has an impaired capacity to respond and thereby grow and develop; consequently, the ability to respond to stressful environmental factors decreases. Environmental stresses such as intense family conflicts, loss of family, and/or other biological factors such as drug abuse and malnutrition continue to interact and shape the individual. Symptoms of schizophrenia are a response of a person's vulnerability to environmental stress.

—— Clinical Manifestations[2,3,17,24,25,47]

A. Division of the symptoms of schizophrenia into two groups facilitates research into pathophysiology and treatment

1. *Positive symptoms*: It is hypothesized that there are normal brain structures. There is good treatment response to medications in the presence of positive symptoms. The positive symptoms are considered florid or strongly emotional and excessive, active.

   a. *Hallucinations* are the experiences of sensory perception without a stimuli.

   (1) Voices are heard commenting in general.

   (2) *Command hallucinations* ("You are . . . ," "You do . . . ,") may make obscene and/or threatening remarks or command the patient to engage in a violent act.

(3) *Tactile and olfactory hallucinations* may indicate temporal lobe epilepsy or the presence of a tumor. Cocaine abuse may cause tactile hallucinations.

(4) *Visual hallucinations* are noted in hysteria and schizophrenia, but can also be indicators of organic disorders (e.g., delirium).

b. *Delusions* are false beliefs which are not altered by reason. There are delusions of persecution, grandeur, impending destruction, somatic signs, and/or using religious ideas or symbols. Example: "I am a researcher and have to tell others about files being kept; they can't be translated because I'm the only one who knows."

c. *Associated behaviors* (e.g., agitation, difficulty sleeping, angry outbursts, assaultiveness, self mutualization, suspiciousness, and other behaviors) in response to or related to hallucinations or delusions

2. *Negative symptoms*: It is hypothesized that there is a structural brain abnormality, e.g., altered ventricular size. Treatment response is poorer. The symptoms or signs are deficits in social and vocational functioning.

   a. *Asocial behavior* (e.g., withdrawal from friends, listening to music all day and refusing to respond, aloofness, lack of social manners)

   b. *Inability to work* (e.g., not completing simple tasks, forgetting and abandoning plans)

   c. *Passivity* (e.g., complaints of no energy, apathy, boredom)

   d. *Inability to care for self* (e.g., poor personal hygiene, wearing inappropriate clothing, urinating in the street, not combing hair)

   e. *Problems of impulse control* range from grabbing another's food, to smoking all of cigarettes, to attempting suicide or striking out at a person or destroying furniture.

   f. *Peculiar mannerisms*, lack of coordinated movements

   g. *Alogia* (e.g., inability to reason or solve problems, lack of input and judgment, concreteness)

   h. *Flattened, blunted, inappropriate affect*

   i. *Loosening of associations* (i.e., making of tangential, rambling, evasive, circumstantial statements)

   j. *Problems in communicating clearly* (i.e., poverty of speech, echolalia, blocking, neologisms, overinclusiveness)

— Clinical manifestations of types[2,24,44,47]

1. *Catatonic schizophrenia* is characterized by a *stuporous state*, in which a person is mute, negative, or complains in response to a request, is immobile, displays waxy flexibility, and may retain urine and feces; or an *excited state*, in which the person is assaultive, aggressive, hyperactive, or agitated.

2. *Disorganized schizophrenia* is characterized by incoherence, inappropriate behaviors, and regressive behavior.

3. *Paranoid schizophrenia* is characterized by delusions of persecution or grandeur.

4. *Undifferentiated schizophrenia* is characterized by a variety of symptoms found in several types.

5. *Residual schizophrenia* is characterized by a history of previous episodes and such remaining signs as social withdrawal, emotional blunting, eccentric behaviors, illogical thinking, and loosening of associations.

— Course of Illness[5,22,24,42,44,47]

A. Early signs, usually beginning in adolescence and developing over few months or days include:

1. Blocking or cutting off conversation; not responding as usual to friends, appearing aloof
2. Expressing various concerns regarding body symptoms (e.g., back pain, digestive symptoms)
3. Forgetting and abandoning plans or life goals
4. Disregarding social customs and talking about abstract ideas such as love, creation, equality

B. Diagnosis
Schizophrenia may first be identified when signs are associated with a psychotic episode that may be precipitated by a loss, separation, rejection, by use of a hallucinogenic drug or alcohol, or by other major stressful events such as going away to college.

C. Active phase or psychotic state.
There are positive symptoms for a period of at least one week to months.

D. Residual phase
There are negative symptoms throughout the life span.

E. Exacerbations and remissions
These generally occur over a period of 5 years, with increasing severity of negative symptoms. The course of illness is described as subchronic, chronic, subchronic with acute exacerbation (positive symptoms), chronic with acute exacerbations (positive symptoms) in remission. Indications of a recurrence include problems in sleeping, increasing restlessness, lack of appetite, lack of pleasure in anything, depression, and problems in concentrating.

— Risk[1,24,45]

- Suicide: 50% of patients attempt suicide. The suicide mortality rate is 10 times higher than for the general population.
- The overall mortality rate is twice that of the general population.

— Prognosis[22,24,47]

- Schizophrenia is a chronic, disabling disorder.
- Only 20–30% of schizophrenics are able to live minimally sheltered lives.
- Most persons with schizophrenia require an extended range of supportive services.
- Better prognosis is associated with rapid onset of symptoms after 30 years of age, good social and work history, the identification of an associated stressor, and lack of family history.

── Treatment[4–10,12–14,16,18–24,26–27,29–38,40–44,46–48]

A. *Biological/psychopharmacologic interventions* focus on the following:
1. Administration of antipsychotics to provide management in acute, chronic, and maintenance states
   a. Management of insomnia, psychomotor restlessness, aggression, and irritability are achieved in 1–2 weeks.
   b. Depression, anxiety, discomfort in social situations are then lessened.
   c. Hallucinations, delusions, other disorders of thinking are the last to abate, usually in 6–8 weeks.
2. Management of side effects of medication (e.g., hypokinesia, akathesia, dystonia) to increase patient comfort and enhance treatment compliance
3. Preventive management of tardive dyskinesia (TD):
   a. Careful, deliberate initial prescribing of antipsychotics
   b. Frequent and consistent checks for development of TD symptoms
   c. Discontinuation of antipsychotic medication when TD symptoms appear, because there is no effective treatment (although vitamin E may be of some help)
   d. Continued evaluation at periodic intervals to determine the need to continue antipsychotic medication

B. *Behavioral*—Focuses on resolving the psychotic dysfunctions as perceived to be behavioral excesses (e.g., hallucinations), behavioral deficits (such as poor grooming skills), and lack of behavior situation fit
1. Careful analysis of situation to determine stimuli preceding and following behaviors, to identify behaviors needing alteration, and to teach skills needed. Examples of skills taught include
   a. Social skills training (e.g., assertiveness training, job interviewing, problem solving, use of leisure time)
   b. Personal grooming skills
   c. Eating skills, meal planning and preparation
   d. Communication skills (e.g., nonverbal communication, introducing self and others, giving compliments)
2. Token economy programs reinforce desired behaviors using praise or other special incentives such as points or privileges.

C. *Psychosocial/psychotherapeutic/psychoeducational*—Focuses on the following:
1. Helping the patient and/or family manage socioenvironmental stressors and understanding the limitations related to the condition of schizophrenia
2. Assisting in developing and then maintaining self-esteem
3. Managing symptoms related to the disorder while assisting in engaging in activities of daily living to the fullest extent possible
4. Skill development and training may be used. The therapeutic relationship with the patient is particularly important because of the poorly developed self system and dependency needs. The patient needs to experience supportive, accepting, encouraging, advising, and sometimes directive interactions. Group work is difficult primarily because

of the patient's problems with attention and focusing, as well as sensitivity to overstimulation. Group work is valuable for its focus on how to express emotions or problems, on the meaning of words to others, and on ways to give and receive support from others.

D. *Interpersonal/familial*
1. Focuses on assisting families to
    a. Learn how to be supportive without fostering dependency;
    b. Make constructive remarks without increasing feelings of guilt and anger;
    c. Offer feedback about behavior without escalating hostility;
    d. Express own anger in effective ways
2. Family systems-oriented therapy focuses on functional and structural organization and the coalitions in the family and seeks to change the behaviors occurring among the members. Strategic family therapy focuses on achieving change within the family through the therapist's use of directives and paradoxical interventions. Bowen family system theory focuses on the emotional system in the multigenerational family system and seeks to increase the differentiation of the self in the system.

E. *Residential*
1. Short hospitalization assists with problems of dangerousness to self or others, with deviant behaviors that are increasingly abrasive to family and community, and with monitoring the effects of drugs or other therapies; the focus is on crisis and emergency treatment.
2. Milieu therapy assists in changing behavior while in a residential setting and explores and supports the change process in therapy sessions.

F. *Outpatient*—Focuses long-term care in providing medication monitoring and social/vocational skill development; it is best provided through a case management model which provides continuity of care through an assigned clinician responsible for the patient's care. Outpatient services in public or nonprofit centers provide the majority of the care given for the person with schizophrenia.

—— Associated Nursing Diagnoses

Aggression
Communication, impaired
Coping, ineffective individual
Crisis, situational
Depression
Decisional conflict
Family processes, altered
Self-esteem disturbance
Social interaction, impaired
Suicide, potential
Thought processes, altered (delusions, hallucinations, suspiciousness)

■ REFERENCES

1. Allebeck P: Schizophrenia: a life-shortening disease. Schizophr Bull 15(1):81–90, 1989
2. American Psychiatric Association: Diagnostic and Statistical Manual of Mental Disorders, 3rd ed, revised (DSM-III-R). Washington, DC, American Psychiatric Association, 1987
3. Andreasen NC, Flaum M et al: Positive and negative symptoms in schizophrenia: a critical reappraisal. Arch Gen Psychiatry 47(7):615–621, 1990
4. Baker AF: How families cope. J Psychosoc Nurs Ment Health Serv 27(1):31–36, 1989
5. Bellack AS (ed): Schizophrenia: Treatment Management and Rehabilitation. New York, Grune & Stratton, 1984
6. Bigelow DA, Cutler DL et al: Characteristics of state hospital patients who are hard to place. Hosp Community Psychiatry 39(2):181–185, 1988
7. Brady JP: Social skills training for psychiatric patients. I: concept, methods, and clinical results. Am J Psychiatry 141(3):333–340, 1984
8. Brady JP: Social skills training for psychiatric patients, II: clinical outcome studies. Am J Psychiatry 141(4):491–498, 1984
9. Chesla CA: Parents' illness models of schizophrenia. Arch Psychiatry Nurs 3(4):218–225, 1989
10. Coursey RD: Psychotherapy with persons suffering from schizophrenia: the need for a new agenda. Schizophr Bull 15(3):349–353, 1989
11. Eaves L (chairperson): Genetics, immunology and neurology. Schizophr Bull 14(3):21–38, 1988
12. Elkahef AM, Ruskin PE et al: Vitamin E in the treatment of tardive dyskinesia. Am J Psychiatry 147(4):505–506, 1990
13. Gerace L: Schizophrenia and the family: nursing implications. Arch Psychiatr Nurs 2(3):141–145, 1988
14. Glass LL, Katz HM, Schnitzer RD et al: Psychotherapy of schizophrenia: an empirical investigation of the relationship of process to outcome. Am J Psychiatry 146(5):603–608, 1989
15. Gottesman II, Bertelsen A: Confirming unexpressed genotypes for schizophrenia. Arch Gen Psychiatry 46(10):867–872, 1989
16. Greenberg L et al: An interdisciplinary psychoeducation program for schizophrenia patients and their families in an acute care setting. Hosp Community Psychiatry 39(3):277–282, 1988
17. Guelfi GP, Faustman WO, Csernansky JG: Independence of positive and negative symptoms in a population of schizophrenic patients. J Nerv Ment Dis 177(5):285–290, 1989
18. Haley J: Leaving Home: The Therapy of Disturbed Young People. New York, McGraw-Hill, 1980
19. Hogarty GE, Anderson CM, Reiss DJ et al: Family psychoeducational, social skills training, and maintenance chemotherapy in the aftercare treatment of schizophrenia. One year effects of a controlled study on relapse and expressed emotion. Arch Gen Psychiatry 43(7):633–642, 1986
20. Kahn EM, Frederick N: Milieu-oriented management strategies on acute care units for the chronically mentally ill. Arch Psychiatr Nurs 2(3):134–140, 1988

21. Kanas N, Stewart P, Haney K: Content and outcome in a short-term therapy group for schizophrenia outpatients. Hosp Community Psychiatry 39(4):437–439, 1988
22. Kanter J, Lamb HR, Loeper C: Expressed emotion in families: A critical review. Hosp Community Psychiatry 38(4):374–380, 1987
23. Kanter JS: Talking with families about coping strategies. In JS Kanter (ed). Clinical Issues in Treating the Chronic Mentally Ill. San Francisco, Jossey-Bass, 1985
24. Kaplan HI, Sadock BJ: Synopsis of Psychiatry: Behavioral Sciences, Clinical Psychiatry, 5th ed. Baltimore, Williams & Wilkens, 1988
25. Kay SR, Single MM: The positive-negative distinction in drug-free schizophrenia patients. Arch Gen Psychiatry 46(8):711–718, 1989
26. Liberman RP: Psychiatric rehabilitation of chronic mental patients. Washington, DC, American Psychiatric Press, 1987
27. Liberman RP: Social Skills Training for Psychiatric Patients. New York, Pergamon Press, 1989
28. Lyon M et al: Fetal neural development and schizophrenia. Schizophr Bull 15(1):149–160, 1989
29. Madnes C: Strategic family therapy. San Francisco, Jossey-Bass, 1982
30. Malone JA: Schizophrenia research update: implications for nursing. J Psychosoc Nurs Ment Health Serv 28(8):4–9, 1990
31. Manderino MA, Bzdek VM: Social skill building with chronic patients. J Psychosoc Nurs Ment Health Serv 25(9):18–23, 1987
32. Markowitz JC: Taking issue: "meat-and-potatoes" inpatient psychotherapy. Hosp Community Psychiatry 40(9):877, 1989
33. McGlashan T, Nayfack B: Psychotherapeutic models and treatment of schizophrenia. Psychiatry 51(4):340–362, 1988
34. Minuchin S: Families and Family Therapy. Cambridge, MA, Harvard University Press, 1974
35. Neyland TC, van Kammen DP: Biological mechanisms of schizophrenia. An update. In Hall RCW (ed): Psychiatr Med 8(1):41–52, 1990
36. Olfson M: Assertive community treatment: an evaluation of the experimental evidence. Hosp Community Psychiatry 41(6):634–641, 1990
37. Pelletier LR: Psychiatric home care. J Psychosoc Nurs Ment Health Serv 26(3):22–27, 1988
38. Plant TG: Social skill training: a program to help schizophrenic clients cope. J Psychosoc Nurs Ment Health Serv 27(3):7–10, 1989
39. Rosenstein MJ, Milazzo-Sayre LJ, Manderscheid RW: Care of persons with schizophrenia: a statistical profile. Schizophr Bull 15(1):45–58, 1989
40. Sautter FJ, McDermott BE: Current concepts in the psychosocial management of schizophrenia. In Hall RCW (ed): Psychiatric Medicine 8(1):125–144, 1990
41. Selvini-Pazzoli M, Leccin G, Prata G et al: Paradox and Counterparadox. New York, Jason Aronson, 1978
42. Stein LI, Test MA (eds): The Training in Community Living Model: A Decade of Experience. San Francisco, Jossey-Bass, 1985
43. Stroul BA: Residential crisis services: a review. Hosp Community Psychiatry 39(10):1095–1099, 1988
44. Strome TM: Schizophrenia in the elderly: what nurses need to know. Arch Psychiatr Nurs 3(1):47–52, 1989

45. Suddath RL, Christison GW, Torrey EF et al: Anatomical abnormalities in the brains of monozygotic twins discordant for schizophrenia. N Engl J Med 322(12):789–794, 1990
46. Task Force Report of the American Psychiatric Association: Treatment of Psychiatric Disorders, vol 3. Washington, DC, American Psychiatric Association, 1989
47. Tomb DA: PSychiatry for the House Officer, 3rd ed. Baltimore, Williams & Wilkens, 1988
48. Wong SE, Flanagan SG: Training chronic mental patients to independently practice personal grooming skills. Hosp Community Psychiatry 39(8):874–878, 1988

■ MOOD DISORDERS AND ADJUSTMENT DISORDER WITH DEPRESSED MOOD

Mood disorders[1–24] are a group of mental disorders that present mainly with symptoms of mood disturbance, mania, and depression, with associated changes in thinking and behavior that range from normal to severe.[1]

Mood disorders:
- *Depressive disorders: Major depression, single or recurrent; Dysthymia*
- *Bipolar disorders: Bipolar disorder mixed or manic or depressed; Cyclothymia*

Adjustment disorder with depressed mood

— Incidence[1,11,22]

A. Depressive disorders
- 3% of population has major depression (6 month period)
- 1 in 5 persons will experience depression in their lifetime.
- Only 20–25% of people with depression seek treatment.
- Females outnumber males 2:1.
- Frequently associated with physical illness, especially if depression occurs for the first time after age 40
- 10–65% of people over 65 years of age experience depression. It is frequently not diagnosed in the elderly; is associated with other medical disorders, e.g., cancer, Alzheimer's disease; may be related to pharmacologic treatments for medical conditions (e.g., antihypertensives); can be caused by poor diet; is denied, ignored, or blamed on physical state.

B. Bipolar disorders
- 0.5% of population has a bipolar disorder
- Generally occurs before age of 30

— Risk[3,11,22]

- Suicide: 15% of people who are depressed kill themselves. The risk is thirty times greater for a depressed person who has been hospitalized. There is greater risk for an elderly person placed in a nursing home.

- Suicide attempts: 24% of those with depressive disorders attempt suicide as compared to 18% of those having bipolar disorders and 1% in the general population.
- Relapse: 75% of patients with a depressive disorder relapse in 2 years. Persons with a bipolar disorder have about seven to nine episodes of mania.

—— Contributing Factors[8–12,14,15,22,24]

Research and theories emphasize several factors.
- Female sex vulnerability
- Genetic factors: 50% of bipolar patients have parents with mood disorders; the evidence is not as strong for depressive disorders.
- Age: People born after World War II and between 1960 and 1975 have greater incidence.
- Dysfunction of the biogenic amine system, particularly involving neurotransmitters, norepinephrine, serotonin, and dopamine
- Abnormality in the limbic system, basal ganglia (pituitary, adrenal and hypothalamus)
- Disturbance of steroid hormones
- Stressful life events prior to onset of illness
- Associated health problems or medical disorders involving endocrine or nervous systems, malnutrition, and certain drugs (e.g., antihypertensives, alcohol, analgesics); manic symptoms may be associated with certain drugs (e.g., amphetamines, cocaine, captopril)
- Disturbances in biological rhythms as noted in seasonal affective disorder (SAD), with depression occurring as change in time, light, latitude, and/or climate occurs
- Influence of relationships
- Family functioning
  - Research regarding depression and family functioning reports disturbances in family symptoms in areas of communication, problem-solving abilities, and parenting role.
  - There is insufficient evidence for stating that poor family functioning is the cause of disorder or contributes to relapse or is the effect of having the disorder. However, the patient is more vulnerable when poor family functioning is present.
- Behavioral view
  - Stressors affect the balance between the environment and interactions with others, and scripted negative behavior patterns develop.
  - Person becomes aware of the dysphoria and inability to restore balance, or change, which leads to concern about self, more self-examination, and evaluation.
  - The negative direction continues with further negative criticism of self, more dysphoria, believing self to be cause of the state.
  - Maladaptive thoughts, feelings, and associated behaviors then become reinforced by the environment and the interaction experience.
- Interpersonal view

- Disruption in the development of affectional or attachment bonds in early life results in vulnerability to stressors, because of a lack of positive social relationships and problems with intimacy.
- As a result, problems occur, especially when a significant relationship is terminated or lost, during role transitions, in relationships with differing role expectations, and in relationships when deficits in social skills exist.
- Psychoanalytic view
  - Depression arises from the infant's early experience of the loss of a love object, which creates a block of the libido and regression to an immature mode of thinking and relating.
  - The person experiences loss and frustration, despair, and intense anger that is turned against self.

— Clinical Manifestations of Selected Types[1,8,11,24]

A. Major depression
Major depression is characterized by sadness, apathy, feelings of worthlessness, self-blame, thoughts of suicide, desire to escape, avoidance of simple problems, anorexia, weight loss, lessened interest in sex, sleeplessness, reduction in activity, or ceaseless activity.

1. In infants and older children, symptoms are refusal to eat, listlessness, lack of activity, fear of the death of a parent, and fear of separation from parents.
2. In adolescents, symptoms are social isolation, negative attitude, sulkiness, feelings of being unappreciated, acting out in antisocial ways.
3. The term *psychotic features* indicates a more severe form of depression, having a thought disorder with hallucinations or delusions.

B. Dysthymia
Dysthmia is characterized by a chronic depressed mood (at least 2 years), no pleasure in activities of daily living, sleeping problems, loss of appetite or overeating, problems in concentration, poor self-esteem, hopelessness, and impairment in social relationships.

C. Bipolar disorder, manic
Manic bipolar disorder is characterized by euphoria, hyperactivity, speech pressure, grandiosity, manipulativeness, irritability, mood lability, hypersexuality, delusions, assaultiveness, sleeplessness, inability to perform usual social and work roles, being easily redirected and distracted or intensely goal-focused in activities. Mania slowly increases.

D. Adjustment disorder with depressed mood
Adjustment disorder with depressed mood is characterized by a depressed mood, crying, hopelessness; it is directly related to a disturbance occurring within 3 months after the beginning of an identifiable psychosocial stressor; there is interference with usual functioning, or the symptoms exceed the expected normal response to the stressor.

—— Treatment[2–5,7,10–13,16–19,21–23]

A. Biological/psychopharmacologic

1. Tricyclics, heterocyclic, and monoamine oxidase inhibitors (MAOIs) are specific antidepressant medications (e.g., nortriptyline Aventyl, Pamelor), phenelzine (Nardil).
2. Lithium, especially, and carbamazepine (Tegretol) are specific drugs in the treatment of bipolar disorder.
3. Antipsychotics, e.g., perphenazine (Trilifon) or trifluoperazine (Stelazine) may be used to manage manic behaviors or psychotic features of severely depressed persons.
4. Benzodiazepines may be used briefly to treat anxiety and sleep problems.
5. Electroconvulsive therapy (ECT) is used in severe depression, especially if the patient is highly suicidal, malnourished, or not responding to medication regimens.
6. Light treatment (high intensity) is used in seasonal affective disorder to shift the circadian rhythms by affecting production of melatonin and serotonin.

B. Social learning/behavioral therapy in depressive disorders:

1. Cognitive behavior therapy (CBT) focuses on discovering and changing the automatic negative thinking patterns of the following:
   a. cognitive triad of negative beliefs about self, interpersonal relationships and the future (e.g., inadequacy of self, unsympathetic and increasingly demanding interpersonal environment and a hopeless future)
   b. silent assumptions or rules by which the organization of thoughts, feelings, and behaviors are identified
   c. "Logical errors" (e.g., personalization)
   This is achieved in a therapeutic relationship with a therapist using the relationship to guide the monitoring of thoughts and the identification of themes with use of logic and homework, and to teach alternative views and responses.

C. Interpersonal/familial therapy in depressive disorders
   Interpersonal psychotherapy[12,15] focuses on:
   - The depression itself, understanding it as a clinical condition, then dealing with problems of grief reaction and the mourning process and developing new relationships,[6,20] skills, interests
   - The problem of role disagreement and learning new interpersonal behaviors and communication skills
   - The problem of role transition and learning the many skills required
   - The problem of interpersonal deficits and more specific behavioral learnings to be achieved.

This is achieved in a therapeutic relationship with a therapist who actively uses a variety of skills to assist the patient in problem solving and to facilitate the learning of social skills. Families or significant persons should be assisted in understanding the nature of depression and/or mania, its effect on marital and family roles, the role of stress in increasing dysfunction, and the effects of support. Help is also provided to learn new ways to resolve conflicts instead of confronting the patient.

D. Interpersonal/familial therapy in bipolar disorder
This therapy focuses on ways the patient and/or family can obtain support, on providing education regarding the disorder and its treatment, and in giving direction or counseling regarding interpersonal problems.

E. Psychoanalytic/psychotherapeutic
This method focuses on understanding anger, craving for love, and ambivalence as resulting from past disappointing and disapproving experiences with parents and other significant others; it focuses on understanding the ways this is repeated in here-and-now experiences and the self-defeating ways of attempting to gain self-esteem, unrealistic expectations of self, and overwhelming disappointments. This is achieved in a therapeutic alliance with the therapist, using the relationship to resolve issues of transference and resistance, and to identify defenses and distortions of reality. Long-term therapy is more frequently used with clients when etiological factors are more clearly psychological as related to rules of self or coping techniques. Grief therapy focuses on the bereavement and the associated feelings of loss, ambivalence associated with the lost person or object and guilt; it also provides support and direction as necessary to assist the person to assume greater responsibility for self.

F. Residential
Hospitalization is indicated to prevent suicide or homicide in severe depression or mania. The person may also be incapable and/or resistive to providing shelter, clothing, food, etc., for self. Other indications include crisis (e.g., loss of close family member), and need for diagnostic clarification.

── Associated Nursing Diagnoses

Aggression
Anxiety
Coping, ineffective individual
Crisis, situational
Decisional conflict
Depression
Family processes, altered
Grieving, anticipatory
Grieving, dysfunctional
Self-esteem disturbance
Social interaction, impaired
Suicide potential

■ REFERENCES

1. American Psychiatric Association: Diagnostic and Statistical Manual of Mental Disorders, 3rd ed, revised (DSM-III-R). Washington, DC, American Psychiatric Association, 1987
2. Beck AT, Rush AH, Shaw BF: Cognitive Therapy of Depression. New York, Guilford Press, 1979

3. Beck AT et al: Hopelessness and eventual suicide: a 10-year prospective study of patients hospitalized with suicidal ideation. Am J Psychiatry 142(5):559–563, 1985

4. Beck AT et al: Relationship between hopelessness and ultimate suicide. A replication with psychiatric outpatients. Am J Psychiatry 147(2): 190–195, 1990

5. Bellack AS, Hersen M, Himmenoch JM: Social Skills Training for Depression: A Treatment Manual. In J Suppl Abstracts Service. Courte Madera, CA, Selected Press, 1981

6. Bowlby J: Loss, Sadness and Depression. New York, Basic Books, 1980

7. Brenners DK, Harris B, Weston PS: Managing manic behavior. Am J Nurs 87(5):620–623, 1987

8. Davis T, Jensen L: Identifying depression in medical patients. IMAGE: J Nurs Schol 20(4):191–195, 1988

9. Ellicott A et al: Life events and the course of bipolar disorders. Am J Psychiatry 147(9):1194–1198, 1990

10. Hensley M, Rogers S: Shedding light on "SAD"ness. Arch Psychiatr Nurs 1(4):230–235, 1987

11. Kaplan HI, Saddock BJ: Synopsis of Psychiatry: Behavioral Sciences and Clinical Psychiatry, 5th ed. Baltimore, Williams & Wilkins, 1988

12. Karasu TB: Toward a clinical model of psychotherapy for depression. I: Systematic comparison of three psychotherapies. Am J Psychiatry 147(2):133–147, 1990

13. Karasu TB: Toward a clinical model of psychotherapy for depression. II: An integration and selected treatment approach. Am J Psychiatry 147(3):269–278, 1990

14. Keitner GI, Miller IW: Family functioning and major depression: an overview. Am J Psychiatry 147(9):1128–1137, 1990

15. Klerman GL, Weissman MM: Increasing rates of depression. JAMA 261(15):2229–2235, 1989

16. Klerman GL, Weissman MM, Rounsaville BR et al: Interpersonal Psychotherapy of Depression. New York, Basic Books, 1984

17. Manderino MA, Bzdek VM: Mobilizing depressed clients. J Psychosoc Nurs Ment Health Serv 24(5):23–28, 1986

18. Miller IW, Norman WH, Keitner GI: Cognitive-behavioral treatment of depressed inpatients. Six- and twelve-month follow-up. Am J Psychiatry 146(10):1274–1279, 1989

19. Monti PM, Corriveau D, Curran JP: Social skills training for psychiatric patients: Treatment and outcome. In Curran JP, Monti PM (eds): Social Skills Training. New York, Guilford Press, 1982

20. Parkes CM, Weiss RS: Recovery from Bereavement. New York, Basic Books, 1983

21. Pollack LE: Improving relationships: groups for inpatients with bipolar disorder. J Psychosoc Nurs Ment Health Serv 28(5):17–22, 1990

22. Regier DA et al: The NIMH depression awareness, recognition, and treatment program: structure, aims, and scientific basics. Am J Psychiatry 145(11):1351–1357, 1988

23. Task Force Report of the American Psychiatric Association: Treatment of Psychiatric Disorders, vol. 3. Washington, DC, American Psychiatric Association, 1989

24. Tomb D: Psychiatry for the House Officer, 3rd ed. Baltimore, Williams & Wilkins, 1988

■ DELUSIONAL (PARANOID) DISORDER AND PSYCHOTIC DISORDERS NOT ELSEWHERE CLASSIFIED

■ DELUSIONAL DISORDERS[1-3]

Delusional disorders represent several types, manifested by the type of delusion but not including hallucinations, bizarre delusions, or inappropriate affect[1,2]

Types of delusional disorders[2] are as follows:

- *Ecotomanic type*: Theme is that one is loved by person or superior
- *Grandiose type*: Theme of one of great worth, power, or special relationship with powerful figure
- *Jealous type*: Theme is one of unfaithfulness of sexual partner
- *Persecutory type*: Theme is of one being malevolently treated
- *Somatic type*: Theme is having a physical problem
- *Unspecified type*

— Incidence[1,2]

- 0.03% of population

— Contributing Factors[1,2]

- Deficit in the limbic system or basal ganglia of the brain
- Psychodynamic theory postulates the development of the delusions through the use of mechanisms of reaction formation, projection, and denial as a defense against homosexuality, dependency and affectional needs, or feelings of inferiority and rejection.
- Stress situations involving lowering of self-esteem, increasing distrust, envy, isolation, expectations of mistreatment from others, and other factors leading to a delusional system that is frightening but also partially comforting

— Treatment[1-3]

A. Psychoanalytic
This method focuses on the problem of establishing a trusting relationship and on immediate concrete problems. As trust develops, the patient begins to note how the delusion affects lifestyle, and then the therapist assists in reality testing; the patient may learn how to live with the delusion by recognizing some situations that increase the symptoms; the patient can also learn another way to manage.

B. Biological/psychopharmacological
Antipsychotics may be used in severe agitation; however the patient may refuse them because of the delusion; thus, noncompliance is frequent.

— Associated Nursing Diagnosis

Aggression
Coping, ineffective individual
Thought process, altered: delusions, suspiciousness

■ PSYCHOTIC DISORDERS NOT ELSEWHERE CLASSIFIED[1-3]

Psychotic disorders not elsewhere classified include the following:

A. *Brief reactive psychosis*
This disorder is characterized by an acute episode for a period of less than 1 month of disorganized, bizarre behavior, hallucinations, delusions, marked emotional shifts; it is related to a psychosocial stressor.
1. *Contributing factors* involve inadequate coping mechanisms in dealing with the stressor and the use of psychosis as a defense or escape.
2. *Treatment* is psychodynamic and focuses on the specific stressor, on developing new coping mechanisms, and on ways to build self-esteem.

B. *Schizophreniform disorder*
This disorder is similar to schizophrenia and brief reactive psychosis, except that symptoms last from 1 to 6 months. Symptoms are acute and begin and end abruptly.
1. *Contributing factors* are not known.
2. *Treatment*: Psychotic symptoms are treated with antipsychotics. Psychotherapy focuses on resolving the thoughts and feelings experienced during the psychotic episode.

C. *Schizoaffective disorder*
This condition is characterized by alternating manifestations of mood disorder and schizophrenia disorder. Diagnosis is difficult and the category may be used when establishing another diagnosis is particularly problematic.
1. *Contributing factors* are not known.
2. *Treatment*: Antidepressants and antimania medications are used to manage the psychotic symptoms. Antipsychotics may be necessary to control the symptoms in the acute state.

D. *Induced psychotic disorder* is characterized by shared delusion or having the same delusion as another person.
1. *Contributing factors*: It is found when there is a dyad in which there is a dominant and a submissive person with a mental disorder; few outside contacts with others; and benefits to both persons.
2. *Treatment*: Involves separation of the dyad along with psychotherapy to resolve psychosocial issues and treatment of the dominant person with the mental disorder.

E. *Psychotic disorder (atypical psychosis)*
This diagnosis is used when a more specific diagnosis of the patient's condition cannot be made.

— Associated Nursing Diagnoses

Aggression
Coping, ineffective individual
Crisis, situational
Self-esteem disturbance
Thought process, altered (delusions), (hallucinations)

■ REFERENCES

1. American Psychiatric Association: Diagnostic and Statistical Manual of Mental Disorders, ed. 3, revised (DSM-III-R). Washington, DC, American Psychiatric Association, 1987
2. Kaplan HI, Sadock BJ: Synopsis of Psychiatry: Behavioral Sciences, Clinical Psychiatry, 5th ed. Baltimore, Williams & Wilkens, 1988
3. Tomb DA: Psychiatry for the House Officer, 3rd ed. Baltimore, Williams & Wilkens, 1988

■ ANXIETY DISORDERS AND ADJUSTMENT DISORDERS WITH ANXIOUS FEATURES

Anxiety disorders[1–20] are a group of mental disorders in which anxiety is the main concern.[1]

Anxiety disorders include the following:

- *Panic disorder*
  with agoraphobia
  without agoraphobia
- *Agoraphobia without history of panic disorder*
- *Social phobia*
- *Simple phobia*
- *Obsessive-compulsive disorder*
- *Post-traumatic stress disorder*
- *Generalized anxiety disorder*
- *Anxiety disorder not otherwise specified*

Adjustment disorders include

- *Adjustment disorder with anxious mood*

— Incidence[1,2,9,18]

- 10–15% of the adult population experiences some type of anxiety disorder.
- The most common in the general population are simple phobia, generalized anxiety disorder, and adjustment disorder with anxious mood.
- Persons seeking treatment for anxiety are diagnosed as having:
  Panic disorder—2–5%
  Agoraphobia—0.6%
  Post-traumatic stress disorder—0.5%
  Obsessive-compulsive disorder—0.05%–3%

—— Contributing Factors[6-9,11,12,15,16]

- Research and theories emphasize several factors.
- Genetic factors (e.g., history of drug and alcohol use)
- Neuroanatomical hypothesis or a psychophysiological model, particularly associated and researched in relation to panic disorder, proposes a relationship between the acute panic attack and the brain stem; the anticipatory anxiety and limbic system; and phobic avoidance and the prefrontal cortex. A positive feedback loop exists between the trigger (physiological or cognitive) and the perception of the changes (body or cognitive) and the perception of changes as danger, and the response to physiological symptoms as danger or to cognitive symptoms as danger, and the resulting anxiety or panic.
- Effects of neurotransmitters, norepinephrine, GABAS, and serotonin on brain function
- Increased autonomic nervous system responsiveness
- Childhood trauma (e.g., death of parent)
- Lack of social support system
- Behavior theory and research focuses on the stimuli and conditioned response—anxiety. It also recognizes that learnings occur not only as the result of a fear, but also by observing, imitating, and identifying with another person. Cognitive theory proposes that anxiety experienced is mediated through thinking; thus, having a belief that an experience is dangerous and having a distortion about the situation, bodily sensations, or one's ability to cope, leads to development of panic and phobias.
- Psychoanalytic theory describes the origin of anxiety during early growth and development as
  Impulse or id anxiety (e.g., fear of loss of control over person's helpless state and many needs;
  Separation anxiety (e.g., fear of loss of significant relationship, abandonment);
  Castration anxiety (e.g., fear or bodily mutilation or decrease abilities and skills);
  Superego anxiety (e.g., fear of being found guilty).
  The ego recognizes the anxiety as a signal that an unconscious sexual or aggressive drive is reaching conscious awareness. The panic attack is an experience of acute, intense anxiety. If the anxiety is repressed or placed in the unconscious, then there is no symptom development. However, repression may not be successful, and defense mechanisms (which are unconscious) are used (e.g., use of displacement in phobia; use of isolation, undoing, and reaction formation in obsessive-compulsive disorder, use of denial and undoing in post-traumatic stress disorder).

—— Clinical Manifestations of Selected Types[1,9,16,20]

A. Panic disorder
Panic disorder is characterized by an acute anxiety episode (panic attack) of intense terror and dread, an awareness of palpitations and

tachycardia, chest pain and air hunger, lasting minutes to an hour, with recurrences once a week to once a year.

1.   Diagnosis requires absence of an organic etiological factor. Mitral valve prolapse and thyrotoxicosis are frequently associated with panic disorder because of a genetic component, and their presence needs to be considered in the assessment.

2.   The patient quickly learns strategies to avoid, to flee from, or to manage the symptoms.

3.   Panic disorder is diagnosed with or without agoraphobia.

B.   Agoraphobia
This is characterized by chronic anxiety, fears of being in a situation where escape is difficult, fears of symptoms associated with panic attacks, fears of restricted movement, fears of having no companionship, and/or resorting to simply enduring the situation.

C.   Agoraphobia without history of panic attack
(See description of panic attack)

D.   Social phobia and simple phobia
These phobias are characterized by anxiety associate with specific situations, e.g., claustrophobia (fear of enclosed places) and speaking in public, which results in behaviors that interfere with normal functioning.

E.   Obsessive-compulsive disorder
This is characterized by a persistent idea or impulse that is neither acceptable nor controllable; by anxiety; by a complex ritual or other behavior; and by a disruption in the activities of daily living

1.   Examples of some frequent rituals or behaviors are excessive handwashing, checking, cleaning, counting, hoarding, recurring thoughts about violent acts, and slowness in carrying out tasks.

2.   This disorder is frequently associated with depression.

F.   Post-traumatic stress disorder
It is characterized by the experience of a grave or critical loss or severe trauma (e.g., car crash, rape, earthquake, fires, assaults, war); having dreams and/or recurring thoughts about the experience; avoiding thoughts, feelings, and activities associated with the event; and having symptoms of anxiety, depression, disturbed sleep patterns, and problems with concentration. It is frequently associated with a personality disorder, depression, or substance abuse disorder.

G.   Generalized anxiety disorder
This is characterized by a moderate level of anxiety occurring for more than 6 months, with restlessness, irritability, dry mouth, sweating of palms, G.I. symptoms, insomnia, and problems of concentration.

H.   Adjustment disorder with anxious mood
This is characterized by a chronic, mild level of anxiety associated with specific psychosocial stressors and a maladaptive reaction occurring

within 3 months and lasting less than 6 months, manifested by reduced social or work functioning or considered to be exceeding a normal response to stress.

— Treatment[2–5,7,9–17,19,20]

A. Biological/psychopharmacologic
1. Benzodiazepines (diazepam [Valium]) for a short period only to deal with anxiety or phobia
2. Tricyclic antidepressants (e.g., imipramine [Tofranil]), monoamine oxidase inhibitor (MAOI) (e.g., phenelzine [Nardil]), and benzodiazepines (e.g., alprazolam [Xanax]), in panic disorders
3. Clomipramine (anafranil) for treatment of obsessive-compulsive disorder.
4. Propranolol (Inderal) for social phobia.

B. Social learning/behavioral
1. Focuses on management of the symptoms of anxiety through exposure to the feared object or situation by systematic desensitization, flooding, or implosion; focus on giving up attempts to avoid or control the object or situation; examination of the fear surrounding the physical symptom; assistance to not remain focused on fears, but on the task; and exploration of the reasons for the anxiety
   - Breathing techniques to prevent hyperventilation
   - Relaxation techniques (e.g., meditation, biofeedback)
   - Thought-stopping techniques to manage discomforting ideas
   - Self-statement training to identify negative thoughts about self
2. Cognitive theory focuses on identifying, controlling, and altering the negative automatic thoughts associated with anxiety (cognitive approach). Techniques are similar to the behavioral approach, but are used for a different purpose: Use of imagery, role playing, exposure, etc. assists in identifying the emotion and automatic thoughts which are related to negative statements about self and/or one's abilities. The relationship between the feeling and thinking is explored, and work is begun on modifying the thoughts through increased information about anxiety, use of distraction, reality testing, etc.

C. Psychodynamic
This method focuses on management of the manifest anxiety, which is believed to be a state of being overwhelmed by instinctual fears and needs and/or of having impaired abilities to relate to others. The patient is assisted in identifying conflicts (around sexual or aggressive needs), irrational fears (abandonment, separation), or relationship patterns (seeking approval, affirmation, protection). The meaning of the traumatic event is sought. The defense patterns developed to avoid or to escape the experience of anxiety are explored.

D. Interpersonal/familial
Assistance may be offered to families to identify ways to change the environmental or relationship stresses.

— Associated Nursing Diagnoses

Anxiety
Coping, ineffective individual
Ritualistic behavior
Social interaction, impaired

■ REFERENCES

1. American Psychiatric Association: Diagnostic and Statistical Manual of Mental Disorders, ed. 3, revised (DSM-III-R). Washington DC, American Psychiatric Association, 1987
2. Baker R (ed): Panic Disorder: Theory, Research and Therapy. New York, John Wiley & Sons, 1989
3. Calarco MM: Managing Myra's madness. AJN 89(3):346–349, 1989
4. Clark DM, Beck AT: Cognitive approaches. In Last CG, Hersen M (eds): Handbook of Anxiety Disorders. New York, Pergamon Press, 1988
5. Faustman WO, White PA: Diagnostic and pharmacological treatment characteristics of 536 inpatients with post-traumatic stress disorder. J Nerv Ment Dis 177(3):154–159, 1989
6. Gorman JM et al: A neuroanatomical hypothesis for panic disorder. Am J Psychiatry 146(2):148–161, 1989
7. Harnett DS: Panic disorder: integrating, psychotherapy and psycho-pharmacology. In Hall RCW (ed): Psychiatr Med 8(3):211–222, 1990
8. Horowitz M: Stress Response Syndrome, 2nd ed. New York, Aronson, 1986
9. Kaplan HI, Sadock BJ: Synopsis of Psychiatry: Behavioral Sciences, Clinical Psychiatry, 5th ed. Baltimore, Williams & Wilkens, 1988
10. Karl GT: Survival skills for psychic trauma. J Psychosoc Nurs Ment Health Serv 27(4):15–19, 1989
11. Laraia MT, Stuart GW, Best CL: Behavioral treatment of panic-related disorders: a review. Arch Psychiatr Nurs 3(3):125–132, 1989
12. Mejo SL: Post-traumatic stress disorder: an overview of three etiological variables, and psychopharmacologic treatment. Nurs Pract 15(8):41–45, 1990
13. Perse T: Obsessive-compulsive disorder: a treatment review. Clin Psychiatry 49(2):48–55, 1988
14. Sargent M: Panic disorder. Hosp Community Psychiatry 41(6):621–623, 1990
15. Task Force Report of the American Psychiatric Association: Treatments of Psychiatric Disorders, vol 3. Washington, DC, American Psychiatric Association, 1989
16. Tomb DA: Psychiatry for the House Officer, 3rd ed. Baltimore, Williams & Wilkens, 1988
17. Van Korff M, Eaton WW: Epidemiologic findings in panic. In Baker R (ed): Panic Disorder: Theory, Research and Therapy. New York, John Wiley & Sons, 1989
18. Weissmann MM: Epidemiology of panic disorder and agoraphobia. In Hall RCW (ed): Psychiatr Med 8(2):3–11, 1990
19. Yates WR, Weener RB: Clinical review: advances in anxiety management. J Am Board Fam Pract 2(1):37–42, 1989
20. Zal HM: Panic Disorder: The Great Pretender. New York, Insight Books, 1990

▬ SOMATOFORM DISORDERS

Somatoform disorders[1-5] are a group of disorders characterized by multiple somatic complaints with no actual physical illness, although complaints may closely resemble a physical disease.[1]

Somatoform disorders include:
Body dysmorphic disorder
Conversion disorder
Hypochondriasis
Somatization disorder
Somatoform pain disorder
Undifferentiated somatoform disorder
Somatoform disorder not otherwise specified

── Contributing Factors[1-8]

Research and theories support several possible factors:
- Central nervous system dysfunction in arousal that affects perception—perhaps an increase in body sensation
- Repression of aggressive impulses towards others, developed as the result of past experiences of loss and rejection, which are displaced into physical symptoms
- In conversion disorders it is hypothesized that repression of conflicts between aggressive or sexual impulses and prohibition against these impulses results in anxiety which is converted into physical symptoms.
- Use of the defense mechanism of undoing against guilt feelings of "being bad."
- Family cultural factors teaching expression of physical symptoms as pain behaviors to obtain/avoid a particular role, to receive special consideration, or to receive love.

── Clinical Manifestations of Selected Types[1-8]

A. Body dysmorphic disorder
This is characterized by the individual's belief that he/she has a body defect particularly related to his/her appearance (e.g., face) and with increased anxiety.

B. Conversion disorder
Conversion disorder is characterized by abnormal movement, paralysis, or loss of function of a part of the body system; the stressor is identified as a psychological conflict or need. Examples of symptoms are paresthesias and anesthesia, blindness, and pseudocyesis. Symptoms may symbolically represent a psychological conflict, and frequently provide some benefit to the patient.

C. Hypochondriasis
This is characterized by a persistent belief that one has an illness or that the illness has not been discovered; the beliefs are not supported by laboratory or physical findings. Symptoms frequently focus on the

GI tract and cardiovascular systems. The disorder is frequently seen in general medical practice.

D. Somatization disorder
Somatization disorder is characterized by multiple symptoms of fatigue, nausea and vomiting, bowel problems, headaches, fainting, pain in extremities, shortness of breath, problems swallowing, and amnesia. The patient generally presents with a complex medical history and describes problems dramatically and with emotionality.

E. Somatoform pain disorder
Somatoform pain disorder is characterized by an experience of pain for at least 6 months where no cause can be found; it is frequently associated with depression.

—— Treatment[2–8]

A. Psychodynamic
Treatment focuses on management of lifestyle problems and on developing positive coping strategies; psychoanalysis may be used in the treatment of conversion disorder, focusing on understanding unconscious conflicts and symptom development.

B. Social learning/behavioral
Treatment focuses on overall treatment goals and tasks and on pain as symptom management. Concern about the symptom itself may produce a secondary gain of attention and interest from others. Techniques used include stress management, relaxation training, assertiveness training, distracting skills, and improving general health techniques.

C. Biological/psychopharmacologic
Physical examinations are done on occasion to reconfirm the absence of disease, in order to avoid misdiagnosis or to assure the patient of continued care and treatment.
- Anxiety and depression, when present, are treated with antianxiety or antidepressant drugs.

D. Interpersonal/familial
Treatment focuses on fostering stress reduction, sharing with others, coping with illness, and moving towards less expression of physical problems and complaints.
- Support is given to the family to decrease the attention and concern about the symptom.

—— Associated Nursing Diagnoses

Anxiety
Coping, ineffective individual

■ REFERENCES

1. American Psychiatric Association: Diagnostic and Statistical Manual of Mental Disorders, ed. 3, revised (DSM-III-R). Washington, DC, American Psychiatric Association, 1987
2. Barsky AJ, Klerman GL: Overview: hypochondriasis, bodily complaints, and somatic styles. Am J Psychiatry 140(3):273–283, 1983
3. Corbin LJ, Hanson RW et al: Somatoform disorders: how to reduce overutilization of health care services. J Psychosoc Nurs Ment Health Serv 26(9):31–33, 1988
4. Kaplan HI, Sadock BJ: Synopsis of Psychiatry: Behavioral Sciences, Clinical Psychiatry, 5th ed. Baltimore, Williams & Wilkins, 1988
5. Mabe PA, Jones LR, Riley WT: Managing somatization phenomena in primary care. In Hall RCW (ed): Psychiatr Med 8(4):117–127, 1990
6. Sartorius N et al: Psychological Disorders in General Medical Settings. Toronto, H Huber & CJ Hogrefe Publishers, 1990
7. Task Force Report of the American Psychiatric Association: Treatment of Psychiatric Disorders, vol. 3. Washington, DC, American Psychiatric Association, 1989
8. Tomb DA: Psychiatry for the House Officer, 3rd ed. Baltimore, Williams & Wilkins, 198

■ DISSOCIATIVE DISORDERS

Dissociative disorders[1–9] are a group of mental disorders presenting as a temporary alteration in conscious awareness, identity, and behavior.[1]

Dissociative disorders include:
Multiple personality disorder
Psychogenic fugue
Psychogenic amnesia
Depersonalization disorder
Dissociative disorder not otherwise specified

— Incidence[1,4]

- Uncommon
- Psychogenic amnesia is the most common of the group.

— Clinical Factors, Clinical Manifestation and Treatment[2–9]

A. Multiple personality disorder
 This disorder is characterized by the presence of two or more personalities, headaches, blank spells, and amnesia for childhood. Usually a variety of symptoms characteristic of other diagnoses are present (i.e., depression).
 1. *Contributing factors* include sexual or physical abuse in childhood. Psychodynamic theory proposes that in exposure to child abuse, the ego manages the pain, anger, fear, sadness, etc. by dissociation or separating a group of thoughts and feelings from the consciousness. Protection is not offered by parents or others and there are no experiences of being cared for and loved.

2. *Treatment*:
   a. Psychodynamic: focuses on the integration of each personality into the whole person by understanding the dissociative process, the experience (most frequently severe abuse) which overwhelms self, and other factors which continue to operate. Hypnosis and amytal interviews are effective.
   b. Antidepressants may be used for treatment of depression.
   c. Residential: Inpatient treatment may be required for self-destructive behaviors, inappropriate behaviors.

B. Psychogenic fugue
This is characterized by a sudden memory loss and leaving home and work; the individual acts like someone else; the fugue may last hours or days. It is triggered by a painful emotional event from which the person wishes to escape. Treatment is supportive.

C. Psychogenic amnesia
Psychogenic amnesia is characterized by abrupt inability to recall pertinent information in the absence of any organic cause. It is frequently associated with physical injury.
1. *Contributing factors*: An emotionally traumatizing event occurs in which the ego uses the defense mechanism of dissociation to cope with the severe anxiety or conflict.
2. *Treatment*: Psychodynamic treatment focuses on brief immediate assistance in recalling of event and managing the anxiety. Hypnosis and/or the amytal interview is usually effective.

D. Depersonalization disorder
This disorder is characterized by the experience of perceiving oneself as unreal, with thoughts and feelings unattached to anything; the environment may be experienced in the same way.
1. *Contributing factors*: Severe stress.
2. Depersonalization can be a symptom of anxiety disorders, mood disorders, and schizophrenia; it may also be indicative of a brain tumor, endocrine disorder, or epilepsy. The diagnosis of depersonalization disorder is not made under these circumstances.

─ Associated Nursing Diagnoses

Aggression
Anxiety
Crisis, situational
Coping, ineffective individual
Suicide, potential

▬ REFERENCES

1. American Psychiatric Association: Diagnostic and Statistical Manual of Mental Disorders, ed. 3, revised (DSM-III-R). Washington, DC, American Psychiatric Association, 1987
2. Anderson G: Understanding multiple personality disorder. J Psychosoc Nurs Ment Health Serv 26(7):16–30, 1988

3. Anderson G, Ross CA: Strategies for working with a patient who has multiple personality disorder. Arch Psychiatr Nurs 2(4):236–243, 1988
4. Kaplan HI, Sadock BJ: Synopsis of Psychiatry: Behavioral Sciences, Clinical Psychiatry, 5th ed. Baltimore, Williams & Wilkins, 1988
5. Kluft RP: An update on multiple personality disorder. Hosp Community Psychiatry 38(4):363–374, 1987
6. Ross CA, Miller SD et al: Structural interview data on 102 cases of multiple personality disorder from four centers. Am J Psychiatry 147(5):596–601, 1990
7. Steele K: Looking for answers: understanding multiple personality disorders. J Psychosoc Nurs Ment Health Serv 27(8):5–10, 1989
8. Task Force Report of the American Psychiatric Association: Treatment of Psychiatric Disorders, vol 3. Washington, DC, American Psychiatric Association, 1989
9. Tomb DA: Psychiatry for the House Officer, 3rd ed. Baltimore, Williams & Wilkins, 1988

▄ PERSONALITY DISORDERS

Personality disorders[1–22] are a group of behaviors and traits that represent life-long patterns of maladaption in school, work, and intimate relationships. They are coded in DSM-III-R on AXIS II, and frequently coexist with other mental disorders. Diagnostic problems are related to reliability, overlapping of criteria for a diagnosis, and lack of research using DSM-III-R.

— Incidence

- 6–10% of the adult population

— Contributing Factors

- Genetic factors as noted in twin studies
- Central nervous system dysfunction may cause a predisposition.
- Biochemical disturbances (i.e., hormone levels, neurotransmitters)
- Disturbance in development, particularly early childhood, involving presence of inconsistent, neglectful, abusive parents

— Clinical Manifestations and Treatment of Selected Types[1–22]

A. Clinical manifestations: Cluster A (odd or eccentric behaviors)

1. *Paranoid personality disorder* is characterized by longstanding mistrust of others and suspiciousness, high sensitivity to others, and emotional restrictiveness. The person seldom seeks treatment, because the problems with intimacy and lack of symptoms do not bring the person into contact with a health agency.
2. *Schizoid personality disorder* is characterized by longstanding withdrawal from social interactions and seclusion.
3. *Schizotypal personality disorder* is characterized by longstanding peculiarities of thinking, perceiving, behaving and communicating. Person may be involved in cults, and occult, or bizarre religious acts.

B. Treatment: Cluster A
1. *Psychodynamic*
   a. Long-term therapy focuses on feeling states underlying the personality disorder, such as weakness, insecurity, vulnerability, inadequacy, and doubt; it also focuses on resolution of conflicts, resolution of transference/countertransference issues of victim or aggressor, and on intense dependency.
   b. Short-term therapy focuses only on increasing the capacity to tolerate the feelings of aloneness or other affective states.
2. *Social learning/behavioral* treatment focuses on targeted behaviors that are maladaptive, using techniques such as social skills training (i.e., introducing self to others).
3. *Biological/psychopharmacologic* approach targets symptoms and behaviors such as cognitive distortion, anxiety, and intense anger, and treats patient with specific medications.
4. *Residential*: A day hospital or half-way house may be indicated at times when the patient is particularly isolated or experiencing increased stress.

C. Clinical manifestations: Cluster B (dramatic, emotional or erratic behaviors)
1. *Histrionic personality disorder* is characterized by a history of very dramatic, seductive, attention-seeking behaviors.
2. *Narcissistic personality disorder* is characterized by a history of an exaggerated sense of uniqueness of self, or of being a special person, a superior view of self, exaggeration of talents, boastful behavior, grandiosity, self-centered or arrogant behavior, need for attention, periods of high achievement, and a sense of entitlement.
3. *Borderline personality disorder* is characterized by a history of instability of affect, impulsivity, periods of intense anger, intense clinging relationships, and unpredictable self-destructive acts. Frequently identified features are self-mutilation, use of suicide gesture as manipulative technique, demanding or entitlement behaviors, treatment regression, countertransference problems, concerns regarding abandonment, engulfment, annihilation, and quasi-psychotic thought.
4. *Antisocial personality disorder* is characterized by a history of disregarding social rules, committing criminal acts, manipulation, and dishonesty.

D. Treatment: Cluster B
1. *Psychodynamic*
   a. *Histrionic personality disorder*: Treatment focuses on unresolved dependency needs; the anger when needs are not met; the use of sexual display to have opposite sex become substitute mother; the process of analyzing events to the point of giving step-by-step instruction; analyzing "emotional storms."
   b. *Narcissistic personality disorder*: Treatment focuses on the negative transference and grandiose, self-sufficient position as defense against feelings of rage, envy, and inferiority, or focuses on the developmental arrest when parents do not empathize with the child and idealization does not then occur.
   c. *Borderline personality disorder*: Treatment focuses on resolving the failure of the attachment experience in early childhood that results

in inadequate sense of self (history of abuse is frequent), or focusing on the transference between therapist and patient around issues of omnipotence, submission, idealization, and then on making connections among feelings, motivations, and action in the present. Emphasis is also given to decreasing the gratification found in self-destructive behaviors (i.e., promiscuity, drug abuse, self-mutilation, suicide attempts, manipulation).

   d. *Antisocial personality disorder*: Treatment focuses on issues of intimacy, limit setting, responsibility for self, and defenses against loss. The patient frequently attempts to outwit the therapist, and the therapist may unwittingly take the position of morally condemning or forming a protective alliance with patient.

   e. Short-term therapies focus on feeling states in the here and now and strategies to deal more effectively with them.

2. *Social learning/behavioral*: Treatment focuses on targeted maladaptive behavior and teaches new strategies and/or behaviors (i.e., social skills training such as asking for help). The process may be more formalized through the use of contracts. Cognitive therapy may be used to decrease criticism of self and/or to lessen anxiety.

3. *Biological/psychopharmacologic*: Treatment may use medications to treat target symptoms and behaviors such as brief psychotic states, depression, intense anger, anxiety, and depersonalization.

4. *Interpersonal/familial*: Family members need to be involved in the treatment of the member who has a borderline personality disorder, because of the tendency towards overinvolvement, neglect, or abuse as the family copes with their feeling states.

5. *Residential*: Hospitalization is indicated to set limits on self-destructive acts, for brief psychotic periods, and for depression.

   a. The borderline personality disorder patient's use of defense mechanisms, splitting, and identification, contributes to developing confused, chaotic interpersonal relationships in the system, e.g., family, hospital, or community.

      (1) Splitting is an unconscious process in the patient which is played out among others and results in development of polarized groups (i.e., good or bad); focuses on the community or the individual; focuses on the incompetent person or highly skilled person; focuses on being the sensitive, caring person or the punitive person.

      (2) The staff's response to the conflict may be related to views of treatment outcomes. If structured change in the self system is the goal, then the staff needs to respond to the patient's regression in a positive, caring manner. If a more adaptive behavior change is the goal, then the staff actively sets limits on regressive behavior. Staff members have varying responses to the patient's needs for "help" or "to be protected." Unresolved dependency needs of the staff also create conflict as rules are applied or the patient is nurtured.

      (3) *Management*
         - Recognition of splitting as a human process which offers the patient a protection, keeping good and bad images of self and the other separate
         - Providing for staff education regarding splitting and its

consequences of rejection or idealization of others through discussion, clinical supervision, and consultation
- Consistent, frequent staff meetings which encourage openness and support of each other
- Monitoring for signs of splitting as punitiveness, indulgence, protectiveness, or understanding by only one person
- Meeting with patient, "good object" staff, and the "bad object" staff as indicated

b. *Self-mutilation*: The borderline personality disorder may include self-mutilation—the causing of harm to one's body without conscious intent to kill one's self. Skin cutting, occular injuries, and genital injuries are the most common. Self-mutilation may also be associated with other mental disorders.

(1) Explanations are varied. Sexual and religious explanations are given by patients. Biological factors are not known. Psychological factors reflect a view of the behavior as a personality disorder, impulse control disorder, or intolerance of affect.

(2) Treatment: There is no single approach. Treatment is difficult because of the continued acts of self-mutilation and the reaction of the therapist and staff to the acts (guilt, rage, sadness, betrayal, etc.). A careful description of the behavior in its situational context may lead to pattern and risk factor identification and perhaps to a way of dealing with the strong impulses.

E.   Clinical manifestations: Cluster C (anxious or fearful behaviors)

1. *Obsessive-compulsive personality disorder* is characterized by a long history of orderliness, obstinateness, emotional restrictiveness, indecisiveness, perfectionism, and inflexibility.

2. *Passive aggressive personality disorder* is characterized by a history of resistance to most expectations involved in social and work settings, and by procrastination, forgetfulness, and inefficiency.

3. *Dependent personality disorder* is characterized by a history of having others make decisions for self, subordination of own needs, and close attachments to others.

4. *Avoidance personality disorder* is characterized by a history of hypersensitivity to rejection, low self-confidence, and a desire for uncritical acceptance.

F.   Treatment: Cluster C

1. Psychodynamic

a. Obsessive-compulsive personality disorder: Treatment focuses on a defensive pattern of control to deal with the unacceptable aggressive impulses or focuses on the developmental arrest occurring as the child seeks autonomy and acceptance from the mother, and on problems with feelings of tenderness. The pattern is difficult to identify because of the many techniques used by the patient to maintain control such as intellectualization, questioning, distracting, evading, colluding).

b. Passive-aggressive personality disorder: Treatment focuses on the defensive behaviors arising from the dependency needs that the person believes are going to be met but are not, then the therapy focuses on the resultant anger and resentment that increases as the patient seeks revenge.

   c. Dependent personality disorder: Treatment focuses on the defensive structure protecting self from abandonment and on separation anxiety; it seeks to decrease unrealistic demands and gives explanations of how to be responsible for self.

   d. Avoidant personality disorder: Treatment focuses on the fear and guilt related to unconscious sexual, dependent, or aggressive impulses and the defensive pattern of avoidance.

   e. Short-term therapies focus on specific feelings and behaviors, and alternative ways to cope with them.

2. Social learning/behavioral: Treatment focuses on developing new behavior patterns to deal with the stress of daily living. Techniques include assertiveness training to assist in expression of aggression; social skills training (e.g., decision making); and stress management to decrease anxiety and avoidance of certain situations.

3. Biological/psychopharmacologic: This approach utilizes drug treatment to target symptoms and behaviors such as panic attack or phobia, depression, increased anxiety, or anger.

4. Residential: When a compulsive or specific fear or thought prevents a person from functioning, a brief period of hospitalization or placement in crisis bed may be indicated.

⎯ Associated Nursing Diagnoses

Aggression
Anxiety
Coping, ineffective individual
Depression
Manipulation
Powerlessness
Ritualistic behavior
Self-esteem disturbance
Social interaction, impaired
Suicide potential
Thought processes, altered

▬ References

1. Adler G: Borderline Psychopathology and Its Treatment. New York, Aronson, 1985
2. American Psychiatric Association: Diagnostic and Statistical Manual of Mental Disorders, ed. 3, revised (DSM-III-R). Washington, DC, American Psychiatric Association, 1987
3. Aronson TA: A critical review of psychotherapeutic treatments of the borderline personality. J Nerv Ment Dis 177(9):511–528, 1989
4. Braverman BG, Shook J: Spotting the borderline personality. AJN 87(2):200–203, 1987
5. Favazza AR: Why patients mutilate themselves. Hosp Community Psychiatry 40(2):137–145, 1989
6. Feldman MD: The challenge of self-mutilation: a review. Compr Psychiatry 29(3):252–269, 1988

7. Freeman SK: Inpatient management of a patient with borderline personality disorder: a case study. Arch Psychiatr Nurs 2(6):360–365, 1988
8. Gabbard GO: Splitting in hospital treatment. Am J Psychiatry 146(4):444–451, 1989
9. Gorton G, Akhtar S: The literature on personality disorders 1985–88: trends, issues, and controversies. Hosp Community Psychiatry 41(1):39–51, 1990
10. Johnson M, Silver S: Conflicts in the treatment of the borderline patient. Arch Psychiatr Nurs 2(5):312–318, 1988
11. Kaplan HI, Sadock BJ: Synopsis of Psychiatry, 5th ed. Baltimore, Williams & Wilkins, 1988
12. Kernberg O: Severe Personality Disorders: Psychotherapeutic Aspects. New Haven, CN,, Yale University Press, 1984
13. Kohut H: Restoration of the Self. New York, International University Press, 1977
14. Nighorn S: Narcissistic deficits in drug abusers: a self-psychological approach. J Psychosoc Nurs Ment Health Serv 26(9):22–26, 1988
15. Piccinimo S: The nursing care challenge: borderline patients. J Psychosoc Nurs 28(4):22–27, 1990
16. Ronningstam E, Gunderson J: Identifying criteria for narcissistic personality disorder. Am J Psychiatry 147(7):918–922, 1990
17. Runyon N, Allen CL, Ilnicki SH: The borderline patient on the med-surg unit. AJN 88(12):1644–1650, 1988
18. Sarason TG, Sarason BR: Abnormal Psychology, 6th ed. Englewood Cliffs, NJ, Prentice-Hall, 1989
19. Task Force Report of the American Psychiatric Association: Treatment of Psychiatric Disorders, vol 3. Washington, DC, American Psychiatric Association, 1989
20. Tomb DA: Psychiatry for the House Officer, 3rd ed. Baltimore, Williams & Wilkins, 1988
21. Widiger TA, Frances AJ: Personality disorders. In Talbott JA, Hales RE, Yudofsky SC (eds): Textbook of Psychiatry. Washington, DC, American Psychiatric Press, 1988
22. Zanarinic MC, Gunderson JG, Frankenburg FR, Chauncey DL: Discriminating borderline personality disorder from other AXIS II disorders. Am J Psychiatry 147(2):161–167, 1990

Administration of Drug Therapy

/7

A major responsibility of the nurse is to administer medication in collaboration with the physician and the patient. The degree of the nurse's involvement in the administration of medications is influenced by the varying conditions of the patients and the health care systems. Careful assessment, diagnosis, and evaluation contribute to the effectiveness of medication administration, teaching, and supportive processes.

— Areas for Nursing Assessment[1-34]

The nurse should observe and evaluate
1. Baseline data for future assessment of changes: blood pressure in standing and sitting position, temperature, pulse, respiration, weight, physical examination (done by nurse or physician); CBC, urinalysis, blood chemistry screens, ECG, and other tests as indicated and ordered by physician or psychiatric nurse
2. Signs/symptoms of other medical problems
3. Signs/symptoms of side effects, toxicity, tardive dyskinesia (see specific drug groupings in this chapter)
4. Use of other prescribed drugs, over-the-counter drugs, alcohol, and street drugs: Many potentially dangerous drug interactions may be averted.
5. Effect that the medication is having on the disorder and health
6. Changes in patient's pattern of eating (e.g., a person begins a 3-day fast and then a fad diet to lose weight) or in the taking of fluids
7. Changes in elimination pattern, particularly constipation and polyuria
8. Changes in activity (exercise and work patterns): Resuming daily activities is an indication of improvement.
9. Changes in sleep pattern (e.g., patient sleeping most of day)
10. Changes in feeling, thought and perception (e.g., voices reported returning at night, suspicious manner)

11. Changes in self-concept (e.g., expressing fears of medication harming one's body; being able to ask specific questions about the medication)
12. Changes in important interpersonal relationships, including ability to communicate with nurse and others
13. Changes in ability to function socially (e.g., acknowledging the presence of another, saying "Good morning")
14. Changes in sexual functioning (e.g., impotence related to some drug use can be very frightening)
15. Changes in daily routine which lead to increased stress
16. Major life events increasing stress
17. Ways the patient learns new material
18. Areas for patient education, including readiness for self-medication

—— Related Nursing Diagnoses

Ineffective individual coping
Thought processes, altered (delusions, auditory hallucinations, suspiciousness)

—— Knowledge About Medication Needed by Patient

WHAT	Name of drug
	Dosage
	Side effects
	Cost
WHEN	Time(s) to take
	What to do when dose is missed
	How long to take
WHERE	Obtaining drug
	Administering at home, hospital, clinic
WHY	Effect of drug and how soon effect is noticed
	Effect when drug is stopped
HOW	Route of administration
WHO	Name of physician, nurse, case manager
	Name and number of person to call in emergency
UNDER WHAT CIRCUMSTANCES	Laboratory or other tests required
	Food restrictions
	Alcohol restrictions
	Activities to avoid
	Monitoring of vital signs, blood pressure, other symptoms
	Other medication restrictions

—— Factors That May Affect the Process of Change in Lifestyle Required by Medication

1. Dysphoric responses to the medication: feelings of being in space, slowed down, confused, fearful, and nervous

2. Sedative and anticholinergic effect; constipation, dry mouth, blurred vision, urinary retention, and palpitations when on antidepressants
3. The "highs" experienced with some medication; e.g., benzotropine (Cogentin)
4. Leveling of the mood swings (some patients may prefer the manic state)
5. Impairment of sexual functioning
6. Daily oral dosage versus long-acting I.M. injection
7. Food restrictions
8. Alcohol restriction
9. Effect of medication on work: "not being as sharp," slight hand tremor, needing time for clinic appointments
10. Support network: availability, beliefs of others about taking medication

▬ ANTIPSYCHOTIC DRUGS[1-34]

Antipsychotic drugs are effective in the treatment of psychoses (Table 7-1)

— Indications

Schizophrenia
Bipolar disorder, manic
Psychosis related to organic disorder
Alcohol withdrawal
Nausea and vomiting

TABLE 7-1   Antipsychotic Drugs

	Representative Drugs		Daily PO Doses	PRN I.M.	Depot I.M.
Major Groups	Generic Name	Trade Name	(Range)	Dose	Dose (Range)
Phenothiazines					
Aliphatics	Chlorpromazine	Thorazine	300–2,000 mg	12.5–50 mg	
	Triflupromazine	Vesprin	100–300 mg		
	Promazine	Sparine	40–1,000 mg		
Piperazines	Fluphenazine	Prolixin			
	hydrocholoride	hydrochloride	2.5–30 mg	2.5–5 mg	
	decanoate	decanoate			12.5–100 mg q̄ 1–4 wks
	enanthate	enanthate			12.5–100 mg q̄ 1–2 wks
	Perphenazine	Trilafon	16–64 mg		
	Trifluoperazine	Stelazine	10–100 mg		
Piperidines	Mesoridazine	Serentil	75–400 mg		
	Thioridazine	Mellaril	50–800 mg		
Non-phenothiazines					
Butyrophenones	Haloperidol	Haldol	2–100 mg	2–5 mg	
	decanoate	decanoate			100–300 mg q̄ month
Thioxanthenes	Thiothixene	Navane	6–100 mg		
Dibenzoxazepines	Loxapine	Loxitane Daxolin	25–250 mg		
Indolics	Molindone	Lidone Moban	25–400 mg		
Dibenzodiazepine	Clozapine	Clozaril	100–900 mg		

—— Pharmacodynamics

1. Blocks dopamine receptors in the pathways concerned with extrapy-ramidal, endocrine, and antipsychotic activities
2. Blocks noradrenergic receptors

—— Pharmacokinetics

1. Absorbed from GI tract and metabolized by a complex process in the liver
2. Serum levels peak in 30 minutes following IM injection and 100 minutes after oral dosage.
3. Half-life: 1-2 days; Drug is stored in body fat.
4. Serum levels to guide administration of the drugs are not useful, due to the complex metabolism, storage in body fat, and individual unknown factors.
5. A steady state may be reached in 5-10 days.

—— Administration

1. All antipsychotic drug are equally effective in relieving psychosis.
2. Target or positive symptoms are hallucinations, delusions, assaultive-ness, agitation, sleep alteration, mannerisms.
3. "Neuroleptic drugs that are usually effective when given in the range of 30 mg/day or less are called high-potency; those that are usually effective when more than 400 mg/day are given are termed low-potency; and those intermediate in dosage are termed medium-potency. Although the dose of the neuroleptic drug must be individualized, in general, a dosage of 400–800 mg/day of chlorpromazine, or its approximate equivalent (e.g., 8–15 mg/day of haloperidol), is adequate for many clients."[24, pp. 802–803]
4. High-potency and low-potency refers to an antipsychotic drug equivalency to 100 mg of chlorpromazine (CPZ) e.g., high-potency: flu-phenazine (Prolixin), haloperidol (Haldol), trifluoperazine (Stelazine), thiothixene (Navane); and low potency: thioridazine (Mellaril), chlorpromazine (Thorazine).
5. The effectiveness of low-potency versus high-potency drug in agitated or withdrawn clients is a myth and not supported by research.
6. Four to six weeks should be allowed for a drug trial.
7. The choice of drug for treatment is related to side effects produced and psychiatrist's preference.
8. Identification of antipsychotic drug successfully used in the past is also used to determine choice of medication.
9. Dosage may be divided throughout the day or given at bedtime.
   a. Bedtime is preferable, since sedative effect assists in establishing a normal sleep pattern, and compliance is better.
   b. There are fewer extrapyramidal/anticholinergic effects experienced by the patient.
10. Polypharmacy (use of more than one antipsychotic drug) has not proven to be effective nor harmful; it is not recommended.

Side Effects of Antipsychotic Drugs

Side Effects	Drugs Having Greatest Effect	Drug Having Least Effect
Sedative and hypotensive	Chlorpromazine (Thorazine)	Trifluoperazine (Stelazine) Haloperidol (Haldol) Thiothixene (Navane)
Extrapyramidal	Trifluoperazine (Stelazine) Fluphenazine (Prolixin) Thiothixene (Navane)	Thioridazine (Mellaril) Mesoridazine (Serentil) Clozapine (Clozaril)
Anticholinergic	Thioridazine (Mellaril) Mesoridazine (Serentil)	Trifluoperazine (Stelazine) Haloperidol (Haldol) Thiothixene (Navane)

—— Treatment of Acute Psychosis

1. Obtain baseline vital signs.
2. Administer antipsychotic drug (haloperidol [Haldol] or chlorpromazine [Thorazine]) in a small test dose.
3. Observe for an hour and then give daily in divided doses equivalent to 300-400 mg CPZ.
4. Increase dosage every 3-4 days, remembering that most patients respond to doses equivalent to 1500 mg CPZ.
5. Rapid effect is achieved by the hourly administration of haloperidol (Haldol) 5 mg I.M., until sedation or control of violent behavior is achieved.
   a. Monitor blood pressure for hypotension before each dose; withhold dose if BP is 90 systolic or below.
   b. Monitor sleep state to achieve a 6- to 7-hour period.
   c. Monitor for dystonia occurring 1–48 hours after beginning of treatment; treat with an anticholinergic or antihistaminergic agent.
   d. Monitor the patient for a decrease in danger to self and others.
   e. Total dosage should not exceed 50 mg in 12 hours.

—— Maintenance Antipsychotic Drug Treatment

1. Recommended time periods:
   a. First or second psychotic episode: 6 months
   b. Three or more psychotic episodes: indefinitely, with trial withdrawal every 4–5 years
2. When reducing the dosage or discontinuing the drug, the physician tapers the dosage slowly to prevent dyskinesia or relapse.
3. Compliance is a major problem in long-term treatment.

▬ LONG-ACTING (DEPOT) ANTIPSYCHOTIC DRUGS

1. Indicated in maintenance treatment of schizophrenia to deal with problems of compliance

2. Administered every 1–4 weeks
3. Given deep I.M. or using Z track injection technique to prevent the drug from irritating tissue
4. Concentrate forms are light-sensitive and therefore must be kept in dark bottles or packaging.
5. Add concentrate to liquid or food just before administration to insure potency; avoid using liquids containing tannic acid (tea), caffeine (coffee, cola), and pectinates (apple juice).

— Contraindications

Contraindications include comatose states, glaucoma, prostatic hyperplasia, myocardial infarction or other severe cardiac problems, seizures, ingestion of drugs that would interact with antipsychotic drug to cause CNS depression.

— Precautions

1. Discontinue prior to surgery.
2. Be aware that the seizure threshold can be lowered by these drugs, especially in patients who have a history of epilepsy.

— Examples of Drug Interactions

1. Alcohol, barbiturates, and other CNS drugs: potentiate sedation, hypotension
2. Antiparkinsonian drugs and tricyclics: increase anticholinergic effects (i.e., dry mouth, postural hypotension, urinary retention, constipation)
3. Antacids: interfere with absorption rate
4. Epinephrine: Neosynephrine may be administered to raise the blood pressure when it is dangerously low. Epinephrine is *not* used, because it causes further lowering of blood pressure.

— General Responses to Treatment

1. Sedative effect may be noted 30–60 minutes following I.M. administration; it lasts 2–3 hours.
2. Cooperation increases and disruptive behavior decreases within a day to a week of administration of dosage.
3. Thought disorder generally disappears within 6 weeks or more following initial dose.
4. Failure to respond may be caused by the following:
   a. underdosage
   b. insufficient trial of drug (minimum 2 weeks)
   c. undiagnosed organic disorder
   d. noncompliance

— Side Effects

1. Drowsiness and sedation
   a. Tolerance develops in about 2 weeks.
   b. Activities such as driving a car or repairing delicate equipment

should be avoided because alertness and muscular coordination are impaired.

c. Give at bedtime to minimize problems.

2. Orthostatic hypotension

   a. Symptoms: systolic blood pressure 90 or below, dizziness, weakness; although tolerance develops rapidly in some patients, orthostatic changes may persist with continued therapy. The danger exists that the patient could fall and sustain injuries.

   b. Monitor blood pressure standing and sitting before and after the first dose and the first few days of treatment—and periodically, if problems persist.

   c. Instruct the patient to change positions slowly to prevent hypotension

   d. Lower head and raise feet slightly if hypotension occurs.

3. Anticholinergic side effects

   a. Symptoms and treatment

     (1) Dry mouth: Rinse mouth frequently with water, use sugarless candy or gum.

     (2) Blurred vision: Physostigmine drops may be indicated.

     (3) Bowel problems may range from constipation to paralytic ileus: Increase fluids, bulk in diet, and exercise. Laxative or stool softener may be indicated.

     (4) Urinary problems may range from urinary retention to bladder paralysis: Advise the patient to empty bladder every 3–4 hours. Bethanechol (Urecholine) may be prescribed.

   b. Central anticholinergic syndrome

     (1) Cause: Patient is taking several drugs with anticholinergic effects; e.g., taking antipsychotic, antiparkinsonian and antidepressant drugs at the same time.

     (2) Symptoms: agitation; restlessness to confusion; disorientation; hallucinations to coma; flushed, dry skin; fever; dilatation of pupils.

     (3) Treatment: Stop drug. Administration of physostigmine is controversial, because newer information does not recommend using it for anticholinergic syndrome since cardiac problems can occur.

4. Extrapyramidal symptoms (EPS)

   a. Dystonia: spasms of muscles of jaw (most common), face, neck, back, eyes, arms, and legs

     (1) Occurs within 5 minutes to first few days of treatment in about 10% of patients

     (2) Symptoms: opening of jaw, protrusion of tongue, oculogyric crisis (fixed upward gaze from spasm of the oculomotor muscles), torticollis (pulling of head to the side from spasms of cervical muscles), opisthotonus (hyperextension of back from spasms of back muscles)

     (3) Treatment: administration of anticholinergic agent, e.g., benztropine (Cogentin), or an antihistaminergic agent (e.g., diphenhydramine [Benadryl]), orally or parenterally for more rapid relief.

   b. Akathisia

     (1) Occurs within 6 hours to 60 days

(2) Symptoms: continuous motor restlessness that may not be noted because restlessness may be erroneously attributed to psychosis or resistance to antipsychotic drug

(3) Treatment: reduction of antipsychotic drug; perhaps treatment with propranolol (Inderal)

c. Parkinsonian effects

(1) Occur in about 15% of patients in the first week to 4 weeks.

(2) Symptoms: shuffling gait, mask-like facial expression, drooling, tremor

Akinesia: lack of body movement, especially in arms; frequently not treated because it is not striking and patient seldom complains

Cogwheel rigidity (overlying racheting during passive flexion at a joint)

Rabbit syndrome (chewing tremor)

(3) Treatment: anticholinergic drug

5. Endocrine or metabolic effects

a. Symptoms: weight gain (indicates need for exercise and dietary adjustments); menstrual irregularities and excessive secretion of mammary gland in females (indicates need for dosage adjustment); decreased libido, impotence, impaired ejaculation in males (which patient may be too embarrassed to report); decreased thermoregulatory ability—complaints of being too hot or too cold (care should be taken in use of ice bag or hot water bottle and in regulation of temperature of seclusion room); glycosuria

b. Treatment: generally consists of changing to another antipsychotic drug and lowering the dosage

6. Examples of skin effects

a. Symptoms: rashes which generally clear up after few weeks; phototoxicity or severe sunburn occurring with use of phenothiazines

b. Treatment: sunscreens and adequate clothing recommended for patients on phenothiazines

7. Opthalmologic effects

a. Phenothiazine lens disease is partially reversible and does not affect visual acuity.

b. Toxic retinopathy is irreversible pigmentation of retina progressing to blindness related to thioridazine (Mellaril) dosage over 800 mg/day or mesoridazine (Serentil) dosage over 400 mg/day.

c. Prevention: eye examination every 3–12 months and minimal dosage of drugs.

—— Withdrawal Syndrome

1. Sweating, diarrhea, nausea, vomiting, insomnia, restlessness, tremor
2. May be associated with cholinergic rebound, CNS stimulation, emerging tardive dyskinesia, or great sensitivity to stress

—— Tardive Dyskinesia

1. Generally occurs after at least 3 months to years of use of antipsychotics
2. Risk is also associated with high-level antipsychotic drug dosage, fe-

male sex, age 50 years or older, and presence of organic brain syndrome.
3. Symptoms: Most common are abnormal movements of jaw, tongue, and lips, including grimacing. Movements may involve neck, trunk, pelvis, etc., in severe cases.
4. Treatment
   a. No known effective treatment
   b. Use of antipsychotic drugs only as necessary and at minimum dose
   c. Monitoring for symptoms (AIMS test can be used)
   d. Evaluating neuroleptic medication every 6 months for possible reduction
   e. When symptoms appear, reduce and/or discontinue antipsychotic drug; some patients experience disappearance of symptoms within months after discontinuation of the drug.
   f. Advantages and disadvantages of neuroleptic drugs must be discussed with the patient.
   g. It is suggested that the patient's agreement to take neuroleptic drugs with full knowledge of the possible effects of tardive dyskinesia be documented.

—— Life-Threatening Effects

1. Agranulocytosis
   a. Symptoms: rapid onset of sore throat and fever
   b. Occurs in first 3–8 weeks of treatment
   c. Prevention: Teach the patient to report sore throat and fever promptly. CBC is ordered to rule out disease.
   d. Treatment: Stop the drug immediately; use reverse isolation technique; administer antibiotics.
   e. Mortality rate is 30%.
2. Neuroleptic malignant syndrome (NMS) (Differentiate from catatonia.)
   a. Symptoms: muscular rigidity (initial), hyperpyrexia, autonomic nervous system dysfunction (i.e., hypertension, hypotension), diaphoresis, altered states of consciousness
   b. Risk factors: dehydration, prolonged agitation, and prior treatment with lithium; current lithium treatment combined with high-dose, high-potency neuroleptic drug.
   c. Although some patients recover completely, mortality is reported at 12% and is related to respiratory failure, renal failure, and cardiovascular collapse.
   d. Treatment: discontinuance of antipsychotic drugs, Bromocriptine (Parlodel) 15–80 mg per day; maintenance of electrolyte balance, treatment of complications, behavior control
3. Lethal catatonia (differentiate from NMS)
   a. Symptoms: extreme psychotic excitement (initial), fever, muscular rigidity
   b. Treatment: Antipsychotic medication, supportive measures
4. Laryngeal spasm: treat with I.M. diphenhydramine (Benadryl) or I.V. benztropine (Cogentin).
5. Hyperpyrexia
   a. Caused by suppression of hypothalamus by antipsychotic drugs, heat, humidity, and exercise

   b. Symptoms: extremely high body temperature, lack of sweating, and dysfunctional central nervous system
   c. Treatment: use of treatment principles for heat stroke, with techniques to lower body temperature and to maintain respiratory and cardiovascular systems.

— Overdose

1. Symptoms: increased sedation, hypotension, and extrapyramidal signs, seizures
2. Treatment: gastric lavage, antiparkinsonian drugs, I.V. fluids, and norepinephrine for decreased blood pressure; anticonvulsants.

■ CLOZAPINE (CLOZARIL) — ANOTHER MORE RECENT ANTIPSYCHOTIC DRUG
— Indications

Treatment-resistant schizophrenia

— Pharmacodynamics

Clozadine binds to dopamine receptors and blocks serotonin histaminergic, adrenergic, and cholinergic activities.

— Pharmacokinetics

1. Absorbed from GI tract; generally not secreted in urine and feces because it is almost completely metabolized
2. Half-life: 8–12 hours

— Administration

Previously, this drug was distributed through Sandoz Pharmaceuticals as part of the Clozaril Patient Management System (CPMS) because of the risk of seizures. Close monitoring is still recommended.
   a. Weekly CBC is drawn and results shared.
   b. Medicine is dispensed following analysis of test results and clinical change.

— Side Effects and Management

1. Sedation: Warn patient about driving a car or operating other equipment that requires alertness.
2. Agranulocytosis (1–2% incidence)
   a. Symptoms: sore throat, fever
   b. Prevention: WBC weekly
   c. Treatment: discontinue drug, symptomatic treatment
3. Seizures (1–5% incidence that is dose-related): seizure precautions (see Chapter 5)
4. Hypotension: orthostatic vital sign monitoring three times per day
5. Potential for hypothermia: monitor room temperature, provide warm blankets and clothing as needed

6. Pruritus: cool water bath and calamine lotion
7. Nausea: Provide crackers, have patient focus on deep breathing.
8. Hypersalivation: Low-dose anticholinergics may be indicated.

ANTICHOLINERGIC/ANTIPARKINSONIAN DRUGS[1–34]

ANTICHOLINERGIC/ANTIPARKINSONIAN DRUGS

Anticholinergic and antiparkinsonian drugs (Table 7-2) are used to alleviate the side effects of antipsychotic drugs. Representative drugs include trihexyphenidyl (Artane), benztropine (Cogentin), biperiden (Akineton), and procyclidine (Kemadrin).

— Indications

Antipsychotic drug-induced extrapyramidal symptoms
a. Acute dystonic reactions
b. Akathisia
c. Parkinsonian syndrome

— Pharmacodynamics

Reduce cholinergic activity by inhibiting the effect of acetylcholine.

— Pharmacokinetics

1. Absorbed from GI tract and excreted in the urine
2. Effects of benztropine (Cogentin) or biperiden (Akineton) are noted within 30 minutes after I.M. or I.V. injection and in 30–60 minutes after oral dose; they last up to 24 hours. (There is no significant difference in rate of effect between I.M. or I.V. administration.)

— Administration

1. Dosage is kept at a minimum level because of the side effects. If symptoms of dry mouth and blurred vision are experienced, dosage is not increased.

TABLE 7-2 Anticholinergic/Antiparkinsonian Drugs

	Representative Drugs		*Daily PO Doses*	*One-Time PRN Dose*
Major Classes	*Generic Name*	*Trade Name*	*(Range)*	*I.M. or I.V.*
Anticholinergics	Trihexyphenidyl	Artane	2–15 mg	1–2 mg
	Benztropine	Cogentin	0.5–6 mg	2 mg
	Biperiden	Akineton	2–10 mg	
	Procyclidine	Kemadrin	5–30 mg	
Dopamine agonist	Amantadine hydrochloride	Symmetrel	100–300 mg	
Miscellaneous	Diphenhydramine hydrochloride	Benadryl	25–100 mg	10–50 mg

2. Drug is discontinued slowly so as not to produce extrapyramidal syndrome.
3. Contraindications: closed-angle glaucoma, prostatic hyperplasia
4. Caution: during pregnancy and lactation

—— Examples of Drug Interactions

1. *Antidepressants and antipsychotics*: increased blurred vision, dry mouth, constipation, and other anticholinergic activities
2. *Monoamine oxidase inhibitors*: potentiate neurological symptoms.

—— General Responses to Treatment

1. Relief of acute dystonia will occur within 30 minutes after I.M. injection of benztropine (Cogentin).

—— Side effects

Dry mouth, blurred vision, constipation, drowsiness, nausea, nervousness, and urinary retention (see *side effects of antipsychotics* in this chapter)

—— Overdose or Atropine Intoxication with Biperiden (Akineton) or Benztropine (Cogentin)

1. Symptoms: dilated pupils, flushed face, tachycardia, decreased bowel sounds, urinary retention, confusion, anxiety
2. Treatment: lavage, supportive measures (administration of physostigmine is controversial)

Amantadine (Symmetrel)

1. Used in the treatment of parkinsonian syndrome and for extrapyramidal reactions because of lower incidence of anticholinergic effects
2. Has antiviral activity, which is helpful in a hospital environment
3. Some patients experience insomnia; therefore, give early in day or at dinner time and not at bedtime.

Diphenhydramine (Benadryl)

Infrequently used in treatment of extrapyramidal symptoms because of sedative effects

■ ANTIDEPRESSANT DRUGS[1–34]

Antidepressant drugs (Table 7-3) are used to treat affective disorders.

■ Tricyclics (TCAs):

Amitriptyline (Elavil)
Desipramine (Norpramin)
Imipramine (Tofranil)
Nortriptyline (Aventyl, Pamelor)
Protriptyline (Vivactil)
Doxepin (Sinequan)
Maprotiline (Ludiomil)

TABLE 7-3   Antidepressant Drugs

Major Groups	Representative Drugs		Daily PO Doses (Range)
	Generic Name	*Trade Name*	
Tricyclic antidepressants	Amitriptyline	Elavil	75–300 mg
	Desipramine	Norpramin	75–300 mg
	Imipramine	Tofranil	75–300 mg
	Nortriptyline	Aventyl, Pamelor	50–200 mg
	Protriptyline	Vivactil	15–60 mg
	Doxepin	Sinequan	75–300 mg
	Maprotiline	Ludiomil	75–225 mg
Monoamine oxidase inhibitors	Isocarboxazid	Marplan	10–30 mg
	Phenelzine	Nardil	15–90 mg
	Tranylcypromine	Parnate	10–30 mg
Miscellaneous	Trazodone	Desyrel	50–600 mg
	Fluoxetine	Prozac	20–80 mg
	Clomipramine	Anafranil	25–250 mg
	Amoxapine	Asendin	100–600 mg

—— Indications

Major depression
Bipolar disorder, depressed or mixed
Psychotic depression
Panic disorder
Agoraphobia
Chronic pain

—— Pharmacodynamics

Believed to cause an increase in norepinephrine and/or serotonin in CNS

—— Pharmacokinetics

1. Absorbed from GI tract, metabolized in liver, and excreted by the kidney
2. Serum levels peak in 2–8 hours
3. Half-life may extend for 3 days
4. Serum therapeutic levels:
   Amitriptyline (Elavil) 100–250 mg/ml
   Desipramine (Norpramin) 150–300 mg/ml
   Imipramine (Tofranil) 150–300 mg/ml
   Nortriptyline (Aventyl, Pamelor) 50–150 mg/ml
   Protriptyline (Vivactil) 75–250 mg/ml
   Doxepin (Sinequan) 100–250 mg/ml
   Maprotiline (Ludiomil) 150–300 mg/ml
5. Steady state plasma level may take 5–14 days to achieve.

—— Administration

1. Initial dosage is low and is gradually increased as tolerated by patient.
2. A maintenance dose may be given at bedtime, thereby reducing drowsiness, dry mouth, etc., during the day and assisting sleep at night.
3. Generally, prescriptions are written for short intervals initially (i.e., one week) to decrease overdose potential, then monthly, then at 2- to 3-month intervals.
4. Antipsychotic medications may be added when treating psychotic depression.
5. Lithium may be continued when treating bipolar disorder.
6. Six weeks should be allowed for drug trial.
7. Medication should be continued 3–4 months after the patient is free from depression, because of the risk of relapse in first 4 months.
8. Following the acute phase, the dosage is tapered slowly to prevent cholinergic reversal, i.e., nausea, vomiting, headache, sweating, pain in neck area.

—— Contraindications

Closed-angle glaucoma, agitated states, urinary retention, certain cardiac disorders

—— Cautions

1. Urinary retention—Monitor closely.
2. Surgery—Discontinue prior to surgery.
3. Suicide—Potential for suicide is greater as the patient begins to feel more energetic and as depression lifts as a result of drug treatment and other therapies.
4. Abuse of amitriptyline (Elavil) by drug abusers
5. Do not use, or use with caution, during first 3 months of pregnancy and lactation, because of potential harm to fetus or newborn.
6. Seizure disorders—All antidepressants lower seizure threshold.

—— Example of Drug Interactions

1. Many interactions are reported; therefore, refer to a current list of drug interactions or to pharmacist when other drugs are being given.
2. Antipsychotic drugs: increase anticholinergic and sedative effects
3. Alcohol, barbituates, cold medications: CNS depression
4. Heavy smoking, birth control pills, lithium: decreases tricyclic antidepressant (TCA) plasma levels
5. Antihypertensives: blocking of antihypertensive effect when used in conjunction with clonidine (Catapres), methyldopa (Aldomet), and guanethidine (Ismelin)
6. Anticholinergics: toxic psychosis
7. Anticoagulants: increases anticoagulant effect

—— General Responses to Treatment

1. Drowsiness may occur and subside after initial period. Patient is warned about driving a car or operating a vehicle that requires alertness.

2. Maximum clinical response is noted in 2–4 weeks (up to 6 weeks for elderly patients)
   a. Sleep pattern and appetite improve first.
   b. Psychomotor activity increases before the patient speaks about feeling better.
   c. Mood and other symptom improvement occur approximately 3 weeks later.
3. Frequently medication dosage is lowered or discontinued prematurely, causing a relapse.

— Side Effects (partially treated by adjustment of dosage)

   a. Drugs with high sedating effect: amitriptyline (Elavil), doxepin (Sinequan), trazodone (Desyrel)
   b. Drugs with high anticholinergic effects (dry mouth, constipation, retention of urine, blurred vision): amitriptyline (Elavil), doxepin (Sinequan), imipramine (Tofranil). Treatment: sugarless candy and gum, increase fiber and fluids. Bethanechol (Urecholine) may be prescribed in some cases.
   c. Orthostatic hypotension, frequently resulting in falls, particularly in the elderly; patients do not become tolerant of this effect. Nortriptyline (Pamelor) has least effect.
   d. Precipitation of manic episode
   e. Cardiovascular effects (tachycardia)
   f. Skin rashes: dermatological measures
   g. Weight gain: caloric restrictions and increased exercise may be recommended

— Overdose

1. Symptoms: cardiac arrhythmia, convulsions, low blood pressure, respiratory depression, mydriasis, delirium. May be fatal.
2. Treatment: lavage, supportive treatment to maintain respiratory function and adequate blood pressure and to control seizures and cardiac arrhythmias

■ MONOAMINE OXIDASE INHIBITORS (MAOIs): ISOCARBOXAZID (MARPLAN), PHENELZINE (NARDIL), TRANYLCYPROMINE (PARNATE)

— Indications

Atypical depression
Treatment failures with TCAs
Panic disorders

— Pharmacodynamics

MAO inhibitors work by blocking the MAOI enzyme that assists in oxidation of intracellular catecholamines; the process is irreversible and the body takes 2 weeks to produce more MAOI enzyme.

—— Pharmacokinetics

Absorbed from GI tract and metabolized in liver

—— Administration

1. Advise dietary restriction of tyramine-rich foods (see *tyramine-induced hypertension crisis*).
2. Initial dosage is low and is gradually increased as tolerated by the patient.
3. Administer before 3–4:00 P.M. to avoid insomnia.
4. Four weeks should be allowed for drug trial.
5. Allow 1–2 weeks after discontinuing drug before beginning another antidepressant.

—— Contraindications

Liver disease, hypertension, cardiovascular disease, pheochromocytoma, cerebrovascular disease, pregnancy, and lactation

—— Cautions

Discontinue prior to surgery.

—— Examples of Drug Interactions

1. Foods rich in tyramine or tryptophan, sympathomimetic drugs, or excessive ingestion of chocolate or caffeine may cause hypertensive crisis.
2. Drug-free intervals of 1–2 weeks are recommended by drug manufacturers before changing from one MAOI to another MAOI, from an MAOI to a TCA, or from a TCA to an MAOI, to prevent hypertensive crisis or seizures. However, TCA and MAOI have been used in combination for treatment-resistant patients.
3. Psychotropic agents: potentiation of MAOI effect
4. Anticholinergics potentiate anticholinergic effect.
5. Antihypertensive drugs: hypotension
6. Insulin or oral hypoglycemics: additive hypoglycemic effect
7. Levodopa (Larodopa, Sinemet—as combination with carbidopa) potentiate MAOI effect.
8. Sympathomimetics (ephedrine (Tedral, Broncholate), phenylpropanolamine (Dexatrim), pseudoephedrine (Sudafed), phenylephrine (nose drop preparations), and amphetamines): hypertensive crisis, excess CNS stimulation

—— General Responses to Treatment

1. Clinical response may not be seen for 4 weeks.

—— Side Effects (partially treated by adjustment of dosage)

1. Drowsiness (and in some cases, brief stimulation): Warn patient about driving a car or operating other equipment that requires alertness.

2. Insomnia: Arrange dosage schedule so that medication is not administered after dinner.
3. Orthostatic hypotension: Advise patient to change positions slowly, wear support hose, and maintain adequate fluid intake; warn patient of danger of falls.
4. Impotence: Refer to physician for dosage adjustment.
5. Constipation: Increase bulk and fluids in diet, and exercise.
6. Weight gain, edema: Instruct in dietary and exercise management
7. Precipitation of manic attack: monitor
8. Hepatotoxicity: Monitor by periodic liver function tests.

—— Tyramine-induced Hypertensive Crisis

1. Prevention: Advise dietary restriction of tyramine-rich foods (aged cheese, beer, wine, liver, fava beans, packaged soups, meat extracts, pickled and smoked meats, fish, poultry). Continue dietary restrictions for 2 weeks after MAOI is discontinued.
2. Symptoms
   a. Occur 30 minutes to 24 hours after eating foods containing tyramine
   b. If headache, neck stiffness, nausea, or vomiting occur, advise patient to seek medical treatment.
   c. As crisis progresses, symptoms of severe headache, increased BP, chest pain, and collapse occur.
3. Treatment:
   a. Sublingual nifedepine
   b. Chlorpromazine (Thorazine) may be given to the patient to take as an emergency treatment. Teach patient that headache may be caused by the hypotension from chlorpromazine (Thorazine) as well as by hypertension from tyramine-rich foods.
   c. Phentolamine (Regitine) I.V. lowers blood pressure.

—— Overdose

1. Symptoms: coma, increased respirations, tachycardia, and hyperthermia. Note that there is a 1- to 6-hour lag before serious symptoms appear.
2. Treatment is symptomatic; dialysis can also be used.

▬ TRAZODONE (DESYREL)
—— Indications

Affective disorder

—— Response

Therapeutic effect may be noted in 1–2 weeks. Trazodone differs from TCAs in that the side effects do not include most cardiac or anticholinergic effects.

— Caution

Prompt treatment needed for priapism (prolonged or inappropriate penis erection).

— Side Effects

Headache, orthostatic hypotension, GI distress, sedation

■ FLUOXETINE (PROZAC)
— Indications

> Affective disorders
> Obsessive-compulsive disorders
> Bulemia

Note
1. Therapeutic effect may not be noted for 2–4 weeks.
2. Differs from TCAs in that side effects include less daytime sedation and anticholinergic effects

— Side Effects

> Precipitation of mania, weight loss, GI distress, insomnia

■ CLOMIPRAMINE (ANAFRANIL)
— Indication

> Obsessive-compulsive disorder

Note: Therapeutic effect may be noted in 7–14 days. Withdrawal of drug may cause the return of symptoms.

— Side Effects

> Dry mouth, drowsiness, tremor, dizziness, constipation

■ ANTIMANIC DRUGS[1-34]

Antimanic drugs (Table 7-4) are used to treat bipolar disorders.

■ LITHIUM SALTS – LITHIUM CARBONATE
— Indications

> Bipolar disorder, manic phase, and as prophylaxis for schizoaffective disorder
> Major depression
> Periodic impulsive aggressiveness

— Pharmacodynamics

Lithium is believed to be related to a group of neurotransmitters acting through a second messenger system.

TABLE 7-4   **Antimanic Drugs**

Major Groups	Representative Drugs Generic Name	Trade Name	Daily PO Doses (Range)
Lithium salts	Lithium carbonate	Lithane Lithonate Eskalith Lithobid	300–2,400 mg
	Lithium citrate	Cibalith-S	
Anticonvulsants*	Carbamazepine	Tegretol	1,200–1,600 mg
	Clonazepam	Klonopin	2–16 mg
Calcium channel inhibitors*	Verapamil	Isoptin Calan	160–480 mg
Alpha adrenergic agonist*	Clonidine	Catapres	(Clonidine dosage is still investigational)

* Not FDA approved use

—— Pharmacokinetics

1. Absorbed from GI tract and eliminated by kidneys
2. Excreted in breast milk and may be found in sweat and feces
3. Serum levels peak in 2 hours; half-life is about 24 hours.
4. Steady state plasma level reached in 5–8 days of administration
5. Therapeutic index (Narrow): Adult 0.6 to 1.2 mEq/L and in elderly 0.4 to 0.6 mEq/L

—— Administration

1. Obtain data on renal function, cardiac states, thyroid function.
2. Adequate kidney function, sodium balance and hydration are essential to lithium excretion.
   a. Sodium balance is affected by low-salt diets, fad diets, and diet pills that lead to reduction in food and fluid intake. Excessive use of foods and drugs that are high in sodium also affect sodium levels (e.g., diet sodas, antacids, and corned beef).
   b. Encourage the patient to consume 2–3 quarts of fluids per day because urination may be more frequent as kidneys excrete lithium.
   c. Coffee, tea, and colas in large amounts (over 10 cups per day) may also promote the excretion of lithium because of the diuretic effect of the caffeine in these drinks. The stimulant effects from caffeine may interfere with mood stabilization.
3. Given 2–4 times a day because of its rapid excretion from body; may be given at mealtime to minimize tendency to cause gastric upset
4. Periodic serum lithium levels are drawn as frequently as necessary to assure maintenance of therapeutic dosage level.
   a. Serum levels are drawn 12 hours after last dose of lithium

    b. Initially, serum levels are monitored weekly.
    c. Maintenance serum levels may be monitored every 2–3 months.
5. Serum creatinine and TSH (thyroid-stimulating hormone) are checked 2–4 times a year.

—— Contraindications

Cardiovascular disease, renal disorders, epilepsy, dehydration
Pregnancy (increased number of birth defects)

—— Cautions

1. Fever and/or diarrhea: The amount of lithium required will be less, and danger of toxicity will be greater.
2. Breast-feeding: Infant may develop toxicity.
3. Surgery: Lithium may be restarted the following day.

—— Examples of Drug Interactions

1. Antipsychotic drugs: neurotoxicity
2. Diuretics or steroids: electrolyte imbalance
3. Antidepressant drugs: increased risk of manic relapse
4. Nonsteroidal anti-inflammatory drugs; e.g., ibuprofen (Motrin, Advil): lithium toxicity
5. Note: Aspirin, acetaminophen, and Clinoril do not affect serum levels of lithium; however, because Clinoril has not been studied adequately, it should be used cautiously in lithium patients.

—— General Responses to Treatment

1. Lag time of 5–10 days before therapeutic effect
2. In acute mania, because of the lag period, an antipsychotic may be administered to achieve psychomotor control. Observe for neurotoxicity.
3. Recommended trial period of 4–6 weeks
4. Geriatric patients require less lithium, probably because the kidneys of people in this age group have a decreased ability to excrete it.
5. Because drowsiness may be experienced, extra precautions need to be taken if the patient is driving or handling mechanical equipment.

—— Side Effects

1. Subsiding after 1–2 weeks: nausea, vomiting, diarrhea, thirst, weight loss, hand tremors and muscle weakness, polyuria (may wet the bed at night), swelling in hands and feet, decrease in sexual functioning
2. Related to long-term use
    a. Fine hand tremor: lithium-induced tremor is related to voluntary movement and is not relieved by antiparkinsonian drugs. Treatment consists of decreasing lithium dosage in cases where tremor is more troublesome. Beta-blockers have also been effective; i.e., Propanolol (Inderal), 10–40 mg bid; Atenolol (Tenormin) 50 mg per day; Nadolol (Corgard) 80–240 mg per day.

b. GI distress, pain, and diarrhea: caused by presence of unabsorbed lithium irritating the large intestine. Treated by changing type of lithium, by having smaller, more frequent doses, and by taking the drug with meals

c. Weight gain: Approaches include dietary instruction about avoiding high-calorie drinks, having a sufficient amount of sodium intake, and increasing exercise.

d. Polyuria and polydipsia: caused by blockage of antidiuretic hormone (ADH), resulting in decreased ability to concentrate urine; symptoms are polyuria, thirst, weight gain, and nocturia; not considered a reason to discontinue lithium. A diuretic such as chlorothiazide (Diuril) may be used as treatment.

e. Depressed thyroid function: There is an asymptomatic enlargement of the thyroid after long-term use of lithium. Symptoms of hypothyroidism are tiredness, coldness in extremities, headache, myxedema, decreased T_3 and T_4, and increased TSH. Treating by discontinuing lithium and using thyroid medications.

f. Acne and psoriasis: Dermatological treatments may be used.

—— Toxicity

1. Causes: kidney disease, severe dehydration, overdosage of lithium
2. Symptoms
   a. early: muscle weakness, diarrhea, nausea, lack of coordination, fine tremor, slurred speech
   b. moderate (1.5–2.5 mEq/L serum level): vomiting, severe diarrhea, coarse tremor, lack of coordination, hypotension, seizures
   c. severe (above 2.5 mEq/L serum level): nystagmus, seizures, coma, oliguria, anuria, cardiac arrhythmias, muscle hyperirritability
3. Treatment: discontinuance of lithium, administration of fluids, correction of fluid and electrolyte imbalance, and protection of kidney function; hemodialysis when lithium level is greater than 3.0 mEq/L

—— Neurotoxicity (life-threatening)

1. Causes: neuroleptics, anticonvulsants
2. Symptoms: confusion, disorientation, slurred speech; absence of nausea, vomiting and diarrhea; lithium level is low-moderate.
3. Treatment: discontinuance of lithium or anticonvulsant

■■ ANTICONVULSANTS

Carbamazepine (Tegretol)

—— Indications

Convulsive disorders; temporal lobe epilepsy; bipolar disorder, manic phase; trigeminal neuralgia

—— Pharmacodynamics

Unknown

—— Pharmacokinetics

1. Absorbed from GI tract and metabolites eliminated in urine and feces
2. Serum levels peak in 2–8 hours.
3. Therapeutic range 6–12 mcg/ml

—— Administration

1. Initial dose is low, 400 mg daily, and is increased slowly to reduce side effects (i.e., drowsiness, dizziness, nausea and vomiting). Maximum dose of 1,600 mg daily.
2. Contraindications: history of bone marrow depression; renal, hepatic, or cardiovascular disease.
3. Cautions
   a. Development of aplastic anemia or agranulocytosis; recommended monitoring of CBC every 3–6 months and for symptom of fever, bruising, sore throat
   b. Development of hepatotoxicity: liver function tests every 3–6 months recommended.

—— Examples of Drug Interactions

1. Anticoagulants: carbamazepine (Tegretol) affects the metabolism of oral anticoagulants; therefore, dosage requirements need careful monitoring.
2. Cimetidine (Tagamet), erythromycin (E-mycin), diltiazem (Cardizem), verapamil (Isoptin, Calan): toxicity, with signs of neuromuscular disturbance appearing first

—— General Responses to Treatment

1. Advise patient to use caution when handling machinery or driving.
2. Side effects: drowsiness, dizziness, nausea, vomiting, blurred vision and photosensitivity; increasing dosage slowly, as tolerance develops, may help relieve these side effects.
3. Toxicity
   a. Symptoms: altered level of consciousness, from drowsiness to coma; motor restlessness, from tremors to more gross movements; nausea; vomiting
   b. Treatment: induction of vomiting; supportive measures

Clonazepam (Klonopin)
—— Indications

1. Seizure disorder
2. May be useful for acutely manic patient

—— Administration

1. May be used in acute mania to achieve behavior control when an antipsychotic drug cannot be used.

2. Discontinuation of drug may cause withdrawal symptoms (i.e., abdominal muscle cramps, sweating, nausea, convulsions).
3. Contraindications: pregnancy and lactation (effects are unknown); liver disease
4. **Caution:** May increase seizures when seizure disorder exists.

── Examples of Drug Interactions

Antipsychotics, anxiolytics, antidepressants: CNS depression

── General Responses to Treatment

1. Decreased alertness: Advise care in driving or handling equipment where alertness is needed.
2. Abruptly discontinuing the drug may cause status epilepticus.
3. Side effects: drowsiness, ataxia

── Overdose

1. Symptoms: drowsiness, confusion, decreased reflexes
2. Treatment: lavage, supportive measures

■ ALPHA-ADRENERGIC AGONIST ── CLONIDINE (CATAPRES)
── Indications

Antihypertensive
Acute mania (under study)
Note: Consult with most recent literature for additional information.

── Side Effects

Drowsiness, hypotension, depression

■ CALCIUM CHANNEL INHIBITORS ── VERAPAMIL (ISOPTIN, CALAN)
── Indications

Acute mania (under study)
Essential hypertension
Note: Consult the most recent literature for additional information.
Verapamil acts as a calcium channel blocker.

── Side Effects

Constipation, congestive heart failure, atrial ventricular block

■ ANTIANXIETY DRUGS[1-34]

Antianxiety drugs (*Anxiolytics*, Table 7-5) are used in the treatment of anxiety disorders and insomnia, in alcohol detoxification, and to reduce preoperative anxiety.

TABLE 7-5   Antianxiety Drugs

Major Classes	Representative Drugs		Daily PO Doses (Range)
	Generic Name	Trade Name	
Benzodiazepines	Alprazolam	Xanax	0.5–10 mg
	Clorazepate	Tranxene	15–60 mg
	Chlordiazepoxide	Librium	15–200 mg
	Diazepam	Valium	2–40 mg
	Lorazepam	Ativan	2–6 mg
	Oxazepam	Serax	30–120 mg
Azaspirodecanedione	Buspirone	BuSpar	15–60 mg
Antihistamines	Diphenhydramine	Benadryl	25–200 mg
	Hydroxyzine	Atarax	50–400 mg
		Vistaril	

▬ BENZODIAZEPINES

Alprazolam (Xanax)
Chlorazepate (Tranxene)
Chlordiazepoxide (Librium)
Diazepam (Valium)
Lorazepam (Ativan)
Oxazepam (Serax)

— Indications

Anxiety disorders
Relief of symptoms of anxiety associated with life crises (e.g., heart attack and other major medical conditions, death of a loved one)
Seizure disorders
Alcohol withdrawal
Panic disorder
Skeletal muscle relaxation

— Pharmacodynamics

Depressant effect on the CNS through the limbic system through the neurotransmitter, GABA

— Pharmacokinetics

1. Absorbed rapidly in the GI tract, metabolized in the liver, and also excreted in the urine
2. Serum levels peak in 1–3 hours, but in 1 hour for diazepam (Valium).
3. Half-life: 5–15 hours for oxazepam (Serax), 10–20 hours for lorazepam (Ativan), 12–15 hours for alprazolam (Xanax), 30–100 + hours for diazepam (Valium), chlorazepate (Tranxene) and chlordiazepoxide (Librium)
4. Steady-state plasma level may take about two weeks.
5. Lipid-soluble; effects of the drug may be noted for a longer period of time in the obese and in the elderly who have less muscle tissue

—— Administration

1. Benzodiazepines are divided into two major groups because of their metabolism in the body.
   a. Short-acting: oxazepam (Serax), lorazepam (Ativan), and alprazolam (Xanax); given t.i.d. or q.i.d. orally
   b. Long-acting: diazepam (Valium), clorazepate (Tranxene), chlordiazepoxide (Librium). Given t.i.d., q.i.d., or h.s., orally.
2. Lorazepam (Ativan) is the *only* benzodiazepine which is consistently and rapidly absorbed by I.M. administration.
3. Specific symptoms are targeted and treated for 1–3 weeks. Drug is usually tapered off in 1–2 weeks and discontinued; Long-acting benzodiazepines used for long periods of time are usually tapered off in 1–3 months.
4. Recommend reevaluation if drug is being used for longer than 4 months.

—— Contraindications

Severe depression; closed angle glaucoma; psychoses

—— Cautions

1. Confusion is common in the elderly.
2. Suicide potential may increase as anxiety is reduced.
3. Pregnancy and lactation: safety not proven
4. Misuse or abuse, particularly after use for sedation
5. In continuous therapeutic dose of long-acting benzodiazepines (diazepam [Valium], clorazepate [Tranxene], chlordiazepoxide [Librium]): toxicity may develop due to the slow metabolism of the drug.

—— Examples of Drug Interactions

1. Alcohol, barbituates, and other sedative-hypnotics: potentiate sedative effects
2. Antidepressants: potentiate symptoms such as sedation, dry mouth, blurred vision, rapid pulse, flushed face, urinary retention
3. Antihypertensives and diuretics: potentiate antihypertensive effects

—— General Responses to Treatment

1. Sedative and calming effects are experienced 30–60 minutes after oral dose.
2. I.M. administration of lorazepam (Ativan) produces sedation within 15–20 minutes. This drug is very useful in psychiatric emergencies.
3. Sedation occurs at low dosage levels; therefore the patient should be warned about handling machinery or engaging in activities requiring quick action.
4. There is no antipsychotic effect.

—— Side Effects (treated by adjustment of dosage)

Faintness and dizziness; drowsiness; paradoxical reaction (i.e., violence related to disinhibiting effect); anterograde amnesia

—— Tolerance, Dependence, Withdrawal

1. Generally does not occur when drug is taken for *short* time—1–2 weeks
2. Development of dependence is related to dosage level, length of time taken, half-life of drug, and psychological factors.
3. Withdrawal symptoms: nervousness; weakness; depression; sensitivity to bright lights, noise, touch; vomiting; sweating; muscle cramps; anorexia; and convulsions. Symptoms may occur in 2–3 days with short-acting group and in 7 days with long-acting group.

—— Overdose

1. Symptoms: coma, confusion, diminished reflexes, hypotension
2. Treatment: lavage and maintenance of respiratory and cardiovascular functions. If other drugs (e.g., alcohol) are involved, the threat to life is more serious.

■ AZASPIRODECANEDIONE – BUSPIRONE (BUSPAR)
—— Indications

Anxiety disorder
This drug has less dependence, fewer drug interactions, particularly no additive effects with alcohol; therefore, it is preferred for initial anxiety presentations.

—— Pharmacodynamics

Unknown, but may affect serotonin receptors

—— Pharmacokinetics

1. Absorbed in GI tract, metabolized rapidly and excreted in urine
2. Serum levels peak in 40–90 minutes

—— Administration

1. Lag time for antianxiety effects may be 1–3 weeks; therefore it cannot be used when reduction of anxiety is desired within hours.
2. New drug and still controversial

—— Cautions

Pregnancy and nursing mothers

—— Examples of Drug Interactions

1. Monoamine oxidase inhibitors: increases blood pressure
2. Other interactions are not known because of lack of data.

— General Responses to Treatment

1. There are *no* sedative, anticonvulsant, or muscle relaxation effects.
2. Patients who have received prior treatment with benzodiazepines may complain because there are no sedative effects
3. Is not addictive

— Side Effects

Nausea, headache, dizziness, nervousness (treated by adjustment of dosage)

— Overdose

1. Symptoms: GI symptoms, dizziness, drowsiness
2. Treatment: lavage, supportive measures

■ ANTIHISTAMINES — DIPHENHYDRAMINE (BENADRYL), HYDROXYZINE (ATARAX), VISTARIL

— Indications

Mild symptoms associated with anxiety (i.e., insomnia, nervousness)
Lack of tolerance for other antianxiety drugs

■ REFERENCES

1. Ballinger BR: New Drugs: hypnotics and anxiolytics. Br Med J 300(6722):456–458, 1990
2. Baraban JM, Worley PF, Snyder SH: Second messenger systems and psychoactive drug action: focus on the phosphoinositide system and lithium. Am J Psychiatry 146(10):1251–1260, 1989
3. Barrett N, Ormiston S, Molyneux V: Clozapine: a new drug for schizophrenia. J Psychosoc Nurs Ment Health Serv 28(2):24–28, 1990
4. Bernstein JG: Handbook of Drug Therapy in Psychiatry, 2nd ed. Littleton, MA, PSG Publishing, 1988
5. Carroll JA, Jefferson JW, Greist JH: Treating tremor induced by lithium. Hosp Community Psychiatry 38(12):1280,1288, 1987
6. Castillo E, Rubin RT, Holsboer-Trachsler E: Clinical differentiation between lethal catatonia and neuroleptic malignant syndrome. Am J Psychiatry 146(3):324–328, 1989
7. Drugs for psychiatric disorders. The Medical Letter on Drugs and Therapeutics. 31(786):13–20, 1989
8. Garza-Trevino ES et al: Efficacy of combinations of intra-muscular antipsychotics and sedative-hypnotics for control of psychotic agitation. Am J Psychiatry 146(12):1598–1601, 1989
9. Georgotas A, Cancro R (eds): Depression and Mania. New York, Elsevier Science Publishing, 1988
10. Guttmacher LB: Concise Guide to Somatic Therapies in Psychiatry. Washington, DC, American Psychiatric Press, 1988
11. Hamilton D: Clozapine: a new antipsychotic drug. Arch Psychiatr Nurs 4(4):278–281, 1990

12. Hansten PD: Drug Interactions: Decision Support Tables. Spokane, WA, Applied Therapeutics, 1987
13. Harris E: The antidepressants. AJN 88(11):1512–1518, 1988
14. Harris E: The antipsychotics. AJN 88(11):1508–1511, 1988
15. Harris E: Lithium in a class by itself. AJN (2):190–195, 1989
16. Hooper JF, Herren CK, Goldwasser H: Neuroleptic malignant syndrome: recognizing an unrecognized killer. J Psychosoc Nurs Ment Health Serv 27(7):13–15, 1989
17. Jackson RT, Haynes-Johnson V: Nutritional management of patients undergoing long-term antipsychotic and antidepressant therapies. Arch Psychiatr Nurs 2(3):146–152, 1988
18. Kaplan HI, Sadock BJ: Comprehensive Textbook of Psychiatry, 5th ed, vol. 2. Baltimore, Williams & Wilkins, 1989
19. Kaplan HI, Sadock BJ: Synopsis of Psychiatry: Behavioral Sciences and Clinical Psychiatry, 5th ed. Baltimore, Williams & Wilkins, 1988
20. Keck PE et al: Risk factors for neuroleptic malignant syndrome. Arch Gen Psychiatry 46(10):914–918, 1989
21. Kiloh LG, Smith JS, Johnson GF: Physical Treatment in Psychiatry. Boston, Blackwell Scientific Publications, 1988
22. Lieberman J, Kane J, Johns C: Clozapine: guidelines for clinical management. J Clin Psychiatry 50(9):329–338, 1989
23. Loebl S, Spratto GR, Woods AL: The Nurse's Drug Handbook, 5th ed. New York, John Wiley & Sons, 1989
24. Lohr M: Psychopharmacology. In McFarland GK, Thomas MD: Psychiatric Mental Health Nursing. Philadelphia, JB Lippincott, 1991
25. Malseed RT: Pharmacology: Drug Therapy and Nursing Considerations, 3rd ed. Philadelphia, JB Lippincott, 1990
26. Middlemiss MA, Beeber LS: Issues in the use of depot antipsychotics. J Psychosoc Nurs Ment Health Serv 27(6):36–37, 1989
27. Physician's Desk Reference, 54th ed. Oradell, NJ, Medical Economics, 1990
28. Rosenstock IM: Adoption and maintenance of lifestyle modifications. Am J Prev Med 4(6):349–352, 1988
29. Sullivan G, Luckoff D: Sexual side effects of antipsychotic medication: evaluation and interventions. Hosp Community Psychiatry 41(11): 1238–1241, 1990
30. Tomb DA: Psychiatry for the House Officer, 3rd ed. Baltimore, Williams & Wilkins, 1988
31. United States Pharmacopoeial Convention, Inc. Drug Information for the Health Care Professional, 9th ed. Rockville, MD, United States Pharmacopoeial Convention, 1989
32. Wagner R: Sandoz agrees to sell Clozapine without the monitoring system. Psychiatr Times 8(1):1, 1991
33. Whall AL et al: Tardive dyskinesia movements over time. Appl Nurs Res 2(3):128–134, 1989
34. Young LY, Koda-Kimble MA (eds): Applied Therapeutics: The Clinical Use of Drugs, 4th ed. Vancouver, WA, Applied Therapeutics, 1988

Index

Numbers followed by an f indicate a figure; t following a page number indicates tabular material.

Abuse, definition of, 238. *See also* Substance use disorders
Acetylcholine, 4
Active listening, 182
Activity area restriction
  definition, 195
  purpose, 196
  specific nursing interventions, 196
Adjustment disorder with depressed mood, 262
Adjustment disorders with anxious features
  associated nursing diagnosis, 272
  clinical manifestations, 270–271
  contributing factors, 269
  definition, 268
  incidence, 268
  treatment, 271
Advocacy
  definition, 179
  purpose, 179
  specific nursing interventions, 179–180
Affective state, assessment, 43
Aggression
  defining characteristics, 55
  definition, 53
  evaluation/outcome criteria, 61
  general principles, 53
  goals and nursing interventions for, 57–61
  model of, 54t
  nursing assessment, 56
  related factors, 55
Agoraphobia, 270
AIDS dementia complex, 235–236
Alcohol abuse, 241–244. *See also* Alcohol use disorders
  complications, 241
  patterns, 241
  treatment, 242–244
Alcohol use disorders
  alcohol abuse, 241–244
  alcohol dependence, 241–244
  alcohol intoxication, 240–241
  alcohol withdrawal, 241

contributing factors, 238–239
  delirium, 241
  effects, 240
  incidence, 239–240
Alcohol treatment programs, 243–244
Aliphatics, 285t
Alogia, 254
Alpha adrenergic agonist, 300t, 305
Alprazolam (Xanax), 306t, 306–307
Altruism, and group therapy, 225
Alzheimer's disease, 234
Amantadine hydrochloride (Symmetrel), 293t, 294
Ambiguous response, 73
Ambivalence, 43
American Law Institute test, of insanity, 2
Amitriptyline (Elavil), 295t
Amnestic syndrome, 236
Amoxapine (Asendin), 295t
Amphetamine use disorders
  abuse/dependence, 245
  effects, 244
  incidence, 244
  intoxication, 244
  treatment, 250
  withdrawal, 244–245
Anger, and grief reaction, 116
Antianxiety drugs, 305–309, 306t
  and alcohol abuse, 242
  antihistamines, 309
  azaspirodecanedione, 308–309
  benzodiazepines, 306–308
Anticholinergic drugs, 293–294, 293t
  administration, 293–294
  drug interaction examples, 294
  indications, 293
  overdose, 294
  pharmacodynamics, 293
  pharmacokinetics, 293
  response to treatment, 294
  side effects, 294
Anticonvulsants, 300t, 303–305
Antidepressant drugs. *See* Monamine oxidase inhibitors; Tricyclics
Antihistamines, 306t, 309

Antimanic drugs, 300t, 301–305
  alpha adrenergic agonist, 305
  anticonvulsants, 303–305
  calcium channel inhibitors, 305
  lithium salts, 301–303
Antiparkinsonian drugs, 293–294, 293t
  administration, 293–294
  drug interaction examples, 294
  indications, 293
  overdose, 294
  pharmacodynamics, 293
  pharmacokinetics, 293
  response to treatment, 294
  side effects, 294
Antipsychotic drugs, 285–293, 285t
  administration, 286
  contraindications, 288
  drug interaction examples, 288
  indications, 285
  life-threatening effects, 291–292
  long-acting drugs, 287–288
  maintenance drug treatment, 287
  overdose, 292
  pharmacodynamics, 286
  pharmacokinetics, 286
  precautions, 288
  response to treatment, 288
  side effects, 287, 288–290
  tardive dyskinesia, 290–291
  treatment of acute psychosis, 287
  withdrawal syndrome, 290
Antisocial personality disorders,
    278–280
Anxiety
  characteristics, 66–68
    extreme (panic), 67–68
    mild, 66
    moderate, 66–67
    severe, 67
  definition, 6, 65
  disorders
    associated nursing diagnosis, 272
    clinical manifestations, 269–271
    contributing factors, 269
    definition, 268
    incidence, 268
    treatment, 271
    types, 268
  evaluation/outcome criteria, 71
  general principles, 65
  interpersonal approach, 10
  normal, 65
  nursing assessment, 68
  patient outcomes and nursing
    interventions, 68–70
  process anxiety, 65
  related factors, 66

  state anxiety, 65
  trait anxiety, 65
Anxiety syndrome, organic, 236
Anxiolytics
  abuse/dependence, 250
  effects, 249
  intoxication, 249
  treatment, 250
  withdrawal, 249–250
Aphasia, 41
Assertiveness training
  definition, 180
  purpose, 180
  specific nursing interventions,
    180–181
Asocial behavior, and schizophrenia,
    254
Assessment. *See* Nursing assessment
Atypical psychosis, 267
Automatism, 41
Avoidance personality disorder,
    280–281
Azaspirodecanedione, 306t, 308–309

"Bad trip," 247
Barbituates, 249–250
Bargaining in grieving, 116
Behaviorist approach, 12–13
  theoretical basis, 12
  therapy, 12–13
Behavior theory, and alcohol abuse,
    239
Behaviorism, 12
Bender-Gestalt Test, 45
Benzadrine, 244–245. *See also*
    Amphetamine use disorders
Benzodiazepines, 306–308, 306t
  abuse of, 249–250
  administration, 307
  alcohol use and, 242
  cautions, 307
  contraindications, 307
  dependence, 308
  drug interaction examples, 307
  indication, 306
  overdose, 308
  pharmacodynamics, 306
  pharmacokinetics, 306
  response to treatment, 307
  side effects, 308
  tolerance, 308
  withdrawal, 308
Benztropine (Cogentin), 293t, 294
Bibliotherapy, 224
Biperiden (Akineton), 293t, 294

Bipolar disorders
  clinical manifestations, 262
  contributing factors, 261
  definition, 260
  incidence, 260
  manic, 262
  risk, 260
  treatment, 263–264
Blocking, 44
Blunting, 43
Body dysmorphic disorder, 273
Borderline personality disorder,
  278–280
Brain structure abnormalities, and
  schizophrenia, 253
Brief reactive psychosis, 267
Buspirone (BuSpar), 306t, 308–309
Butyrophenones, 285t

Calcium channel inhibitors, 300t, 305
Canatonic stupor, 41
Cannabis use disorders, 245
  treatment, 250
Carbamazepine (Tegretol), 300t,
  303–304
Catalepsy, 41
Cataplexy, 41
Catatonic excitement, 41
Catatonic schizophrenia, 254
Catharsis, and group therapy, 225
Chlorazepate (Tranxene), 306t,
  306–307
Chlordiazepoxide (Librium), 306t,
  306–307
Choreiform movements, 41
Circumstantiality, 44
Clarification, as communication
  technique, 182
Clinical specialist, in mental health
  nursing, 20
Clomipramine (Anafranil), 295t,
  300–301
Clonazepam (Klonopin), 300t, 304–305
Clonidine (Catapres), 300t, 305
Clozapine (Clozaril), 292–293
Cocaine use disorders
  abuse, 246
  effects, 246
  incidence, 245
  treatment, 250
  withdrawal, 246
Cognitive behaviorism, 12
Cognitive therapy, 13
Command hallucinations, 253

Communication
  breakdown, 24
  impaired
    characteristics, 74
    definition, 73
    evaluation/outcome criteria, 76–77
    general principles, 73–74
    nursing assessment, 74–75
    patient outcomes and nursing
      interventions, 75–76
    related factors, 74
  skills, 23–24
  techniques, 181–183
Compulsive motor behavior, 41
Condensation, 44
Confrontation, 28–29
  as communication technique, 182
Confusion, acute
  characteristics, 161
  definition, 160
  evaluation/outcome criteria, 164
  general principles, 160
  nursing assessment, 162
  patient outcomes and nursing
    interventions, 162–164
  related factors, 160–161
Consciousness, levels of, 5
Consensual validation, 182
Contracting, therapeutic, 183
Conversion disorder, 273
Coping
  defensive
    characteristics, 81
    definition, 79–80
    evaluation/outcome criteria, 83
    general principles, 80
    nursing assessment, 81
    patient outcomes and nursing
      interventions, 82–83
    related factors, 80–81
  ineffective individual
    characteristics, 86
    definition, 84
    evaluation/outcome criteria, 89
    general principles, 84–85
    nursing assessment, 86–87
    patient outcomes and nursing
      interventions, 87–89
    related factors, 85–86
Corrective reexperiencing, and group
  therapy, 225
Crises
  intervention
    definition, 184
    purpose, 184
    specific nursing interventions,
      184–185

Crises (*contd.*)
  situational
    characteristics, 93
    definition, 92
    evaluation/outcome criteria, 96
    general principles, 92–93
    nursing assessment, 94
    patient outcomes and nursing
      interventions, 94–96
    related factors, 93
Crossed transaction, 73

Decisional conflict
  characteristics, 98–99
  definition, 98
  evaluation/outcome criteria, 100
  general principles, 98
  nursing assessment, 99
  patient outcomes and nursing
    interventions, 94–100
  related factors, 98
Decision making
  definition, 185
  purpose, 185
  specific nursing interventions,
    185–187
Defective hedonic capacity theory, 3
Delirium, 232–233
  alcohol withdrawal, 241
  clinical manifestation, 232
  contributing factors, 232
  risk, 233
  treatment, 232–233
Delusions
  characteristics, 166–167
  definition, 44, 166, 254
  delusional syndrome, organic, 236
  disorders, 266–267
  evaluation/outcome criteria, 169
  general principles, 166
  nursing assessment, 167
  patient outcomes and nursing
    interventions, 167–169
  related factors, 166
Dementia, 233–236
  clinical features, 233–234
  contributing factors, 233
  treatment, 234–236
Demerol, 247–248
Denial, 8, 79–80, 81. *See also* Coping,
    defensive
  grief reaction and, 116
  ineffective, 80–81
Dependence, definition of, 238
Dependent personality disorder,
    280–281
Depersonalization disorder, 43, 226

Depression
  characteristics, 103–104
  definition, 43, 102
  disorders, 260–264
    clinical manifestations, 262
    contributing factors, 261
    incidence, 260
    major depression, 262
    risk, 260
    treatment, 263–264
  evaluation/outcome criteria, 105
  general principles, 102
  nursing assessment, 104
  patient outcome and nursing
    interventions, 104–105
  related factors, 103
Description, as communication
    technique, 182
Desipramine (Norpramin), 295t
Despair, 12
Diathesis stress theory, 3
Diazepam (Valium), 306t, 306–307
Dibenzodiazepine, 285t
Differentiation, 15
Diphenhydramine (Benadryl), 293t,
    294, 306t, 309
Discharge planning
  definition, 187
  purpose, 187
  specific nursing interventions,
    187–188
Disorganized schizophrenia, 254
Dissociative disorders
  associated nursing diagnosis, 276
  clinical manifestations, 275–276
  definition, 275
  treatment, 275–276
  types, 275
Disulfiram (Antabuse), 242
Dopamine, 3
Doxepin (Sinequan), 295t
Draw a Person Test, 45
Drug abuse. *See* Drug therapy;
    Substance abuse disorders
Drug therapy
  antianxiety drugs, 305–309
  anticholinergic/antiparkinsonian
    drugs, 293–294
  antidepressant drugs, 294–301
  antimanic drugs, 301–303
  antipsychotic drugs, 285–293
  areas for nursing assessment,
    283–284
  knowledge about medication, patient,
    284
  lifestyle changes and, 284–285
  related nursing diagnoses, 284

DSM-III-R (Diagnostic and Statistical Manual of Mental Disorders), 44–45
Durham Rule, of insanity, 2
Dysfunctional communication, 14
Dysthymia, 262

Echolalia, 44
Echopraxia, 41
Ecotomanic delusional disorder, 266
Ecstasy, 43
Education. *See* Family education; Patient education
Ego, 6
Ego defenses, 5
Ego development approach, 10–12
    Erikson's eight developmental stages, 10–12
    theoretical basis, 10
    therapy, and, 10–12
Elation, 43
Electra complex, 7
Emotional cut-off, in family approach, 15
Empathy, 27–28
Epinephrine, 4
Euphoria, 43
Existential factors, and group therapy, 225
Existential groups, 16
Exultation, 43

Family approach, 13–15
    Bowen system theory, 14–15
    interactional framework, 14
    structural framework, 13–14
Family education
    definition, 191
    purpose, 191
    specific nursing interventions, 192–194
Family processes, altered
    characteristics, 109
    definition, 108
    evaluation/outcome criteria, 111
    family outcomes and nurse interventions, 110–111
    general principles, 108
    nursing assessment, 109–110
    related factors, 108–109
Family projection process, 14
Fear, 43

Flashback, 247
Flat affect, 43
Flight of ideas, 44
Fluoxetine (Prozac), 295t, 300
Focusing, as communication technique, 182
Functional analysis, 12

Games, 73
Generalist, in psychiatric mental health nursing, 20
Generativity, 12
Genetic factors, 3
    and schizophrenia, 253
Gestalt groups, 16
Grandiose type delusional disorder, 266
Grief counseling
    definition, 209
    purpose, 209
    specific nursing interventions, 209–210
Grieving
    anticipatory
        characteristics, 115
        definition, 114
        evaluation/outcome criteria, 116
        general principles, 114
        nursing assessment, 115
        outcomes and nursing interventions, 115–116
        related factors, 114
    dysfunctional
        characteristics, 117–118
        definition, 116
        evaluation/outcome criteria, 121
        general principles, 116–117
        nursing assessment, 118
        outcomes and nursing interventions, 118–120
        related factors, 117
Group treatment
    adjunctive groups, 224
    client-centered groups, 15
    cohesiveness in, 225
    effective characteristics in, 226
    existential groups, 16
    Gestalt groups, 16
    influencing factors, 225
    initiating, 226
    interpersonal groups, 15–16
    interventions, 228
    phases in, 227–228
    psychoanalytic groups, 16, 224–225
    therapeutic groups, 223–224
    transactional analysis, 15

Hallucinations
  characteristics, 171
  definition, 43, 170
  evaluation/outcome criteria, 173–174
  general principles, 170–171
  nursing assessment, 172
  patient outcomes and nursing
    interventions, 172–173
  related factors, 171
  types of, 253–254
Hallucinogen use disorders
  effects, 246–247
  hallucinosis, 236, 247
  incidence, 246
Hallucinosis, 236, 247
Heroin, 247–248
Histrionic personality disorder, 278–280
Humanistic-Existential approach, 13
Humor, as communication technique,
  182
Huntington's chorea, 234
Hydroxyzine (Atarax, Vistaril), 306t
Hyperkinesia, 41
Hypnopompic hallucinations, 43
Hypnotics, 249–250
  abuse/dependence, 250
  effects, 249
  intoxication, 249
  treatment, 250
  withdrawal, 249–250
Hypochondriasis, 44, 273–274
Hypogogic hallucinations, 43

Id, 5
Identification, as defense mechanism, 8
Identity, 11
Illusion, 43
Imipramine (Tofranil), 295t
Imitative behavior, 225
Impervious response, 73
Impulse control, and schizophrenia, 254
Impulsiveness, 41
Inadequate response, 73
Indolics, 285t
Induced psychotic disorder, 267
Initiative, 11
Insanity, definition of, 1–2
Integrity, 12
Intelligence testing, 45
Interpersonal approach, 9–10
  anxiety, 10
  stages of growth and development, 9
  theoretical basis, 9
  therapy, 10
Interpersonal learning, 225
Intimacy, 11

Introjection, 8
Intoxication. *See* Substance use disorders
Irritability, 43
Isocarboxazid (Marplan), 285t
Isolation, 8, 11

Jealous type delusional disorder, 266

Knowledge assessment, 42

Lability, 43
Lifestyle changes, and medication,
  284–285
Lithium carbonate, 300t
Lithium citrate (Cibalith-S), 300t,
  301–303
Lithium salts, 300t, 301–303
  administration, 302
  cautions, 302
  contraindications, 302
  drug interaction examples, 302
  indications, 301
  response to treatment, 302
  pharmacodynamics, 301
  pharmacokinetics, 301
  side effects, 302–303
Lorazepam (Ativan), 306t, 306–307
Lysergic acid (LSD), 246–247. *See also*
  Hallucinogen use disorders

McNaughton Rule of insanity, 2
Manipulation
  characteristics, 124–125
  definition, 123
  evaluation/outcome criteria, 126
  general principles, 123
  nursing assessment, 125
  patient outcomes and nursing
    interventions, 125–126
  related factors, 124
Maprotiline (Ludiomil), 295t
Marijuana. *See* Cannabis use disorders
Memory, in mental status examination,
  42
Mental disorder classification, 2
Mental health
  defined, 2
  Jahoda's six cardinal aspects of, 1
  Maslow's view, 1
  problems, 2

Mental illness
  behaviorist approach, 12–13
  defined, 1
  ego development approach, 10–12
  family approach, 13–15
  group approach, 15–16
  humanistic-existential approach, 13
  interpersonal approach, 9–10
  neurobiological approach, 3–4
  prevalence of, 2
  psychodynamic approach, 5–9
  statistics regarding, 2
  stress-adaptation approach, 4–5
Mental status examination
  affective state, 43
  alertness, 44
  functioning, 42–43
  general appearance, 41
  judgment, 44
  motor behavior, 41
  objective, 40
  perception, 43
  speech, 41
  thought process and content, 44
Mescaline, 246–247. *See also*
    Hallucinogen use disorders
Methadone, 248
Methaqualone, 249–250
Milieu therapy
  definition, 194
  purpose, 184
  specific nursing interventions,
    194–195
Minnesota Multiphasic Personality
    Inventory, 45
Mistrust, 10
Monoamine oxidase inhibitors, 295t,
    297–301
  administration, 298
  cautions, 298
  contraindications, 298
  drug interaction examples, 298
  indications, 297
  overdose, 299
  pharmacodynamics, 297
  pharmocokinetics, 298
  response to treatment, 298
  side effects, 298–299
  tyramine-induced hypertensive crisis,
    299
Monogenic bioamine theory, 3
Mood disorders
  associated nursing diagnosis, 264
  clinical manifestation, 262
  contributing factors, 261–262
  incidence, 260
  risk, 260–261

treatment, 263–264
  types, 260
Mood syndrome, organic, 236
Morphine, 247–248
Motor behavior, in mental status
    examination, 41
Multigenerational transmission process,
    14–15
Multiple personality disorder, 275
Music therapy, 224
Mutism, 41

Narcissistic personality disorder,
    278–280
Neologisms, 44
Neurobiological approach, 304
  genetics, 3
  neurotransmitters, 3–4
  therapy, 4
Neurotic anxiety, 6
Neurotransmitter abnormalities, and
    schizophrenia, 253
Neurotransmitters, 3–4
Norepinephrine, 4
North American Nursing Diagnosis
    Association (NANDA) list, 49–51
Notriptyline (Aventyl, Pamelor), 295t
Nuclear family emotional system, 15
Nursing assessment
  action observations, 38–39
  awareness observations, 39–40
  conceptual framework, 33, 34f
  discharge planning, 40
  DSM-II-R in, 44–45
  environment, 34f
  initial parameters, 36
  interaction observations, 37–38
  mental status examination, 40–44.
    See also Mental status
    examination
  process of, 33–40
  process recordings, 35
  psychological testing, 45
Nursing diagnoses
  characteristics of, 49
  definition, 49
  framework for discussing, 52
  NANDA list of, 49–51
Nursing process, in assessment, 33–40
  diagnosis, 35
  evaluation, 40
  guidelines, 35
  intervention, 40
  planning, 40
  process recordings, 35

Observation
  as communication technique, 182
  in nursing assessment. *See* Nursing
    assessment
  in suicide prevention, 196–197
Obsession, 44
Obsessive-compulsive personality
    disorder, 270, 280–281
Oedipus complex, 7
Offering hope
  definition, 210
  purpose, 210
  specific nursing interventions,
    210–211
Olfactory hallucinations, 254
Operant conditioning, 12
Opiod use disorders
  abuse/dependence, 248
  effects, 247
  incidence, 247
  intoxication, 247–248
  overdose, 247–248
  treatment, 250
  withdrawal, 248
Organic mental syndromes and disorder
  associated nursing diagnosis, 236–237
  clinical manifestations, 232–236
  contributing factors, 232–236
  incidence, 231–232
  listed, 231
  treatments, 232–236
Orientation, in mental status
    examination, 42
Overdose
  alcohol, 240–241
  amphetamines, 244
  barbituates, 249–250
  opiates, 247–248
Oxazepam (Serax), 306t, 306–307

Panic disorder, 269–270
Paranoid personality disorder, 277, 278
Parataxic mode, 9
Parkinson's disease, 234
Passive aggressive personality disorder,
    280–281
Patient education
  definition, 188
  purpose, 188
  specific nursing interventions,
    188–191
Perception assessment, 43
Persecutory type delusional disorder,
    266
Perseveration, 44

Personality disorders
  associated nursing diagnoses, 281
  clinical manifestations, 277–281
  contributing factors, 277
  definition, 277
  treatment, 277–281
Personality syndrome, organic, 236
Personality testing, 45
Personality types, and alcohol abuse,
    238–239
Phases, in nurse-patient relationship,
    20–23. *See also* Therapeutic
    relationship
Phencyclidine (PCP)
  abuse/dependence, 249
  effects, 248
  intoxication, 248–249
  psychosis, 249
  treatment, 250
Phenothiazines, 285t. *See also*
    Antipsychotic drugs
Phenelzine (Nardil), 295t
Phobia, 44
Piperazines, 285t
Piperidines, 285t
Pleasure principle, 5
Post-traumatic stress disorder, 270
Powerlessness
  characteristics, 128–129
  definition, 127
  evaluation/outcome criteria, 131
  general principles, 127–128
  nursing assessment, 129–130
  patient outcomes and nursing
    interventions, 130–131
  related factors, 128
Preconscious, 5
Preludin, 244–245. *See also*
    Amphetamine use disorders, 244
Prenatal disturbances, and
    schizophrenia, 253
Presence
  definition, 211
  purpose, 211
  specific nursing interventions,
    211–212
Primary process thinking, 5
Procyclidine (Kemadrin), 293t, 294
Projection, 8
Projective response, 73
Protective intervention
  activity area restriction, 195–196
  restraints, 199–201
  seclusion, 197–199
  seizure management, 201–203
  suicide prevention, 196–197
Prototaxic mode, 9

Protriptyline (Vivactil), 295t
Psyche, 5–6
Psychoanalysis, 5–9. *See also* Psychotherapy groups
Psychodynamic approach, 5–9
    defense mechanisms, 7–8
    psychosexual stages of development, 6–7
    theoretical basis, 5–6
    therapy, 8–9
Psychogenic amnesia, 276
Psychogenic fugue, 276
Psychological testing, 45
Psychomotor retardation, 41
Psychosexual stages of development, 6–7
    anal stage, 6–7
    genital stage, 7
    latency stage, 7
    oral stage, 6
    phallic stage, 7
Psychotherapy. *See also* Psychotherapy groups; *specific disorder* defined, 19–20
Psychotherapy groups, 224–225
    insight without reconstruction, 222–225
    personality reconstruction, 224
    problem solving, 225
Psychotic disorder, 267
Punning, 41

Questioning, as communication technique, 182

Rage, 43
Rationalization, 8
Reaction formation, 8
Reality anxiety, 6
Reality orientation
    definition, 203
    purpose, 203
    specific nursing interventions, 203–204
Reality principle, 6
Realization of loss, and grieving, 117
Reflection, as communication technique, 182
Regression, 8
Reinforcement, 12
Remotivation groups, 224
Reorientation groups, 224

Repression, 8
Residual schizophrenia, 254
Respondent conditioning, 12
Restating, as communication technique, 182
Restraints
    definition, 199
    purpose, 200
    specific nursing interventions, 200–201
Rhyming, 41
Rigid complementarity, 74
Ritualistic behavior
    characteristics, 133
    definition, 133
    evaluation/outcome criteria, 135
    general principles, 133
    nursing assessment, 134
    patient outcomes and nursing interventions, 134–135
    related factors, 133
    role confusion, 11
Rorschach Test, 45

Satisfaction, 9
Schizoaffective disorder, 267
Schizoid personality disorder, 277, 278
Schizophrenia
    associated nursing diagnosis, 257
    clinical manifestations, 253–254
        of types, 244
    contributing factor, 253
    course of illness, 255
    definition, 252
    incidence, 252
    prognosis, 255
    risk, 255
    treatment, 256–257
    types, 252
Schizophreniform disorder, 267
Schizotypal personality disorder, 277, 278
Seclusion
    definition, 197
    purpose, 197
    specific nursing interventions, 198–199
Secondary process thinking, 6
Security, 9
Sedatives, 249–250
    abuse/dependence, 250
    effects, 249
    intoxication, 249
    treatment, 250
    withdrawal, 249–250

Seizure management
definition, 201
purpose, 201
specific nursing interventions,
201–203
Self, 13
Self-actualization
in human-existential approach, 13
Roger's process of, 1
Self-awareness, in therapeutic
relationship, 25
Self-disclosure, in therapeutic
relationship, 27
Self-esteem disturbance
characteristics, 137
definition, 136
evaluation/outcome criteria, 139
general principles, 136
nursing assessment, 137
outcomes and nursing interventions,
137–139
related factors, 136
Self-help groups, 242
Self-mutilation, 280
Self-system, 9
Senile dementia. *See* Dementia
Sentence Completion Test, 45
Serotonin, 4
Sexual dysfunction
characteristics, 143
definition, 141
evaluation/outcome criteria, 145–146
general principles, 141–142
nursing assessment, 144
patient outcomes and nursing
interventions, 144–145
related factors, 142–143
Shame and doubt, 11
Sibling position, 14
Signal anxiety, 6
Silence, as communication technique,
182
Social interaction, impaired
characteristics, 149
definition, 148
evaluation/outcome criteria, 151
general principles, 148
nursing assessment, 149
patient outcomes and nursing
interventions, 150–151
related factors, 148–149
Social phobia, 270
Social skills groups, 224
Social skills training
definition, 204
purpose, 204
specific nursing interventions,
204–206

Socializing techniques, 225
Societal regression, 15
Somatic type delusional disorder, 266
Somatization disorder, 274
Somatoform disorders
associated nursing diagnosis, 274–275
clinical manifestations, 273–274
contributing factors, 273
definition, 273
treatment, 274
types, 273
Somatoform pain disorder, 274
Spasms, 41
Speech assessment, 41
"Speed." *See* Amphetamine use
disorders
Stereotypy, 41
Stress-adaptation approach, to mental
illness, 4–5
theoretical basis, 4
therapy, 5
Stress-diathesis model, and
schizophrenia, 253
Stress management
definition, 206
purpose, 206
specific nursing interventions,
206–209
Sublimation, 8
Substance-induced organic mental
disorder, psychoactive, 238. *See
also specific disorder*
Substance use disorders. *See also specific
disorder*
alcohol use disorder, 239–244
amphetamine use disorders, 244–245
cannabis use disorder, 245
cocaine use disorder, 245–246
contributing factors, 238–239
hallucinogen use disorder, 246–247
opiod use disorder, 247–248
phencyclidine, 248–249
sedative-hypnotic-anxiolytic, 249–250
terminology, 238
treatment, 250
Suicide, potential
definition, 152
evaluation/outcome criteria, 158
general principles, 152–153
nursing assessment, 154–155
observation for prevention of,
196–197
patient outcomes and interventions,
155–158
related factors, 153–154
risk factors, 154
Summarization, as communication
technique, 183

Superego, 6
Supportive therapy. *See* Grief
    counseling; Offering Hope;
    Presence
Suppression, 8
Suspiciousness
    characteristics, 175
    definition, 174
    evaluation/outcome criteria, 177
    general principles, 174
    nursing assessment, 175
    patient outcomes and nursing
      interventions, 176–177
    related factors, 174
Symmetrical escalation, 74
Syntaxic mode, 9

Tactile hallucination, 254
Tangentiality, 44
Tangential response, 73
Tardive dyskinesia, 290–291
Thematic Apperception Test, 45
Therapeutic relationship
    communication breakdown and
      distortion, 24
    communication skills in, 23–24
    confrontation, 28–29
    definition and characteristics of, 19
    empathy in, 27–28
    experience and, 27
    phases of nurse-patient relationship,
      20–23
      orientation phase, 20–21
      termination phase, 22–23
      working phase, 21–22
    regard and acceptance in, 28
    self-awareness in, 25
    self-disclosure in, 27
    terms related to, 19–20
    trust development in, 26–27
Therapy. *See also* Drug therapy; Group
    therapy; Therapeutic relationship
    behaviorist approach, 12–13
    ego development approach, 10–12
    family approach, 13–15
    humanistic-existential approach, 13
    interpersonal approach, 9–10
    neurobiological approach, 3–4
    stress-adaptation approach, 4–5
Thioxanthenes, 285t

Thought processes, altered. *See*
    Confusion, acute; Delusions;
    Hallucination; Suspiciousness
Thought process, assessment, 44
Tics, 41
Tolerance, definition of, 238
Transactional analysis groups, 15
Transference, 9
Tranylcypromine (Parnate), 295t
Trazodone (Desyrel), 295t, 299–300
Triangles, in family approach, 14
Tricyclics (TCA's), 294–297, 295t
    administration, 296
    cautions, 296
    contraindication, 296
    drug interaction example, 296
    indications, 295
    overdose, 297
    pharmacodynamics, 295
    pharmacokinetics, 295
    response to treatment, 296–297
    side effects, 297
Trihexyphenidyl (Artane), 293t
Trust, 10
    development, 26–27
Tyramine-induced hypertensive crisis,
    299

Unconscious, 5
Undoing, 8
Ulterior transaction,73
Undifferentiated schizophrenia, 254
Universality, and group therapy, 225

Verbigeration, 41
Verapamil (Isoptin, Calan), 300t, 305
Violence. *See* Aggression, inappropriate

Waist restraints, 200
Waxy flexibility, 41
Weschler Adult Intelligence Scale, 45
Withdrawal, drug. *See* Substance use
    disorders; *specific disorder*
Word salad, 44
Wristcuffs, 200